24.95

D1028962

North Chicago Public Library

North Chicago, IL

Take Care of Your Heart

The Complete Book of Heart Facts

Take Care of Your Heart

The Complete Book of Heart Facts

Ezra A. Amsterdam, M.D.
and Ann M. Holmes

Facts On File Publications
New York, New York ● Bicester, England

Take Care of Your Heart

Library of Congress Cataloging in Publication Data

Amsterdam. Ezra A.
    Take care of your heart.

    Bibliography: p.
    Includes index.
    1. Heart—Diseases.   I. Holmes, Ann M.   II. Title.
RC682.A47   1983   616.1'2   82-12068
ISBN 0-87196-731-6
ISBN 0-87196-732-4 (pbk.)

Printed in the United States of America

10 9 8 7 6 5 4 3 2

Contents

Dedication

In loving memory of our fathers, Howard W. Holmes and Julius Amsterdam, and to our mothers, Elizabeth D. Holmes and Mollie Amsterdam.

Acknowledgments

We wish to express our gratitude to a number of people who assisted us in the research and verification of facts in this book. In particular, we want to thank Donna Holmes, Siobhan T. Holmes, Libby Temple, Kelly Tiernan, and Susan Yarin for their invaluable research assistance. It should be pointed out here that all of the facts presented in the text, especially information presented in Parts I and VII were verified for accuracy (names, addresses, phone numbers, etc., of various organizations) at the time of writing and again just prior to production in September 1982. However, we suggest that readers consult their local chapters of the American Heart Association for assistance if they require additional information. We also want to thank Michael W. Sigall, Ph.D., J.D., for his technical review of Chapter 23, "Heart Attack on the Job: What Are the Legal Issues?" and Mary Lou Welch of the American Heart Association in Dallas, Texas, for her prompt and consistent help throughout the production of this book. The persons who assisted us at a number of American Heart Association affiliates are too numerous to mention, but their cooperation is gratefully acknowledged. The typing services of Elaine Hott and Phyllis Kehoe are also very much appreciated. Finally, a special note of thanks to Mr. Bob Markel, whose patience and continued encouragement made it possible for us to see this work through to completion, and to Eleanora Schoenebaum, for her careful supervision throughout production.

Preface

TAKE CARE OF YOUR HEART is a very informative book written for the consumer. It should prove especially useful for the victim of heart attack and his or her family. This book represents a collaborative effort of one of America's leading cardiologists, Dr. Ezra A. Amsterdam, and an outstanding medical writer, Miss Ann M. Holmes. Dr. Amsterdam is on the faculty of the School of Medicine of the University of California at Davis and Chief of its Division of Cardiovascular Medicine. He is internationally recognized as an outstanding physician, teacher, lecturer and writer. He is also on the editorial boards of many prestigious cardiology journals.

Ms. Holmes is President of TransMedica, Inc., a medical communications company in New York City. I have worked on several medical publications with her in the past. She has a fine understanding of clinical medicine and skillfully relays information in an instructive and absorbing manner to the reader. They have combined their talents to present fundamental information in a concise, useful, easy-to-read style.

The authors have worked for a number of years in developing this volume, yet they have continuously revised it in the process so that the information contained in this book is up-to-date and pertinent. Such new and still experimental techniques as the use of drugs injected into the coronary circulation to dissolve clots during the early phase of a heart attack, developments in the artificial heart program, and the new technique of balloon angioplasty, which is being used increasingly for certain types of patients with angina pectoris, are discussed in this book. Part VII: "Resources, Where to Go for Help" is of particular interest. It contains diverse information on such topics as traveling with a damaged heart, coronary clubs, and obtaining life and health insurance.

The book is explicit in defining terms which are familiar to those in the medical field, yet the patient in the hospital or doctor's office and under some stress often is reticent about asking the physician questions such as "what is angina" or "what is an infarction?" The glossary of terms the authors have included is most helpful in answering questions such as these.

The responsibility thrust upon any individual who is the only witness to a sudden heart attack is sobering and frightening, especially when the victim happens to be a family member or close friend. The authors have described in great detail the particulars of cardiopulmonary resuscitation (CPR), simplifying tne CPR procedure with a step-by-step explanation, along with helpful illustrations.

It is of interest to note that a great many otherwise educated persons fail to realize the importance of recognizing the signs and symptoms of an acute myocardial infarction (heart attack) until they have experienced this type of heart attack first-hand or by observing a close friend or family member with this life-threatening malady. Early recognition is imperative, since the greatest risk to life is in the first minutes to hours. This book serves to make you aware of these symptoms; therefore, should you experience symptoms like those described, immediately contact your own physician or go to the emergency room of a hospital as quickly as possible.

Over the last few years a number of books on heart disease have been written for the general public. As a rule, these tend to be either simplistic and limited in the kinds of information they contain or they have been written in a style and manner that is difficult for the average person to follow. The collaborative effort by Ms. Holmes and Dr. Amsterdam has been extremely successful in overcoming these problems and in presenting medical issues of importance to all of us in a way that makes reading it pleasurable as well as very enlightening.

Elliot Rapaport, M.D.
Professor of Medicine
University of California
School of Medicine, San Francisco;
Chief of Cardiology
San Francisco General Hospital
San Francisco, CA

Dr Rapaport also served as Editor of *Circulation*, the official scientific publication of the American Heart Association, and he was President of the American Heart Association, 1974-1975.

Introduction:
The Case for Keeping Your Healthy Heart Healthy

Is Your Heart Healthy?

It should be! Most of us were born with healthy hearts, which are ready to function exquisitely for us for eighty years or more. Yet very few Americans indeed reach that age without some form of heart disease; in fact, despite the scientific and medical advances of the last two decades, the average life expectancy in 1980 in the United States is only 69 years for men and 76 years for women.

Although the number of deaths attributable to heart disease has declined slightly, the morbidity and mortality rates, as well as the economic burden, remain staggering. Consider, for example, that the American Heart Association estimated that in 1982 in the United States nearly one million persons died as the result of some form of cardiovascular disease—that's over half of all deaths for the year. Such a grim statistic clearly warrants our attention.

What can you do to help yourself? In the following chapters, you will learn how your heart functions, and what steps you can take to help your heart continue to work efficiently for you for many years.

In this book, we have discussed in detail for you the major "risk factors" for coronary heart disease: cigarette smoking, high blood pressure, and a high serum cholesterol level; we have included specific guidelines to help you change your life-style to include daily exercise and a diet prudent in calories and saturated fats. In addition, there are sections to advise you on how to help a child with a heart disease, such as rheumatic heart or congenital heart defects. There's also a special section devoted exclusively to women and heart disease, in which the reported associations between the use of oral contraceptives and the occurrence of stroke and heart attack are discussed.

Finally, we have included in our discussion a look at the newer diagnostic tests used to detect heart disease, such as echocardiography and radioisotopic techniques, and a complete discussion of medical and surgical treatments, as well as methods of rehabilitation, including the return to a fulfilling sex life after a heart attack.

If, after reading this text, you still have some questions, Chapter 26, "Guidelines for Selecting a Physician and a Medical Center," lists some other useful sources. Hopefully, though, you won't ever have to use that guide. Why not start to work right now to improve your chances of avoiding our nation's number one killer: cardiovascular disease. It will undoubtedly be one of the best investments you've ever made!

What You May Be Doing Wrong

Of course, most of us spend little time thinking about our hearts and what we may be doing that is harmful to our health in general and to our hearts in particular. Too many of us continue to smoke cigarettes despite the overwhelming evidence linking cigarette smoking to both lung cancer and heart disease. We also eat too much of the wrong types of foods and ignore warnings about the dangers of high blood pressure.

Until one day it happens. A lifetime of bad habits—cigarette smoking perhaps, overeating of fatty foods, not enough regular exercise—finally catches up with you or your spouse, relative, friend or work associate. (In some cases, none of these risk factors is present, and that adds to the complexity of and frustration over this problem.) One day, when you are simply taking a bus to work, or getting ready to pick up the children at school, or preparing to depart for a vacation, the chest pain starts to build up again, only this time the "heartburn," or whatever it is you have been calling the chest pain, can no longer be ignored, so you call your doctor or go to your local hospital's emergency room, only to learn that you've had a heart attack.

Sometimes, the incident is far worse than that. The victim may collapse suddenly without warning—on the street, in the office, or merely at home, while relaxing in a chair watching television. In a split second—assuming the victim survives this type of "sudden" heart attack, (and the odds are one in two that he or she will not)—the victim's life and the lives of all members of the family are changed dramatically, and often permanently.

To begin with, there is the initial shock of realizing that a loved one has nearly lost his or her life. A career is interrupted or terminated, and there are unanticipated medical costs to deal with. Typically, the victim is a middle-aged man, usually the breadwinner of the family. In addition to these problems and economic burdens, there are children to consider; their lives are often profoundly affected by such a catastrophic event. The greatest tragedy, however, is to realize that many of these heart attacks, and the hundreds of thousands of deaths that occur annually as a result, might have been avoided.

Regrettably, Americans are rather crisis-oriented; few of us are interested in preventive approaches to problems. True, in the last few years we have initiated programs to conserve energy and other natural resources, but such steps are only our reactions to dwindling supplies.

Fortunately, preventive health measures have been introduced and more and more of us, particularly parents, are paying closer attention to the importance of diet, regular daily exercise and other important health measures. "An ounce of prevention is worth a pound of cure" may be a trite expression, but it is perhaps nowhere better applied than in medicine and health care. If you follow the preventive steps outlined here, which may help to avoid heart disease, you can, in many instances, reduce your chances of having a heart attack and the costly, frequently complex medical treatments that accompany it.

The point we wish to make here is quite simple. Don't wait for the medical crisis—a heart attack—to strike you, or any member of your family. A prominent cardiologist and epidemiologist, William B. Kannel, M.D., Director of the noted Framingham (Massachusetts) Heart Study (National Heart, Lung and Blood Institute) has spent over thirty years supervising this study, in which the cigarette smoking, cholesterol (fat) levels, and blood pressure patterns of over 5,000 men and women in that town were monitored. Based on his observations from the Framingham Study, Dr. Kannel concluded that a heart attack is a medical failure, *not* the first indication for treatment. This may seem rather obvious, but how many people have you known, perhaps people close to you, who have ignored the public health warnings, their doctor's advice, maybe even their own early-warning signs, such as a recurring chest pain or shortness of breath, until the crisis—the heart attack—strikes? Then, and only then, do many of us start to correct a lifetime of poor habits. Yet simple precautionary measures could have been taken beforehand; then, perhaps, that life-threatening heart attack might have been avoided.

Before you learn more about the details of how to take care of your heart, it is most important for you and your family to understand how your heart functions. After all, it's easier to keep any piece of equipment or machinery functioning in top form if you understand how it works. So it is with your heart. You've undoubtedly heard that you should stop smoking, cut down on your intake of some dietary fats, and exercise more, but do you really understand why? If your teenage son or daughter asks you why they shouldn't smoke, could you give them more than a trite response, such as, "It's bad for you," "Because I said so," or "They say you might get lung cancer"? Do you have any hard facts at hand to help you explain? And how would you respond, for example, if your spouse asked: "Why are we having skim milk instead of regular milk?" or "What's the point of serving margarine—how can a little butter hurt?" The changes many of us should make in our living habits are really rather simple, subtle ones, but you should learn the potential importance of these changes, and what the easiest methods are for achieving them. Don't wait for your parent, spouse, or even you, yourself, to have a heart attack first, and then decide it's time to get more exercise, lose weight, or cut down on smoking. Remember Dr. Kannel's words: A heart attack is a medical failure, *not* the first indication for treatment.

Luckily, most of us are born with healthy hearts. Read on to discover how your heart works, and what you can do to help keep it healthy.

A GUIDE TO HEART FACTS

.The American Heart Association has prepared a statistical summary of facts pertaining to cardiovascular disease, which is an "umbrella" term that includes all diseases of the heart and blood vessels such as atherosclerosis, heart attack, stroke, diabetes, high blood pressure, congenital heart defects, rheumatic heart disease, diseases of the valves, and arrhythmias. One quick look at Figure 1 should convince you that you should do all you can, starting today, to help keep your heart healthy.

Prevalence

Approximately 39,950,000 Americans have some form of heart or blood vessel disease. These figures break down as follows:

Hypertension (high blood pressure)	34,880,000 (one in six adults)
Coronary heart disease	4,330,000
Rheumatic heart disease (adults) (children)	1,780,000 100,000
Stroke	1,750,000

SOURCE: American Heart Association, "A Guide to Heart Facts," 1981, with permission.

Cardiovascular Disease Mortality

The 1978 estimate of the American Heart Association showed that about 985,800 or 51 percent of all deaths in the United States resulted from cardiovascular disease. (See Figure 2.) In 1977, there were 984,972 deaths attributed to cardiovascular disease, or 52 percent of all deaths that occurred that year. To put that figure in perspective:

Figure 1: Estimated Prevalence of the Major Cardiovascular Diseases (United States, 1978)

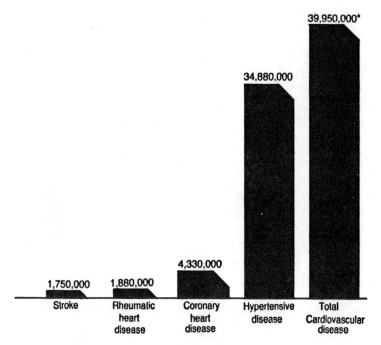

The sum of the individual estimates exceeds 39,950,000 since many persons have more than one cardiovascular disorder.

SOURCE: American Heart Association, with permission.

In 1978, cancer claimed less than half that number, or 396,060 victims; accidents took 107,930 lives. Nearly one-fourth of all persons who die from a cardiovascular disease are under the age of 65.

Heart Attack

Heart attack, which is one type of cardiovascular disease, caused 641,100 deaths in 1978.

Over 350,000 people a year die of a heart attack before they ever reach a hospital; the average victim waits approximately three hours before he or she decides to seek help.

Today, there are over 4,000,000 people in this country who have a history of heart attack and/or angina pectoris.

Figure 2: Deaths Due to Cardiovascular Diseases by Major Type of Disorder

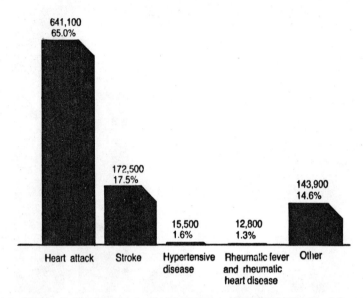

SOURCE: United States National Center for Health Statistics, USPHS, DHEW. Graph from the American Heart Association, "A Guide to Heart Facts," 1981, with permission.

Major Risk Factors

Several decades of study in the United States and Europe have identified three major, potentially reversible factors as increasing the risk of developing coronary heart disease or having a stroke. These are: high blood pressure, high blood cholesterol level, and cigarette smoking.

Today, approximately 34,880,000 people—or more than 10 percent of the population—in this country have hypertension, commonly known as high blood pressure. Even though many effective drugs are available to treat this disease, literally millions of people remain untreated or are inadequately treated. In fact, only a small percentage of those with hypertension have their blood pressure under adequate control.

The higher your blood pressure, the greater your risk for having a heart attack or a stroke. For example, according to the American Heart Association, a man with a systolic blood pressure over 150 mm Hg (millimeters of mercury) has more than *twice* the risk of heart attack and nearly *four* times the risk of a stroke than a man whose systolic blood pressure is 120 mm Hg or less.

Similarly, a man whose blood cholesterol level is 250 mg% or more has about *three* times the risk of heart attack and stroke as a man whose blood cholesterol level is below 194 mg%. (See Figure 3.)

Atherosclerosis is the term for the degenerative process that results in the development of fatty deposits on the inner lining of the walls of the arteries. Many experts believe this process is, in part, caused by a high-cholesterol diet. These fatty deposits result in narrowing of the arterial channel, often to such an extent that blood flow is diminished. Coronary artery atherosclerosis can prevent oxygen-rich blood from supplying the heart muscle with sufficient oxygen, and damage to the heart muscle, such as a heart attack, can occur. Similarly, when atherosclerosis develops in the cerebral (brain) arteries, a stroke or acute brain damage can result. In 1978, atherosclerosis contributed to many of the 800,000 deaths attributed to heart attack and stroke.

The evidence against cigarette smoking is massive. A man who smokes one pack a day runs nearly *twice* the risk of heart attack as his nonsmoking friend.

Finally, it should be noted that some victims of heart attack do not have any

Figure 3: The Danger of Heart Attack and Stroke Increases with the Number of Risk Factors Present

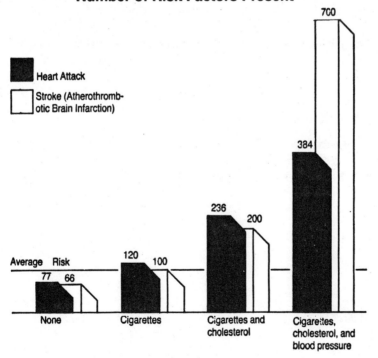

SOURCE: The Framingham Heart Study.

of these major risk factors present—which clearly indicates there is still a great deal to learn about coronary heart disease.

Stroke

In 1978, close to two million Americans were afflicted by stroke and nearly 200,000 died as a result.

Inborn or Congenital Heart Defects

Congenital heart defects are due to abnormalities in the development of the heart prior to birth. In all, there are 35 known types of these defects. Each year, approximately 25,000 babies are born with some type of heart defect, and it was estimated that over 6,000 infants died from these defects in 1978.

Research

Over $300 million in American Heart Association funds have gone into research on the causes and treatments of various types of heart disease since 1949. According to *AHA* statistics, about 60 percent of their national budget is earmarked for research, while the affiliates allocate about 20 percent of their income for research.

The Cost of Cardiovascular Disease

The American Heart Association estimates that in 1981 cardiovascular diseases cost us about $46.2 billion. (See Figure 4.) This total includes treatments, insurance bills, days lost, and so on.

Figure 4: Estimated Economic Costs in Billions of Dollars of Cardiovascular Diseases by Type of Expenditure United States 1981

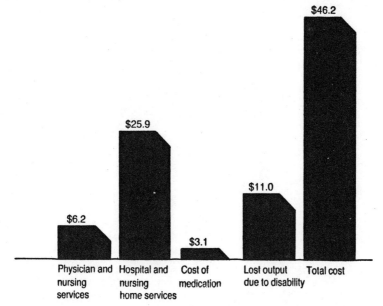

SOURCE: American Heart Association, "A Guide to Heart Facts," 1981, with permission.

PART I
How to Take Care of Your Heart

Risk Factors for Heart Attack: Real or Red Herrings?

In 1977, for the first time since 1964, statistics released from the National Institutes of Health, Washington, D.C. were encouraging in terms of heart disease: annual mortality due to all major cardiovascular diseases, including congenital heart disease, dropped below one million. In particular, cerebrovascular mortality (deaths due to strokes) dropped a dramatic 28.4 percent from 1951 to 1973, whereas the cerebrovascular mortality rates had been extremely stable from 1920 to 1951.

Despite this good news, however, cardiovascular diseases still cause nearly a million deaths a year, and the estimated number of adults in this country who actually have coronary heart disease, hypertensive disease, or suffer stroke is substantially higher than that. The estimated economic costs of cardiovascular diseases are staggering and a sobering reminder that, despite our gains, we still have an uphill fight against heart disease.

What accounts for the decline in cardiovascular mortality? Unfortunately, few topics in cardiology fuel more debate than this one, but we are still uncertain why cardiovascular mortality is declining in the United States, or what factors are responsible for the decrease. Some experts think that the declining death rate due to cardiovascular disease may be related to an increasing number of Americans asserting some control over their "coronary risk profiles."

What factors make up the coronary risk profile? Medical scientists have been probing this subject for years, and, on the basis of several large studies in which the living habits and medical records of thousands of persons were surveyed, they have determined that heart attack victims usually have one or more of the following factors present:

13

The "Big Three"*

Hypertension
   (high blood pressure)
Elevated serum cholesterol and/or triglycerides
   (excessive fatty substances in the blood)
Cigarette smoking

Other Risk Factors

Diabetes
A positive family history
   (a close relative with some form of heart disease)
Obesity
Sedentary life-style (lack of exercise)
Stressful life-style

But the most important question of all still looms large: How significant is each or all of these in the development of coronary heart disease? Will eliminating or controlling them reduce the likelihood of your having a heart attack? Before we discuss these risk factors in detail, let's find out what the current risk-factors controversy is all about.

To begin with, some clinicians doubt the significance of risk factors. They criticize the studies that have defined the importance of these variables for heart attack by saying that the conclusions drawn are based on abuses of logic. On the other hand, proponents of the risk-factor theory stick by the surveys that *implicate* high blood pressure, a high level of cholesterol in the blood and cigarette smoking in the development of coronary heart disease.

The critics emphasize that the relationship of the coronary risk factors to coronary artery disease is one of "association"—not cause and effect. In other words, the studies do link cigarette smoking, high blood pressure, and a diet high in intake of animal fats with a higher likelihood of having a heart attack and/or stroke, but they point out that this is circumstantial *rather than* definitive evidence. In that respect, they are right. Still, the circumstantial evidence implicating the risk factors listed previously, especially the "Big Three," is extremely strong. Therefore, after very careful consideration of the findings of so many studies that linked these factors with heart attack, many clinicians agreed that it would be in our best interest to *modify* our life-styles in order to reduce, to some extent, the presence and degree of these factors, thereby possibly reducing the risk of a heart attack. In our opinion, it is worthwhile to heed these recommendations. Here's why.

---

*The "Big Three" are the most important *potentially reversible* factors. However, other factors such as a positive family history are also significant.

Diet Is at the Heart of the Risk-Factor Controversy

Even the skeptics of the risk-factor theory generally concede that the evidence implicating high blood pressure is overwhelming; the prevalence of stroke and heart attack is markedly higher in people with high blood pressure. Similarly, cigarette smoking is an accepted well-defined risk factor for stroke and heart attack, to say nothing of the extensive evidence demonstrating that lung cancer and cigarette smoking are inextricably linked.

Of the "Big Three," then, diet is the real bone of contention. Is it necessary to reduce your intake of saturated fats to help stave off a heart attack?

Early in 1980 the National Academy of Sciences stirred up scientists, physicians, and consumers alike when it issued statements that, in effect, gave a green light—in terms of diet—to healthy Americans. Specifically, the report said that healthy Americans need not restrict their dietary intake of cholesterol and saturated fats because, in the Academy's opinion, there is no conclusive evidence to show that such steps will have an overall lifesaving benefit.

In our opinion, the evidence suggests that a prudent diet *can* be important in maintaining a healthy heart. For example: Mortality from coronary heart disease rose by 19 percent in this country from 1950 to 1963; then, in 1964, the downward spiral began. Why? Many factors were probably involved, but in particular, two major public health events stand out: In January of that year, the Surgeon General of the United States Public Health Service warned that cigarette smoking may be hazardous to your health. And just a few months later, the American Heart Association (AHA) followed with its recommendations, advocating some dietary changes with the ultimate objective of reducing the incidence of heart attack and stroke by deliberately limiting dietary intake of cholesterol and saturated fats.

Specifically, the AHA stated that Americans should "eat less animal (saturated) fat, increase the intake of unsaturated vegetable oils and polyunsaturated fats, substitute them for saturated fats wherever possible, and eat fewer foods rich in cholesterol."

Since the Surgeon General's warning, the number of adults who smoke cigarettes has fallen off, and thanks to a persistent AHA educational campaign, many Americans also have begun to alter their eating habits. By 1976, the AHA took an even stronger stand. They said: "Although there may be some difference of opinion as to the importance of diet modification in coronary disease and atherosclerosis, the majority of experts believe that modification of diet is justified, especially in high-risk patients."

Finally, the results of a long-range study on the role of diet, cholesterol and death from coronary heart disease were published in the *New England Journal of Medicine*. Specifically, 1,900 men employed by the Western Electric Company in Chicago underwent a physical examination, and their dietary habits were recorded. The following year, the men were divided into three groups, according to how much cholesterol and fat they usually ate. In the 19-year followup, the investigators found that the men who had eaten the least amount of cholesterol and dietary fat had the fewest number of fatal heart attacks.

Despite the findings of this recent study and the Heart Association's thorough review of the evidence, however, no doubt vociferous naysayers will continue to argue that cholesterol has little if any relationship to the development of coronary heart disease. Even those who strongly believe that diets high in saturated fats play a role in the development of coronary heart disease (CHD) also recognize that CHD is a multifactorial disease process; as such, no one will say for certain that the decline in cardiovascular mortality can be traced directly to the warnings issued by the Surgeon General in 1964 or to the AHA's dietary recommendations.

No one can guarantee that if you hold the risk factors in check, you will automatically be assured of a healthy heart. In fact, you have probably heard a friend or business associate say: "My uncle was overweight, never exercised, smoked three packs of cigarettes a day, and he lived to be ninety-one" or "My grandfather didn't drink or smoke. He couldn't afford much beef, he walked to and from work, about five miles a day, and he died of a heart attack when he was forty-six."

The point we wish to emphasize is: The cause of coronary heart disease is multifaceted; many factors come into play, including family history, diet, exercise, stress, and so on. That's why some people can eat two or more eggs every day and still have a normal cholesterol level, while others may have to severely limit their total cholesterol intake. These are unusual conditions, however. Generally speaking, the odds of having a stroke or a heart attack increase in relation to the number and degree of risk factors present. We agree with the majority of medical scientists who say that we should modify our life-styles: Eliminate cigarette smoking; reduce weight if necessary; reduce intake of saturated fats; and get regular exercise. After all, if there *is* a strong chance that modifying smoking and eating habits did contribute to the recent remarkable drop in cardiovascular mortality, doesn't it make sense to adhere to the guidelines set forth by the AHA and the Surgeon General?

The debate over diet—specifically, the significance of cholesterol in coronary heart disease—will continue for some time. Dr. Irvine H. Page, a well-known physician who is Consultant Emeritus to The Cleveland Clinic Foundation, and a postcoronary victim himself, has noted that he still follows his low-cholesterol, low-fat diet because he has no intention of being the smartest man in the cemetery.*

---

*I. H. Page, *The Cholesterol Fallacy*, Cleveland: Coronary Club, *1977.*

Here's How the Risk Factors Add Up

The graph on page 7 shows that the danger of heart attack or stroke increases according to the number of risk factors present. The example given there is that of a forty-five-year old man; note the level of average risk, and then see how his risk for a cardiovascular event rises as each risk factor is added to his coronary risk profile.

In the following pages, you can learn how simple it is to make a few changes in your living habits that may prolong your life. The key is *moderation*, not deprivation. We know you probably can't give up fried foods and cheesecake forever, nor do you have to. The trick is to learn how to balance your calories, and exercise daily—in short, to follow an "even-keeled" life-style. We hope you utilize the guidelines presented here to help you and your family stay healthy.

1
Man Is What He Eats

Man is what he eats. Sound trite? Perhaps, but it also has a distinct ring of truth. Even Shakespeare recognized it.

> I [the gut] am the storehouse of the whole body, and what I receive, I send through the blood to the heart, the brain and even the small inferior veins, and all I am left with for myself is the bran from the flour.
>
> Shakespeare, *Coriolanus*, Act I, scene i.

He was right. Everything you eat, from licorice to liquor to that tiny nibble of chocolate cake passes through the complex maze of the digestive tract. Ultimately, the foods are either utilized by the body's cells and organs, stored for later use, or eliminated.

Knowing this, you would think that we would be far more careful about what, and how much, we eat. But, when it comes to day-to-day nutrition, many of us have a blasé attitude; for the most part, we blithely ingest all that is placed before us, be it three nutritionally balanced meals a day, or a big breakfast, coffee break, luncheon, cocktails and hors d'oeuvres, dinner, and a midnight snack.

The indifference is interesting because many Americans do have some knowledge of sound nutritional principles. Nevertheless, we keep right on eating . . . and eating . . . virtually anything and everything that comes before us!

In the following chapter, you will learn ways to help you and your family eat a balanced diet daily, and we will explain the potential significance of diet in the development of coronary heart disease.

Despite our seeming lack of attention to our daily diets, one thing is certain: the United States Government does care about our eating habits–and with good reason. For example, despite widespread promotion of numerous products to alleviate "tired" or "iron-poor" blood, iron deficiency remains one of this country's most common medical disorders. In fact, it has been estimated that approximately 5 percent of American women have mild iron deficiency anemia.

18

Other studies also show that even with our abundant food supply, one child in five still does not get enough vitamin C each day, and only one in nineteen receives an adequate supply of iron. Similarly, studies conducted among schoolchildren have revealed that those who eat a nutritious breakfast regularly generally do better in school than those who have a skimpy breakfast. What's more, some experts now believe that myriad other medical and behavioral problems such as fatigue, increased irritability, and headache may be linked to dietary problems.

The U.S. Government has also become increasingly concerned about the prevalence of obesity in this country, as well as the association of diets high in animal fat with the incidence of numerous diseases, in particular, coronary heart disease. According to most surveys, approximately 20 percent of the adult American population is overweight. In July 1976, Dr. Theodore Cooper, then Assistant Secretary for Health, testified before the Senate Select Committee on Nutrition and Human Needs, stating that these adults were "overweight to a degree that may interfere with optimal health and longevity." Committee Chairman Senator George McGovern said that "the eating patterns of this century represent as critical a public health concern as any now before us."

Unfortunately, although we live in the most diet-conscious country in the world, with perhaps more foods to choose from than any other nation, the fact remains that few of us actually associate diet with disease. Nevertheless, our excess consumption of fats, especially saturated fats, as well as cholesterol, refined sugar, salt, and alcohol has been linked to six of the ten leading causes of death: heart disease, cerebrovascular disease, cancer, diabetes, arteriosclerosis and cirrhosis of the liver.

What evidence supports this assertion? Interestingly enough, researchers began to investigate diet as a possible cause of several diseases many years ago. As early as 1904, for example, a noted Russian researcher, Dr. Ilia Metchnikov, who worked at the Pasteur Institute in Paris, said that "premature senility and death" were, for the most part, disorders caused by man's "new diet." Essentially, Metchnikov was commenting on the impact of the Industrial Revolution on our eating habits.

Shortly after the introduction of machines designed to refine foods, many products, such as grain and sugar, were processed in mills, where some of the "natural" ingredients, such as fiber, were removed. As time wore on, the processes of refining and manufacturing food became more sophisticated. Ultimately, virtually every type of food could be channeled through the mills, refined, processed, preserved, frozen and made reheatable—all for economy and convenience.

Research continued and, about 1950, epidemiologists and medical researchers began to notice an alarming change in disease and death rates. For no apparent reason, it seemed that the incidence of heart disease, colon cancer, diverticulitis and lung cancer, to name a few, were climbing at a steady rate. To find out why, several major studies were established to assess several possible causes for this new trend in disease and mortality rates. Among other factors, diet was evaluated, and, in many cases, the change in our eating habits could be linked to the altering pattern of disease.

Among other things, these studies established that our current diets contrast sharply with those of our forebears. For example, it has been estimated that today every man, woman and child consumes an average of 125 pounds of fat, 188 pounds of meat and 100 pounds of sugar annually. Our consumption of beef has increased significantly, rising sharply from 55 pounds per person in 1940 to 117 pounds in 1974, an increase of 113 percent. Fat constitutes 42 percent of our total caloric intake—27 percent more than our grandparents consumed in 1910. At the turn of the century, approximately 40 percent of the average daily diet was derived from fresh fruits, vegetables and whole-grain products. Now, only 20 percent of our total calories are consumed in these foods.

Table 1.1. How Our Eating Habits Have Changed (1910–1976)*

Beef	+90%	
Chicken	+179%	
Turkey	+820%	
Tuna, canned	+1,300%	(1926–1976)
Fish, fresh and frozen	+42%	(1960–1976)
Potatoes, fresh	−74%	
Potatoes, frozen	+465%	(1960–1976)
Fresh fruits	−33%	
Frozen vegetables	+44%	
Butter	−76%	
Margarine	+681%	
Wheat flour	−48%	
Soft drinks	+157%	(1960–1976)
Sugar, other sweeteners	+33%	(1909–1976)
Corn syrup	+244%	(1960–1976)
Food colors	+995%	(1940–1977)

* 1910-1976, unless otherwise indicated.
SOURCE: "The Changing American Diet," Center for Science in the Public Interest, 1755 "S" Street, N.W., Washington, D.C. 20009.

In terms of linking diet with coronary heart disease, the evidence accumulated over the last thirty years is massive. Dr. Ancel Keys, noted researcher and nutritionist, has spent years studying the role of diet in disease, particularly heart disease. Dr. Keys' studies have revealed that Japanese peasants have a very low incidence of heart disease; concomitantly, their diets are low in saturated fats. When some of these people moved to Hawaii, however, their dietary intake of saturated fats increased somewhat as did their incidence of coronary heart disease. But the worst findings evolved when the Japanese moved to the continental United States, where they readily adopted our diet—and our incidence of coronary heart disease.

Other extensive studies have been carried out to learn more about the relationship between diet and coronary heart disease. Herewith, a sampling of those surveys.

The International Atherosclerosis Project. In his study, autopsies were performed on more than 31,000 persons aged 10 to 69 who died between 1960 and 1965 in 15 cities throughout the world. Specifically, the degree of atherosclerosis of the aorta and the coronary arteries was measured, and was found to vary considerably, depending on the population autopsied. For example, populations with diets high in cholesterol and saturated fats, such as in New Orleans, Louisiana, and Oslo, Norway, showed the most severe atherosclerotic lesions (fatty deposits in the arteries), while populations that consumed low saturated fat and low-cholesterol diets, such as Durban Bantu in Africa, showed the least.

The Seven-Nation Study. Also known as the International Cooperative Study on the Epidemiology of Cardiovascular Disease, 12,000 men aged 40 to 49 in 18 different towns in Finland, Greece, Italy, Japan, the Netherlands, the United States, and Yugoslavia were followed. After five years, the study showed that men in the United States and eastern Finland had the highest rates of heart attacks—more than eight percent and 12 percent, respectively, had coronary heart disease. On the other hand, the five-year incidence rate was less than two percent among some of the male populations in Greece, Japan and Yugoslavia. A closer look at the diets of these populations showed that the highest intake of saturated or animal fats was found in the diets of the Finnish population (22 percent) and the American men (19 percent).

The Framingham Heart Study. Although a serum cholesterol level between 220 and 250 mg% has been considered acceptable by many physicians, this study revealed that men aged 45 to 54 had a 48 percent higher incidence of coronary heart disease with serum cholesterol levels in that range than men of the same age with serum cholesterol levels less than 220 mg%.

Figure 1 shows that a man with a blood cholesterol level of 250 mg% or greater has approximately *three* times the risk of heart attack and stroke as a man whose blood cholesterol level is less than 194 mg%.

Figure 1.1: Relationship of Heart Attack or Stroke to Level of Cholesterol

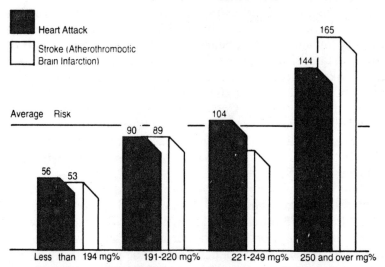

Heart Attack

Stroke (Atherothrombotic Brain Infarction)

Average   Risk

56   53   90   89   104   144   165

Less than 194 mg%   191-220 mg%   221-249 mg%   250 and over mg%

Data from the Framingham Heart Study show that risk of a heart attack or stroke increases as level of cholesterol in the blood increases.
SOURCE: The Framingham Heart Study.

A NEW CONCEPT: THE U.S. GOVERNMENT SETS NUTRITIONAL GOALS

Dr. Jeremiah Stamler, international authority in epidemiology, nutrition, and cardiovascular disease, says we are in the midst of a coronary epidemic. Dr. William Kannel, Director of the Framingham Heart Study, calls coronary heart disease "the curse of the twentieth century."

Today, it is still estimated that approximately one in three men and one in six women in the United States will die from stroke or heart disease before the age of 60. Yet based on the overwhelming evidence accumulated over the last two decades or so, a 1971 report prepared by the Department of Agriculture suggested that considerable improvement in our health could be achieved by improving our eating habits. In that report, the Department estimated that revising our daily food intake could result in a 25 percent reduction in heart and vascular (circulatory) problems.

Based on the studies that show the impact of nutrition on health—cardiovascular status in particular—the U.S. Senate Select Committee on Nutrition and Human Needs established six specific dietary goals for the United States; they also outlined seven ways to help you accomplish these goals.

The U.S. Dietary Goals are:

1. Increase consumption of complex carbohydrates (fruits, vegetables).

2. Decrease consumption of simple carbohydrates.

3. Reduce overall consumption of fats.

4. Specifically, consumption of saturated fats should account for about 10 percent of your total energy intake; that should be balanced with an equal intake of polyunsaturated and mono-unsaturated fats.

5. Reduce cholesterol consumption to 300 mg per day.

6. Drastically reduce salt consumption to about three grams per day.

The Senate Select Committee made the following recommendations also to help you improve your diet:

1. Increase consumption of fruits, vegetables, and whole grains.

2. Decrease consumption of meat and increase consumption of poultry and fish.

3. Decrease consumption of foods high in fat and partially substitute polyunsaturated fat for saturated fat.

4. Substitute nonfat milk for whole milk.

5. Decrease consumption of butterfat, eggs, and other high-cholesterol sources.

6. Decrease consumption of sugar and foods high in sugar content.

7. Decrease consumption of salt and foods high in salt content.

Working Toward Dietary Goals

What steps in particular should you take to achieve the U.S. Dietary Goals? The most important step is moderation. Cut down on your intake of saturated or animal fats, reduce your intake of refined and processed foods, and increase your intake of fresh fruits and vegetables, whole-grain breads and cereals, and polyunsaturated fats. (See Figure 2.) You may not be certain about how to do this without arousing family rebellion! Fortunately, most of the dietary changes that are called for are subtle—chances are, your spouse and children won't even notice—and you can feel good that you are doing all that you can to help keep their hearts healthy.

Before we show you how to adapt your present eating habits so you can achieve the new national dietary goals, including pointers on getting you through the supermarket aisles, providing snacks for your children, and eating out in a restaurant, let's take a moment to brush up on some basic nutritional principles. Take a look at the quiz in the box, and then read on to ascertain your "nutrition I.Q."

How Experts View Diet in Coronary Heart Disease

This survey on coronary heart disease (CHD) was conducted by Dr. K. R. Norum, Chairman of the Nutrition Research Institute at the University of Oslo, Norway. Overall, 92 percent of the 208 medical scientists questioned in twenty-three countries responded. Here's what these experts think:

	YES	NO	UNCERTAIN
Is there a connection between diet and coronary heart disease?	188	1	4
Is there a connection between level of cholesterol in the blood and development of coronary heart disease?	189	2	2
Is our knowledge of diet and CHD sufficient for recommending a moderate change in the diet for the population in an affluent society?	176	16	1
Is your own personal diet influenced by your knowledge?	175	16	2
Should we carry out some type of screening programs to detect persons at high risk CHD?	152	31	10
Do you smoke?	26	162	5

Reprinted with permission, *Nutr. & Metab.* 22: 1–7 (1978)

Figure 1.2: U.S. Dietary Goals

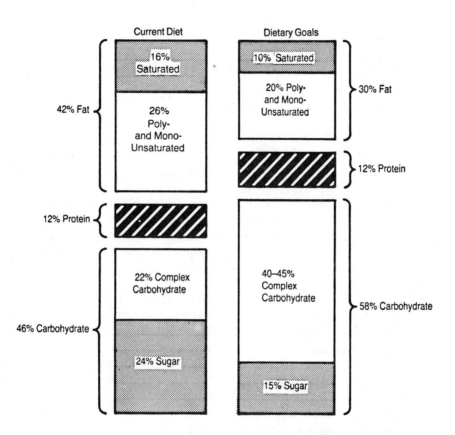

The column on the left shows the composition of our diet today and the column on the right outlines current dietary objectives: reduce dietary intake of saturated fats by 6% and of poly- and monounsaturated fats by 6%. Protein intake is satisfactory; no change is recommended. Sugar intake should be reduced by 9%; intake of complex carbohydrates (fruits and vegetables) should be increased by 18% to 23%.

SOURCE: "Changes in Nutrients in the U.S. Diet Caused by Alterations in Food Intake Patterns." B. Friend. Agricultural Research Service. U.S. Department of Agriculture, 1974. Proportions of saturated versus unsaturated fats based on unpublished Agricultural Research Service data.

Brush Up on Basic Nutritional Principles

Is nutrition old-hat to you?   Do you feel that you are fairly up-to-date in your knowledge and understanding of sound nutritional principles? Let's test your knowledge.

	TRUE	FALSE
1. A plain baked potato is fattening.	☐	☐
2. Foods high in carbohydrates should be virtually eliminated from any weight-reducing diet.	☐	☐
3. Margarine has fewer calories than butter.	☐	☐
4. Low-calorie foods include mushrooms, spinach, avocados, lettuce, and carrots.	☐	☐
5. High-calorie foods include butter, peanuts, bananas, raisins.	☐	☐

Your nutrition score. Here are the answers. A plain baked potato—without butter, margarine, or sour cream—is a mere ninety calories, and it contains important vitamins, such as B_6. Even the fiber of the potato skin will help your digestion.

Several fruits, such as bananas, are high in carbohydrates (about twenty-two grams per banana), but this hardly means that bananas, or any other fruit, should be eliminated if you are on a diet.

A big "error" in diet planning creeps in with regard to margarine. Margarine and butter contain the same number of calories (approximately fifty calories per pat), but margarine has less cholesterol than butter. (If the margarine is labeled "diet" margarine, then it also has fewer calories than butter.)

All of the foods listed in question 4 are low calorie, *except* avocados. Half of an average-sized avocado is about 280 calories, far more than one cup of fresh sliced mushrooms, which contains about twenty calories.

In the last question, everything listed is high in calories, *except* bananas. The average banana has approximately 85 calories.

We will review nutrients, beginning with the most basic element: water.

---

1. *About water.* Overall, 60 percent of your total body weight is water. Some of this water is contained within the body's cells, some is outside the cells, and some makes up the fluid portion of the blood. Generally, six to eight full glasses of water a day are recommended for good health. As of December 1977, eleven countries had reported a correlation between the incidence of coronary heart disease and the hardness of the drinking water: the harder the water, the lower the incidence of coronary heart disease. Still,

the relationship between hardness of water and coronary heart disease has not been established. The primary difference between soft and hard drinking water is the higher content of magnesium and calcium salts in hard water.

2. *About vitamins.* Vitamins are catalysts, or stimulants, involved in complex biochemical processes. Adequate vitamin intake promotes normal body function. Inadequate intake of even one, say vitamin B, can result in various abnormalities such as diarrhea.

   Ideally, you shouldn't need a vitamin supplement, but your doctor may recommend a daily multivitamin tablet, particularly if you cling to a strict vegetarian diet or if you are pregnant. Remember, taking more vitamins than indicated won't make you healthier.

3. *About minerals.* Minerals are necessary for a wide variety of the body's functions. For example, calcium helps build and maintain strong bones, and iron is essential for blood cell formation, among other things.

   Numerous substances, including sodium, zinc, even copper, are vital elements. Overall, fourteen minerals make up approximately 5 percent of your total body weight; the average 175-pound man carries about eight pounds of minerals, including enough iron for two or three hairpins, enough phosphorus to comprise several matchsticks, and enough salt to fill a small shaker!

4. *About proteins.* Proteins are the building blocks of the body's tissues. Essentially, a protein molecule looks like a long chain—every link is an amino acid. Twenty amino acids are necessary to maintain good nutrition. Of these, twelve can be synthesized by the body from the raw materials in certain foods such as meat, fish, milk, whole-grain cereals, beans, and lentils. The remaining eight amino acids, referred to as the "essential amino acids," must be present in the diet.

   Surprisingly, most Americans are very aware of the importance of protein and consume more than required to maintain good health. For example, most adults need approximately 70 to 75 grams of protein a day, or about 1 gram per kilogram of body weight (1 kilogram = 2.2 pounds).

5. *About carbohydrates.* Your energy comes from carbohydrates (sugars and starches). Sugars include table sugar (sucrose), milk sugar (lactose), and fruit sugar (fructose). Besides providing energy, certain sugars are vital to the formation of molecules that ultimately form genes, the complex chemicals that control heredity and are, in effect, the blueprint plan for human

development. Carbohydrates are also derived from starchy foods, such as potatoes, cereals, rice, pastas, breads, turnips, and beets. Numerous calorie guides show the carbohydrate content of many foods.

6. *About fats.* Most of us dread the very word *fat*, but, actually, fat in the diet is essential to life. Fats are the most concentrated source of food energy, providing more energy—nine calories per gram—than any other foodstuff utilized by the body. Fats are classified into three categories, based on their chemical composition: saturated (animal) fats, polyunsaturated fats, and mono-unsaturated fats.

Since fats are essential, why do doctors ask you to cut your saturated-fat intake? First, fats are calorie-packed; they contain nearly twice as many calories per gram as carbohydrates or proteins. For example, if you compare equivalent portions of steak and mussels, they are equal in protein content, but the steak contains twice the number of calories, and approximately eighteen times the amount of fat! Second, saturated, or animal, fats are a primary source of cholesterol, and many studies have identified an elevated serum cholesterol as a risk factor for coronary heart disease. Polyunsaturated fats, on the other hand, tend to depress your blood cholesterol levels, while mono-unsaturated fats have no effect. Since cholesterol has received so much attention in the last few years, we are going to discuss it in detail to help you understand what it is and why it may be significant in terms of the development of coronary heart disease.

A PROFILE OF YOUR BLOOD LIPIDS

Fats are a necessary part of any balanced diet. They help the body utilize protein and they carry the fat-soluble vitamins: A, D, E and K. Fats also go a long way in suppressing appetite. The problem is that most Americans consume far too much in animal fats; in fact, the U.S. Senate Select Committee on Nutrition and Human Needs said that most Americans generally consume 42 percent of their total caloric intake in the form of fats (16 percent saturated and 26 percent poly- and mono-unsaturated). According to their recommendations, it would be better to reduce our dietary fat intake to 30 percent of our total caloric intake (10 percent in the form of saturated fats and 20 percent in the forms of poly-and mono-unsaturated fats).

Why? The data discussed in this section show that a diet high in saturated fats is inextricably interwoven with coronary heart disease. But, you might ask, just how does the excess intake of saturated fats damage the heart? How does fat manage to ride along in the bloodstream, then begin to accumulate—first as streaks, then as clumps (which are referred to as "plaques") on the inside of the coronary arteries, and other arteries as well?

Once fat is digested, it undergoes a very complex range of biochemical processes; the fats are broken down and utilized for their numerous functions such as fuel for energy and cell growth. Excess fat may be stored (much to our dismay), while some is carried into the bloodstream. Over a period of time, fat deposits can build up in the arteries—a process known as atherosclerosis (see Chapter 10 for a more complete discussion of this process and its role in coronary heart disease). Initially, the fatty deposits appear as streaks on the inner lining of the arteries, but, ultimately, the streaks may evolve into clumps of fat and other materials that accumulate on the walls of the arteries. Thus, the arteries, or channels, are narrowed. (It still is not known whether these streaks actually precede the development of plaques, or whether plaques develop independently of the fatty streaks.) Regardless, it is established that these fatty clumps can obstruct blood flow, partially at first, but as the plaque buildup in the artery continues, severe narrowing or total occlusion or obstruction can occur. Unfortunately, plaques are most likely to develop in major arteries, e.g., the coronary, or the cerebral (brain) arteries. When this happens, a heart attack can occur and sometimes that heart attack, even if fatal, is the first and only sign that coronary obstruction is present. Similarly, a stroke may be the first real sign that blood flow to the brain is occluded or obstructed, and signs of kidney disease may appear due to blockage of blood flow in the renal (kidney) arteries. Finally, atherosclerosis can also occur in the aorta, gastrointestinal, leg, and retinal arteries.

To some extent, this clogging of the body's arteries seems to be part of the aging process. However, the life-style of modern industrial society seems to be associated with premature onset of this process. For example, studies show that even infants may have some fat deposits in their arteries, and it has been estimated that by the age of 10, many youngsters have fatty streaks in their arteries.

What do these fatty plugs in the arteries actually contain? For a closer look, pathologists have obtained samples of these atherosclerotic lesions in numerous postmortem studies. (Figure 3 shows a typical occluded artery.) Their findings have helped medical investigators and physicians understand more about what goes on in the coronary arteries, and what you can do that may help to forestall the progression of atherosclerotic disease.

The scientific name for blood fats is *lipids*. There is more than one type of lipid in the blood; you may be aware of cholesterol and triglycerides, while other lipids such as phospholipids, chylomicrons, and lipoproteins may be unfamiliar.

The major classes of blood lipids are cholesterol, triglycerides and phospholipids. All of these combine with a specific group of proteins, *globulins*, to form carrier molecules known as *lipoproteins*. The lipoproteins are

Figure 1.3: Normal and Occluded (Blocked) Coronary Arteries

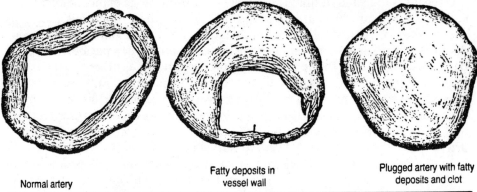

Normal artery

Fatty deposits in
vessel wall

Plugged artery with fatty
deposits and clot

classified into four different types: high-density lipoproteins (HDL), low-density lipoproteins (LDL), very low-density lipoproteins (VLDL), and chylomicrons.

The lipoproteins are composed of varying degrees of cholesterol, triglycerides, phospholipids and proteins.

What Is Cholesterol?

Poor cholesterol. Lately, the word itself conjures up an image of an insidious disease process lurking in the wings. But is the bad press justified? That depends on just how much cholesterol you consume on a daily basis, and your blood's cholesterol level.

Essentially, cholesterol is a fatlike, waxy substance present in living tissue and necessary for good health. Cholesterol is essential to the structure of the body's cells and plays an important role in the production of bile secretions and some hormones such as the sex hormones: estrogens in the female, androgens in the male, and the adrenal gland hormones: hydrocortisone and aldosterone. Infants, in particular, need an adequate intake of dietary cholesterol to insure proper development of the nervous system.

How Is Cholesterol Produced?

The liver can manufacture all the cholesterol that the body needs; however, it may produce excessive amounts, especially when the diet is high in animal fats such as beef, butter, and eggs. (Text continues on page 33.)

Table 1.2. A Guide to Cholesterol Content of Common Foods

	Serving	Cholesterol (mg)
Whole milk	1 cup	33
Cheese:		
Cheddar	1 oz	30
Cottage-creamed (4% fat)	1 cup	31
Swiss	1 oz	26
Light cream	1 Tbsp	10
Sour (cultured) cream	1 Tbsp	5
Ice cream-regular (approx. 10% fat)	1 cup	59
Yogurt-plain (partially-skimmed milk)	8 oz (1 cup)	14
Lean beef	3 oz	77
Poultry (flesh without skin, light meat)	3 oz	43
Fish (lean)	3 oz	43
Shrimp	11 large	96
Tuna (packed in oil, drained solids)	3 oz	55
Lobster	½ cup	62
Liver, beef	3 oz	372
Frankfurters (all beef-30% fat)	1 lb (8 large)	49
Eggs (chicken, whole)†	1 medium	274
Peanut butter	2 Tbsp	0
Bacon, cooked crisp	2 slices	14
Butter	1 Tbsp	31
Imitation (diet) margarine	1 Tbsp	0
Mayonnaise	1 Tbsp	8

†Cholesterol is found only in egg yolk.

Adapted with permission from *The American Heart Association Cookbook*, 3rd edition, New York: David McKay Company, Inc. © 1979 The American Heart Association.

Table 1.3. Contents of Fats and Oils
Fatty Acids
(grams)

	Cholesterol *(milligrams)*	Saturated	Mono-unsaturated	Poly-unsaturated
Butters and margarines (1 tablespoon)				
Butter	31	7.1	3.3	0.4
Imitation margarine (diet)	0	1.0	2.2	2.0
Mayonnaise	8	2.0	2.4	5.6
Vegetable shortening (hydrogenated)	0	3.2	5.7	3.1
Corn oil	0	1.7	3.3	7.8
Safflower oil	0	1.3	1.6	10.0
Soybean oil	0	2.1	3.2	8.1
Olive oil	0	1.9	9.7	1.1
Peanut oil	0	2.3	6.2	4.2
Coconut oil	0	12.1	0.8	0.3

Adapted with permission from *The American Heart Association Cookbook*, 3rd edition, New York: David McKay Company, Inc. © 1979 The American Heart Association.

How Doctors Measure Fats in the Blood

A simple blood test tells all. The amount of cholesterol is measured in milligrams per 100 cubic centimeters of blood. A low/normal level is under 200 (written 200 mg%); the U.S. Senate Select Committee on Nutrition and Human Needs recommends that Americans reduce cholesterol consumption to about 300 mg per day. For many, that means some immediate dietary changes—the average American ingests approximately 600 mg of cholesterol per day!

What Foodstuffs Contain Cholesterol?

Cholesterol is found in animal fats: meats, butter, eggs, and shellfish. The juiciest cuts of beef and steak are often very high in cholesterol if they are marbled or laced with fat. Organ meats, including liver, kidneys, and sweetbreads, also are high in cholesterol.

Shellfish, such as shrimp and lobster, are also high in cholesterol, but the biggest culprit is the egg yolk. It contains 250 mg of cholesterol, compared to 67 mg in a low-cholesterol food such as three or four ounces of chicken.

Why Do Some People Have More Cholesterol Than Others?

Scientists don't know for sure, but several studies show that if your diet is high in cholesterol and saturated (animal) fats, you are apt to have an elevated blood level of cholesterol. When this happens, your risk of having a heart attack may climb, too.

Age, sex, family history, and exercise, as well as your diet, seem to influence your blood level of cholesterol. For example, elevated cholesterol levels are more commonly found in men than in women or children. Presumably, growing children utilize more fully any excess cholesterol that may be ingested, whereas an adult male has little need for it. Thus, it is more likely to remain as stored fat or cholesterol. Of course, adult women don't need any "extra" cholesterol either, but even women who eat more saturated fats than is recommended are less likely than men to have elevated blood cholesterol levels *until* menopause, when their "immunity" to coronary heart disease diminishes.

Exercise as well is known to influence the type of blood cholesterol. Recent studies at Stanford University in Palo Alto, California, showed that long-distance runners and others who engage in habitual strenuous exercise of the aerobic type generally have higher levels of HDLs, which have been associated with lower rates of heart attack than high levels of LDLs.

Finally, genetic predisposition is a factor in your body's ability to manage dietary cholesterol. In particular, two types of lipid, or fat, disorders are relatively common in our society. One, *hypercholesterolemia* means there is too much cholesterol in the blood. The other is *hypertriglyceridemia*, which is an excess of triglycerides in the blood. Even if family members are free of these disorders, it does not necessarily follow that a child's blood lipid levels are normal. Many studies show that the average American child has a serum cholesterol level 50 to 100 mg% higher than levels in children from less developed countries. It's unwise to assume your child is free from any lipid disorder simply because your family history is negative, because many doctors believe that our children's high-saturated fat diet is often a culprit. The box below outlines a statement prepared by the American Heart Association a few years ago. In it, they clearly indicated that most experts agree that the dietary intake of cholesterol and saturated fat should be modified for children and they concluded that such modification seems safe and likely to be beneficial. Remember, modification is the key; before you undertake any drastic dietary changes, we advise you to consult your physician. For most of us, modest changes in diet can "do the trick;" (i.e., keep intake of saturated fats and cholesterol at an appropriate level). In the next several pages, we show you ways to modify your family's diet, so it is healthier . . . better for you and your children.

A reasonable cholesterol for a child (ages 2 to 20) ranges from 160 to 180 mg%. Do you know what your child's cholesterol level is? How about your own?

Phospholipids and Triglycerides

Phospholipids are found in cell membranes and in only very small amounts in deposit fats. *Triglycerides*, called "neutral" fats, are the major component of deposit or storage fats. Triglycerides vary according to the different fatty acids they contain.

A Lexicon of Lipoproteins: HDL, LDL, VLDL

Now to the latest research. What picture immediately comes to mind when we say "bloodstream"? Perhaps you envision a passive conduit . . . a moving fluid pathway that delivers oxygen and other nutrients in a "ho-hum" fashion to the body's organs and cells. But nothing could be more inaccurate! Blood is a very active transport system . . . a complex biochemical and metabolic labyrinth in which highly specialized processes are taking place all the time. One of the most stimulating findings in the last decade has to do with such processes.

HDL: A "Good" Fat in the Blood

For a change, having a high level of one type of cholesterol in your blood
(Text continues on page 36)

Coronary Heart Disease Often Begins in Childhood

What you can do to help

In July 1978, the American Heart Association, relying on a committee report, "Value and Safety of Diet Modification to Control Hyperlipidemia in Childhood and Adolescence," recommended that children in families with a high risk of cardiovascular disease undergo blood tests and be placed on a corrective diet (one low in saturated or animal fats) if the test results showed that they had excessive levels of cholesterol or triglycerides (fats) in their blood.

According to the Heart Association, a high-risk family is defined as follows:
—either or both parents have high blood pressure;
—one or both parent(s) or grandparent(s) has (have) suffered a heart attack or a stroke, or developed peripheral vascular disease (narrowing of veins and arteries in the arms and legs) before the age of 50;
—either parent has hyperlipidemia (a high cholesterol or triglyceride level in the blood).

Following are excerpts from the statement made by the Committee of the American Heart Association (reprinted with permission):

> It is generally accepted that atherosclerosis begins in childhood and undergoes rapid progression in adolescence and young adulthood, even though the serious clinical manifestations do not appear until middle age or later. Many questions remain about the causes of fat deposition in children's arteries and whether these fat deposits lead directly to advanced arterial lesions. However, studies of U.S. men who died from accidental causes have shown that clinically significant lesions begin to appear in the third decade of life, shortly after the childhood years. This observation is one reason why many physicians and scientists believe that prevention, to be effective, must begin in the teenage years and possibly, earlier.
>
> Surveys in the past five years have established unequivocally that U.S. children have higher plasma lipid concentrations than do children in other populations in which adult atherosclerotic disease is less frequent.
>
> Because hyperlipidemia is the most consistent and most frequent risk factor for atherosclerotic disease (other than age and sex), it has received the most attention as a point of attack for the prevention of atherosclerosis. This emphasis remains despite the reservation [described previously] that reduction in morbidity and mortality by lowering plasma lipid concentrations has not been proven conclusively. The relatively small clinical trials that have been completed may have failed to detect a substantial effect because they began in adults in whom atherosclerosis already was well advanced.
>
> Although the evidence does not yet support the recommendation that cholesterol and saturated fat should be reduced in the diet of all children, the public should be advised that such modification appears safe and very likely to be beneficial.

(continued from page 34)
might be good for you. "Indeed," says William P. Castelli, Director of Laboratories for the Framingham Heart Studies, "some cholesterol is actually associated with good health."

While it has been recognized for some time that the *total* serum cholesterol level is a good predictor of coronary risk for persons under 50 years of age, it is not helpful in predicting risk for older individuals. But now, says Dr. Castelli, "knowledge of the HDL levels is more important than knowledge of total serum cholesterol levels." Several recent studies have confirmed an inverse relationship between high-density lipoproteins and coronary heart disease. For example, several findings indicate that the prevalence rates for coronary heart disease decrease progressively as levels of HDL rise in the blood. In addition, a Cincinnati research team headed by Dr. Charles J. Glueck, University of Cincinnati Medical Center, found that members of long-lived families who reached their eighties and nineties without significant cardiovascular disease all had high levels of HDL in their blood.

How do high-density lipoproteins act to prevent coronary heart disease? Medical scientists are still assessing the possible mechanisms involved, but several hypotheses have been put forth.

All blood fats, including cholesterol, are transported through the bloodstream attached to "packets" or lipoproteins. HDL, one of the "packets," seems to expedite the removal of cholesterol from the cells and its passage to the liver for excretion. Also, HDL seems to help a special enzyme, LCAT (lecithin cholesterol acyl transferase), in converting free cholesterol into esterified cholesterol. Cholesterol ester is a larger molecule than free cholesterol and it moves more slowly; in this form, it's more difficult for cholesterol to move back and forth across cell membranes. Thus, if the cholesterol esters remain outside the cell, the odds favor its pickup by the HDL, which transports it for degradation or elimination.

LDL: Too Much of These Fats in the Blood May Be a Risk

Low-density lipoproteins, which are also called "beta-lipoproteins," are associated with a higher incidence of heart attacks. In the studies previously mentioned, a low level of LDLs in the blood was indicative of an increased risk of heart attack.

Can You Build Up HDLs and Cut Down LDLs?

The answer to that may well be yes, or at least you can try. Here's how.

1. *Regular exercise.* Reports from Stanford University show that long-distance runners have higher HDL levels than sedentary individuals.

2. *Diet.* It would be logical to assume that a low-fat, low-cholesterol diet just might reduce the level of HDL in your blood too. Fortunately, however, the opposite seems to be true. Surprisingly, it is known that a typical Asian diet—one in which fish, vegetables, and cereals are consumed, with little if any meat, and certainly no "junk" foods—seems to raise the level of HDL in the blood.

Findings from the Multiple Risk Factor Intervention Trial, appropriately nicknamed *"MR. FIT,"* also showed that three factors were involved in raising HDL. In this six-year study of 12,000 men aged 35 to 57 in twenty cities, it emerged that weight reduction, decreasing or discontinuing cigarette smoking, and increasing alcohol intake led to increased levels of HDL. This last finding was striking, and has provoked a mixed reaction from physicians.

3. *Drugs.* Certain lipid-lowering agents such as clofibrate and niacin can lower the level of LDL in the blood while raising HDL. Generally speaking, however, doctors only resort to drug therapy after diet and exercise programs have failed to produce the desired results.

VLDL and Chylomicrons

The former transport vehicles (molecules) carry endogenous triglycerides *(endogenous* means produced inside the body) to various muscle sites and to fatty *(adipose)* tissues. The *chylomicrons* are the lightest and largest lipoproteins. They carry exogenous or dietary triglycerides from the intestines into the bloodstream.

Dr. Castelli feels that some American adults may be "misclassified" as high-risk candidates for heart attacks, based on their total serum cholesterol level, because according to new findings, your HDL and LDL blood level may be more significant. It's possible that you could have a total serum cholesterol level of 280 or 300 mg%, quite high by most standards, but if your HDL is in the vicinity of 130 mg% or so, your risk could be significantly lower than suggested by the total cholesterol level.

PUTTING IT ALL TOGETHER

Now You Be the Nutritionist

Using the following pages, you can translate all the scientific information you just read into daily servings. The simplest way to insure that you and your family get enough vitamins, minerals, proteins, carbohydrates, and fats daily is to eat foods from each of the groups listed in the chart on the next page.

(Text continues on page 39)

SELECT FOODS FROM EACH OF THESE FOOD GROUPS DAILY

Food Group	Sources	Daily Servings	Sample Servings
meats and fish	poultry; lean meats such as veal; lean cuts of beef and lamb; fish	2	3 oz chicken, veal or fish
breads and cereals	all whole-grain breads and cereals, rice, pastas, rolled oats	4	1 slice whole-grain bread; 1 cup wild rice; or ½–1 cup cooked cereal (bran, whole-grain)
milk and dairy products	milk, eggs, cheese, butter, ice cream, ice milk	2	8 oz cup milk; ½–1 cup cottage cheese; 1 oz cheese
fats and oils	cooking oils, margarine, mayonnaise	2	1 tablespoon
fruits and vegetables citrus fruits, raw cabbage, tomatoes, salads	oranges, tangerines, lemons, limes, grapefruits, lettuce	2	1 dark green (spinach); or 1 yellow (carrot); 1 citrus (orange)
non-citrus fruits, potatoes, other vegetables and fruits not listed above green, yellow, leafy vegetables	cantaloupe, strawberries, pears, plums, apples, pineapples, grapes green beans, spinach, squash, brussels sprouts, carrots, turnips, cauliflower	2	1 baked potato ½ cantaloupe

(Text continues from page 37)

After you have reviewed the food groups, servings and sample servings, you will probably be surprised to see that if you eat a balanced diet, you can have a considerable amount to eat at meals, and you can include a few snacks too, providing these snacks consist of some cheese, or a fresh fruit, a whole wheat or bran muffin, and so forth. Many individuals routinely complain that they have to "starve" themselves to lose weight; in fact, all you really need to do is eliminate refined sugar products and the excessive saturated fat in your diet, and instead, stick to the foods listed in the food chart on the preceding page, and follow the tips outlined by us. Dr. Amsterdam's suggestions for modifying a family's diet and his 20 specific "tips" to do so appear below.

How I Modified My Family's Diet

—Dr. Ezra A. Amsterdam

Several years ago, while we were entertaining, the dinner conversation turned to the significance of diet in the development of coronary heart disease. I explained the findings of several major studies in detail, and said that I believed it was very important for many of us to modify our life-styles. As soon as the last plate was cleared, however, one perceptive guest quipped: "As always, the advice from the doctor is: Do as I say, not as I do."

At that moment, I realized that I had not helped my own family follow what I believe is very good advice. Instead of serving a main course of fish, fresh vegetables (seasoned with spices instead of salt), and perhaps fresh fruit for dessert, my wife and I had prepared sirloin steaks, vegetables with a cream cheese sauce, fried potatoes, and cheesecake for dessert.

After that evening, my wife and I drew up a new supermarket list, tailored to meet our objective of cutting down our intake of animal fats, sugars, and processed foods, but keeping in mind that we not only had well-established eating habits, but also two young daughters who liked to spot a piece of candy and gleefully and rapidly consume it. We decided that the key was really *moderation*—not deprivation. Accordingly, here are the twenty "tricks" that we instituted in our home that have enabled us to meet the U.S. Dietary Goals, and still keep the family satisfied at mealtimes.

Twenty Ways to Modify a Family Diet

1. Broil or roast meats and fish instead of frying or baking. (Fish can also be poached.)

2. Use margarine instead of butter.

3. Use skim milk instead of whole milk or buttermilk. Give children whole milk, but use skim in recipes.

4. Season with spices—not salt. Use oregano or thyme instead.

5. Use bran or sesame-seed toppings instead of bread crumbs. If ambitious, make bread crumbs from whole-grain breads.

6. Use vinegar or lemon juice with spices instead of heavy oil salad dressings.

7. Serve fresh fruits or yogurt instead of puddings and pies.

8. Use fresh fruits to make your shakes rather than serving sugared sodas.

9. Serve whole wheat breads instead of white, refined-flour breads.

10. Buy tuna packed in water, not oil.

11. Don't overcook vegetables. Vitamins are lost in cooking; the fresher they smell, the more nutritious they are.

12. Don't peel potatoes, cucumbers, apples, pears, and so on. The skin is fiber and the added bulk is good for your digestive tract.

13. Keep nutritious snacks handy. Raisins are advertised as "Nature's Candy," and other fruits such as pineapples and strawberries would satiate any sweet tooth.

14. Let children snack on sunflower seeds and nuts rather than on sweet cookies.

15. Remove the sugar bowl. If you must use sugar, buy raw sugar.

16. Don't baste meats or other foods with butter; use sesame oil. Dip barbecue brush in it and baste as usual.

17. Use yogurt instead of sour cream in recipes.

18. Before serving chicken, turkey, or duck, remove the skin.

19. Trim all excess fat from beef.

20. Buy kosher brands of hot dogs or bologna; these are made from beef, not pork, and are generally less fatty than other brands; they also have fewer additives.

SHOULD YOU BREAK WITH YOUR COFFEE BREAK?

Caffeine is known to affect blood pressure and heart rate and rhythm, but most physicians agree that, for healthy individuals, drinking caffeinated coffee in moderate amounts (two cups per day) is probably harmless. However, a single gram of caffeine can produce certain symptoms such as restlessness, motor agitation, and insomnia. Those who experience such effects should make an effort to reduce their caffeine intake. Remember, other products (tea, cola drinks) also contain caffeine, so you may need to cut down across the board.

Among children, the concern over a high caffeine intake seems warranted. For example, some pediatricians have reported that among their cola-drinking pediatric and adolescent patients, they encounter a fair amount of nervousness, headache, and irritability—a syndrome that is nicknamed "caffeinism." Children who drink three or four bottles of cola per day, or who consume chocolate candy bars, hot chocolate, and the like, may have a rather high caffeine intake, and the result is often an irritable or distracted child. Most people don't realize that the average cola drink can have twice the amount of caffeine as a cup of coffee; thus, a child who only weighs a third to half as much as an adult male ends up consuming relatively more than twice the amount of caffeine in a drink. For this reason, parents should watch their child's intake of colas, chocolate products, and so on, particularly if signs of caffeine overload develop.

2
High Blood Pressure: What You Can Do About It

It's a silent killer. Although serious or painful symptoms are exceptionally rare, the disease is life-threatening. In almost every case, doctors don't know what causes it, but they do know that it can end in debilitating kidney disease, stroke, heart failure, and death.

We're talking about *hypertension*. But if you're like most people, you may not think it is a very serious medical problem. In fact, you may not even consider hypertension a disease; perhaps you think of it as a very mild disorder, just something that your spouse happens to have, for instance, because he or she is the tense, "high-strung" type. Or, you may believe people who make remarks like "He really makes my blood boil," or "I get nervous every time my boss walks into my office," are the ones who are apt to be hypertensive.

But do you really know whether or not "nerves" or just a "hot temper" can cause hypertension? What about anxiety and/or "pressure cooker" jobs? Consider whether each of the following statements is *true* or *false*.

Older people have higher blood pressure than younger persons, and that's always acceptable.

Women tolerate high blood pressure much better than men.

If your doctor takes your blood pressure in his or her office and tells you it's elevated, you don't have to worry because you were "nervous" in the office when it was taken.

Hypertension is harmless unless you have related symptoms.

White males, particularly the aggressive always-on-the-go types, have hypertension more than any other group.

Did you say *"true"* to any of the above statements? Each statement is false. Each is a myth about hypertension that somehow survives despite overwhelming contradictory scientific evidence. Before discussing these myths and the role of hypertension in the development of cardiovascular disease, let's find out how much you know about this disorder. The questionnaire that immediately follows in this chapter was adapted from a nationwide survey.* Answer the questions in the boxes. Then read on and rate your understanding of hypertension, a disease that is far more deadly than many people realize.

Questionnaire on Hypertension

1. *What Does the Term* Hypertension *Mean?* (Circle one or more of the answers below.)

    a. Bad nerves, extreme nervous condition
    b. High blood pressure
    c. Too much tension, pressure
    d. Overanxiety
    e. Hyperactivity
    f. Overexcitement
    g. Other
    h. Do not know

2. *What Does the Term* High Blood Pressure *Mean?*
    a. Heart working harder, pressure on heart
    b. Blood pressure above normal
    c. Heart pumping too fast
    d. Blood flowing too fast
    e. Pressure too high on veins, arteries
    f. Danger signal
    g. Related to stress, anxiety
    h. Arteries, veins constricted
    i. Too much blood, blood too thick
    j. May cause stroke
    k. Numeric reading
    l. Trouble with the heart
    m. Getting dizzy
    n. Hypertension
    o. Too much blood to brain

---

*Adapted from "The Public and High Blood Pressure," A Survey Conducted for The National Heart and Lung Institute, June 1973, Lou Harris and Associates, Inc. *DHEW* Publication No. (NIH) 75–356 Study No. 2313.

      p. Poor circulation
      q. Other
      r. Do not know

3. *Do You Know What Blood Pressure Is Considered Normal for a Person Your Age?* (If so, jot down your age and the corresponding blood pressure.)

4. *What Are the Major Likely Causes of High Blood Pressure?*

      a. Emotional pressure, worry, anxiety
      b. Overweight
      c. Improper diet
      d. Fatty foods (cholesterol)
      e. Overexertion
      f. Alcohol (excessive drinking)
      g. Heredity
      h. Too much salt
      i. Smoking
      j. Hypertension
      k. Hardening of the arteries
      l. Pork
     m. Lack of exercise
      n. Old age
      o. Other
      p. Do not know

5. *Can You Have High Blood Pressure Without Obvious Symptoms?*

      a. Very likely.
      b. Somewhat likely.
      c. Hardly likely.
      d. Not sure.

   Now that you've completed that brief questionnaire, let's see how you measure up against the nationwide survey. In 1973, the National Heart and Lung Institute (a part of the Department of Health, Education and Welfare, Washington, D.C.) contracted with the pollsters Louis Harris and Associates, Inc., New York City, to learn how much the public knew about hypertension and its consequences. Overall, 3,181 individuals 17 years of age or older drawn from 200 locations throughout the continental United States were interviewed. To ensure that this random selection was representative of the total adult civilian population in this country, three "over–samples" were developed. For example, since this cross section of a little more than 3,000 people was unlikely to result in interviews with more than 300 blacks, a separate cross section of 686 blacks was interviewed in 100 locations. Combined with the 209 blacks whom the pollsters did interview in their initial survey, this produced a total of 895 blacks. Similar efforts were also made to ensure that people with low incomes and those who already had been told by a doctor or a nurse that they had high blood pressure were included in a representative way in the statistics.

All of the interviews were conducted in person and in the home of the interviewee. Each interview lasted approximately an hour. Among other things, the survey revealed that less than half of all those interviewed between the ages of 17 and 35 considered high blood pressure very serious and, even more striking, only 51 percent of those who already *knew* they had high blood pressure considered it a very serious disease. So, despite all the publicity and efforts, many people, particularly young people, still need to be educated about this disorder and its medical consequences. Now look at the survey results to see how your knowledge and understanding of hypertension compares with that of your peers.

ANSWERS TO QUESTIONNAIRE ON HYPERTENSION

1. In answering this question, slightly less than one-fourth of the people questioned knew that high blood pressure was synonymous with "hypertension." Overall, 23 percent and 26 percent, respectively, thought that too much tension and pressure, and bad nerves or an extreme nervous condition caused hypertension; thus, nearly half of those interviewed believed that hypertension could in some way be attributed to nerves alone, a fourth apparently had no idea what "hypertension" meant, and only 25 percent gave the correct answer. How did you do?

2. With this question, the respondents fared a little better. In the choices given here, it's correct to check off several answers, such as (a) "heart working harder, pressure on heart," (b) "blood pressure above normal," et cetera. Any of those responses reflects some understanding of the terminology; in fact, it could also be considered correct to check responses *e, f, h, j,* and *l.* Of course, if you recognized the word "hypertension" in the list and checked that one immediately, you're ahead of the game! Answer *g* might also be considered correct, but for our purposes, it's risky to view this choice as indicative of an understanding of hypertension.

   For example, answer *m* "getting dizzy," is a common misconception, since high blood pressure rarely causes dizzy spells. In fact, that's part of the problem with hypertension: it's an insidious disease process that wreaks silent damage. You can have high blood pressure for years and never know it because warning signs such as dizziness are usually absent.

We hesitate to accept, then, answers *m* and *g* as correct, since it might mislead you into thinking that you or others are free of hypertension if you don't get dizzy spells or feel especially anxious, but nothing could be further from the truth!

3. Although a full one-fourth of the interviewees said they knew what was considered normal blood pressure for their age, this finding is somewhat deceptive and discouraging. As it turned out, only 38 percent of those who said they knew what blood pressure reading was considered normal *actually* gave the pollsters the correct answer. So, even if you think you know what blood pressure may be considered normal, check with your doctor to find out if your blood pressure is normal.

4. The answers to this question are a bit more difficult. First, it may be somewhat deliberately misleading to ask an individual "What are the major likely causes of a disease?" when the answer is: "In most cases, we don't know." Still, it is interesting to see how many respondents blamed emotional pressures and anxieties, as well as weight and diet, as the cause of high blood pressure. In fact, in a subsequent question in which those interviewed were asked, "What is the single most important cause of high blood pressure?" a full 40 percent answered, "emotional pressure, worry, and anxiety," and 18 percent blamed "overweight."

While it is true that myriad factors are involved in the development of hypertension, it is also clear that an overestimation of the importance of tension and obesity may be preventing many people from recognizing that hypertension can afflict anyone at any age, of either sex, fat or thin, calm or hysterical. Remember, overt symptoms and characteristics are often not present.

How did you measure up against your peers? If you checked hypertension as the major likely cause of high blood pressure, your answer is correct. (These two terms are synonymous, but in this survey hypertension was listed among the possible answers). All other choices except *f*, *l* and *m* provided here could also be considered correct, depending on the individual (for example, a high-salt diet may cause high blood pressure in one person, but not in another). Smoking, heredity, and overweight are also linked to hypertension—if you do smoke, have a positive family history for high blood pressure, and are obese, you should ask your doctor at your next checkup for a report on your blood pressure.

5. Regrettably, the answers to this question quite clearly show that most people do not realize that hypertension is a serious—and typically asymptomatic—disease. According to those surveyed, over half believed it was very likely that symptoms would be present if you had high blood pressure. The most important point to recognize here is that blatant symptoms—headaches, dizziness, or even fainting spells—occur only late in the disease process. By then, considerable heart, brain, eye, and kidney damage may have occurred, all of which might have been prevented by adequate medical treatment (for a discussion of the drugs used to treat hypertension see Chapter 16).

Was your knowledge and understanding of high blood pressure and its implications as good as you thought—or, like most people, are you just now beginning to realize the seriousness of this disease? The Harris survey revealed some other rather discouraging findings. For example, one-third of the individuals who already had been told that they had high blood pressure, as well as roughly 40 percent of the total public, either believed hypertension did not cause other illnesses and symptoms, or were not sure.

SCOPE OF THE PROBLEM

Why such a fuss over a disease that rarely even has symptoms associated with it?

Consider these points: The American Heart Association estimates that in 1981 the annual cost to the United States due to morbidity and mortality from cardiovascular diseases was approximately $46.2 billion! Direct costs of arteriosclerosis and high blood pressure (hospital and nursing home care, physicians' and other medical professional services, and drugs) totaled an estimated $4.3 billion in 1967. Indirect costs due to productivity losses because of illness and disability from arteriosclerotic and hypertensive diseases in 1967 was an estimated $1.1 billion. The estimated indirect economic costs to the nation, measured in terms of the present value of lifetime earnings lost by those who died that year from arteriosclerotic and hypertensive diseases, amounted to $18.5 billion.*

The American Heart Association estimates that approximately 34,880,000 Americans—more than 10 percent of the adult population—have high blood pressure. Of these, only half are even aware that they have the disease, and of the more than 15 million who have been told that they have high blood pres-

---

*Arteriosclerosis, a report by National Heart and Lung Institute Task Force on Arteriosclerosis, II, June 1971, DHEW Publ. No. (NIH) 72–219, National Institutes of Health, DHEW, Washington, D.C.

sure, only one-fourth are receiving adequate treatment. The remaining group is either left untreated or is not being treated sufficiently to control the disease.

Unfortunately, the therapy now available for high blood pressure has not affected, to any large degree, death rates resulting from stroke and other types of heart disease in which hypertension is involved, because so many cases of hypertension often go undetected or untreated until a stroke or a heart attack actually occurs. It has only been during the last few decades that high blood pressure has gained recognition, and within the last 40 years or so that a number of very effective antihypertensive drugs have been developed. About 1940, researchers began to perceive the significance of hypertension. The major studies, the findings of which will be discussed throughout this book, are summarized below.

The Framingham Heart Study. Since 1949, a general population sample of 5,209 men and women, aged 30 to 62 years and living in Framingham, Massachusetts, has been examined twice a year to determine the relationship of antecedent personal attributes and living habits to the development of cardiovascular disease. According to Dr. William B. Kannel, director of the study, Framingham was selected because it is a microcosm of the United States—people in all walks of life live there—and because the population is stable and was willing to cooperate. Only 2 percent of the participants have been completely lost to the study, and a full 80 percent checked in for every biennial examination. This study clearly shows that elevated blood pressure, at any age and in either sex, is a potent contributor to all types of cardiovascular disease, although the risk varies in relation to the number and level of other risk factors present. (See Figure 2.1.)

The National Health Examination Survey. This study was conducted between 1960 and 1962; overall, 6,672 people were surveyed. Of these, about 15 percent had hypertension. In addition, about 60 percent of the hypertensive persons also had concomitant hypertensive cardiovascular disease. (See Figure 2.2.)

Peoples Gas Company Study (1958–1970). In this survey, 1,329 male employees of the Peoples Gas Company in Chicago, Illinois—aged 40 to 59 and all free of definite clinical coronary heart disease when they entered the study—were assessed to determine the relationship between hypertension and mortality. The study showed that the percentage of deaths due to cardiovascular renal diseases and stroke were highest among men with blood pressures higher than 140/90 mm Hg.

(Text continues on page 49, bottom.)

Figure 2.1: Risk of Cardiovascular Disease Climbs According to the Level of Other Risk Factors

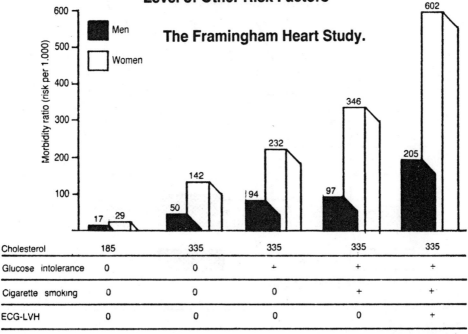

The Framingham Heart Study.

Cholesterol	185	335	335	335	335
Glucose intolerance	0	0	+	+	+
Cigarette smoking	0	0	0	+	+
ECG-LVH	0	0	0	0	+

Level of other risk factors

This chart shows the risks of cardiovascular disease in eight years at systolic blood pressure of 165 mm Hg according to level of other risk factors in men and women age 40. ECG-LVH: ECG stands for electrocardiogram; LVH stands for left ventricular hypertrophy. LVH is a cardiac abnormality that may be detected on the ECG.

SOURCE: W.B. Kannel, "Modest Blood Pressure Rises Can Be Dangerous," *Hypertension*, Vol. 2, No. 3, March, 1976, with permission.

(Text continued from page 48.)

Community Hypertension Evaluation Clinic (CHEC). From 1973 to 1975, more than one million persons at 1,171 different sites were surveyed in this nationwide program. Again, this study demonstrated just how many American adults *are* hypertensive, and that high blood pressure was more common in blacks than in whites. Also, those with undetected, untreated, or uncontrolled hypertension totaled about 55 percent.

**Figure 2.2: Incidence of Hypertension According to the National
Health Examination Survey (1960–62)**

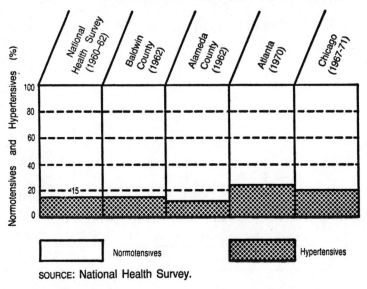

SOURCE: National Health Survey.

What Is Hypertension?

Blood pressure is measured in terms of two factors: the systolic and the diastolic pressures in the arterial system. For example, when your doctor says your blood pressure is "130/85 mm Hg," he or she is telling you the systolic and diastolic pressures, respectively. The number of millimeters a column of mercury rises as a result of the pressure is indicated by "mm Hg."

Quite simply, *systolic* pressure is the maximum pressure put on the arterial system, and occurs during systole—that is, when the heart is pumping and sending blood through the arteries. *Diastolic* pressure, conversely, indicates minimum pressure—that is, when the heart is resting between beats. This period in the cardiovascular cycle is diastole. (See Part II for the anatomy and physiology of the heart.)

What Causes High Blood Pressure?

The major studies we discussed earlier in this section show that high blood pressure is a very common problem among American adults. Why? What causes hypertension, and how is blood pressure controlled? In at least nine out of ten cases, the cause of hypertension is unknown, but many excellent drugs are available for treatment. (See Chapter 16.)

How Is Blood Pressure Regulated?

Just think of a fireman's hose. That may not sound very relevant, but it is! Here's how the hose essentially works: a hydrant supplies the water, the hose transports the water, and the nozzle at the end of the hose determines outflow. It's easy to measure water pressure in the hose. All you have to do is stick a needle into the hose and attach a manometer to the needle. The hose pressure is reflected in the height to which the fluid in the manometer is pushed due to the water running through the hose. Three variables determine the pressure:

1. You could open the hydrant wider so that more water flows through the hose, and pressure is thereby increased.
2. You could tighten the nozzle at the end of the hose so less water would flow through. In a matter of seconds, the backup water would distend the hose noticeably. Sometimes, the hose literally springs from the fireman's hands until the nozzle is shaken loose, permitting the water to flow out.
3. Both of these factors combined—tightening the nozzle and opening up the hydrant even more—will cause an increase in pressure.

Now, back to the cardiovascular system. The hydrant is analogous to the heart because the hydrant pumps water, and the heart is responsible for pumping gallons of blood through the arteries, which are analogous to the hose.

The nozzle represents the arteriolar bed, the very small network of arteries that can become larger or smaller, depending on the response to neural impulses. The walls of the arterioles constrict in response to certain stimuli, so the diameter of the vessel is decreased. Thus, as the arterioles narrow, resistance to blood flow is increased and, ultimately, blood pressure rises.

Why Is High Blood Pressure Dangerous?

The statistics speak for themselves:

The overall death rate from strokes and heart attacks would decline by approximately 20 percent, providing that each person with hypertension had the disease detected early and received prompt and adequate treatment.

Every year, high blood pressure is a factor in 68 percent of all first heart attacks and in 75 percent of all first strokes.

In 1973, it was estimated that high blood pressure was a factor in over 513,000 of the 754,000 deaths due to heart disease that occurred that year.

Left untreated, hypertension can cause brain, eye, heart, and kidney dam-

Figure 2.3: Possible Effects of Hypertension on Major Organs of the Body

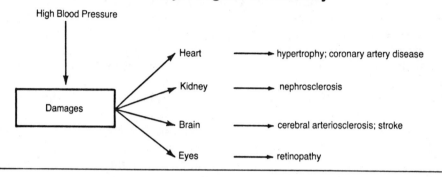

age. (See Figure 2.3.) A report by the National Heart and Lung Institute Task Force on Arteriosclerosis stated that hypertension is the major risk factor for stroke. The Framingham Study showed simillar findngs: hypertension is a risk factor in the development of coronary heart disease, stroke, and congest-

Figure 2.4: Risk of Clinical Manifestations of Coronary Heart Disease According to Hypertensive Status (18-Year Follow-Up, Framingham Heart Study)

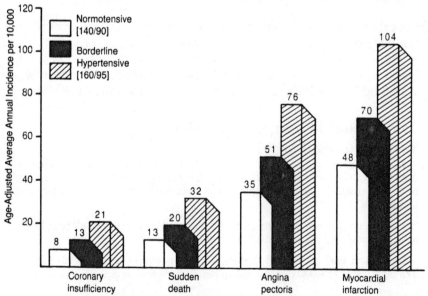

SOURCE: W.B. Kannel, "Prevention of Cardiovascular Disease," Current Problems in Cardiology, vol. 1, no. 4 (1976), with permission.

Figure 2.5: Incidence of Congestive Heart Failure According to Blood Pressure Status (The Framingham Heart Study)

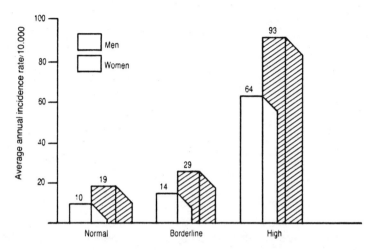

Average annual incidence of congestive heart failure according to blood pressure status at each biennial examination, men and women, 55-64, 16-year follow-up.

SOURCE: W. B. Kannel, "Role of Blood Pressure in Cardiovascular Morbidity and Mortality," *Progress in Cardiovascular Disease*, vol. XVII, no. 1 (1974), with permission.

ive heart failure in particular, and kidney and eye damage may also occur. Figure 2.4 shows that all the known effects of coronary heart disease, including angina, heart attack, and sudden death, were strikingly related to blood pressure status.

Similarly, the Framingham Study found that the incidence of congestive heart failure was highest among people with elevated blood pressure. *(Congestive heart failure* is a condition that can develop if the heart keeps pumping blood under continually high pressure. Like any pump, the heart wears out prematurely and "fails" due to overwork.) (See Figure 2.5.) The Framingham survey also revealed that the incidence of atherothrombotic brain infarction (commonly referred to as *stroke*) was much higher among persons who had high blood pressure. Finally, minor-to-major kidney damage can occur, and the tiniest blood vessels in the eyes may be injured. (See Figure 2.6.)

How does a disease without symptoms or other warnings manage to inflict such damage? The answer is easy to understand if you envision the heart as a pump, and the veins and arteries as a network of pipelines. High pressure means the pump (or heart) works harder to keep the blood flowing. And that means more pressure on the pipelines. The more pressure on the pipelines, the

Figure 2.6: Atherothrombotic Brain Infarction (Stroke)

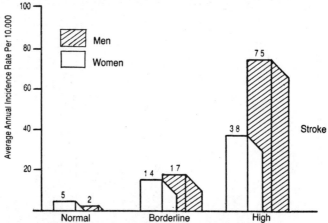

Average annual incidence of cardiovascular disease according to blood pressure status at each biennial examination, men and women 55–64, 16-year follow-up.

SOURCE: W.B. Kannel, "Role of Blood Pressure in Cardiovascular Morbidity and Mortality," *Progress in Cardiovascular Diseases*, vol. XVII, no. 1 (1974), with permission.

more likely they are to undergo degenerative changes and damage. Narrowing or rupture of an artery can occur. If the narrowing is severe enough, it can impair blood flow to an organ, and rupture can cause hemorrhage. Blockage or a hemorrhage in a cerebral artery can cause a stroke. These problems can occur elsewhere too: in a renal artery or coronary artery, and so on.

Now, let's clarify the link between high blood pressure and coronary heart disease. Although it is not known why, it does seem that prolonged high blood pressure "predisposes" the blood vessels to atherosclerosis. Then, plaques form within the arterial linings. These *plaques*, or lumps of fat, ultimately clog the artery and obstruct blood flow, especially within the coronary arteries, and this can cause a heart attack. The medical term for this condition is *atherosclerosis*. This disease will be discussed in Chapter 10. For now, it is enough to say that the insidious process of atherosclerosis is one more reason why hypertension should be detected and controlled as early as possible. Four major organs—the brain, heart, kidneys and eyes—can all be damaged, sometimes permanently, by this silent disease. What can *you* do? Be alert, have regular blood pressure checkups (even schools and "street corner" paramedics will measure your blood pressure, often free of charge), and follow your doctor's advice in keeping your heart and entire cardiovascular system healthy. If you do develop high blood pressure, get treatment, and stick to the program the doctor recommends for you.

Is There More Than One Type of Hypertension?

Hypertension is usually divided into two categories: (1) primary hypertension and (2) secondary hypertension. The vast majority of hypertensive patients—90 percent—have primary or "essential" hypertension. It's referred to as "primary" because the high blood pressure itself is the main disorder rather than a symptom of some other disease. Primary hypertension is the "garden variety" type; it's very common, and anyone can get it, regardless of age, race, or sex.

Secondary hypertension is much rarer, but when it does occur, distinct symptoms may appear and a specific cause such as a tumor on the adrenal gland can be found.

Even though doctors can't pinpoint a precise cause in most cases of hypertension, several factors may play a role in its development, and/or exacerbate the condition. These include: heredity, race, sex, age, emotional factors, obesity, drugs, foodstuffs, exercise, smoking, and other maladies often associated with hypertension, such as diabetes, gout, and fibroid tumors of the uterus. While none of these latter conditions is directly responsible for hypertension, the chances are that if you are diabetic or if you have gout, your doctor will want to check your blood pressure at frequent intervals.

Is Hypertension Hereditary?

There's little doubt that a family history of heart disease plays a role, although the degree of importance varies. For example, a study conducted at Johns Hopkins University showed a 21 percent hypertension rate among daughters with two hypertensive parents, compared to a rate of 4.5 percent when both parents had normal blood pressure. Other surveys have shown that siblings of hypertensives have high blood pressure up to four times as often as siblings of normotensives, and that children of hypertensive parents have high blood pressure up to six times as often as children of parents with normal blood pressures. Of course, because so many factors are involved, it is often difficult to distinguish hereditary from environmental influences.

Race

Many studies support the idea that race is significant in hypertension. (See Figure 2.7.) In a survey of about 2,000 people in Charleston, South Carolina, incidence of hypertension was appreciably higher among blacks than whites, and the blacks also suffered a proportionately higher rate of morbidity and mortality from hypertensive disease. Recently, investigators have also found that there is an association among obesity, hypertension, and uterine fibroid

Figure 2.7: Percent Prevalence of Definite Hypertension by Age in Four Race-Sex Groups

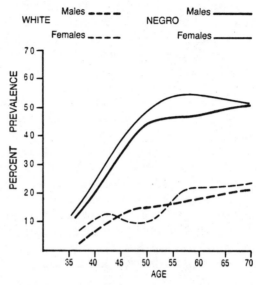

SOURCE: *Journal of the American Medical Association*, Sept. 7, 1970, vol. 213, No. 10, 1637-43.

tumors among blacks, but no such links have been established for white women.

Sex and Age

For some reason, many people are inclined to think that women have far fewer heart attacks than men, and that high blood pressure is mainly a disease of the tense, anxious businessman. However, as many studies have shown, risk is proportional to the level of blood pressure at any age in either sex.

While it is true that the absolute risk for men is greater than that for women at any level of blood pressure, the *relative* risk is equal in both sexes. In fact, in terms of having a stroke or developing congestive heart failure, women enjoy very little advantage over men, relative or absolute.

Look at Figure 2.8 to get a clearer picture. This graph reflects fourteen-year findings in men and women, aged 30 to 49. As you can see, women with blood pressures in the upper 20 percent of the population actually had *more* heart disease than men with the highest pressures.

Today, most doctors are somewhat flexible in evaluating blood pressure in terms of age. One of the best commentaries on this appeared in a British med-

Figure 2.8: Coronary Heart Disease

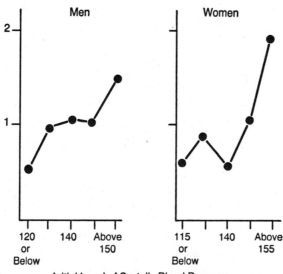

Initial Level of Systolic Blood Pressure

Relative chance of developing coronary heart disease, heart attack, or angina depending upon level of initial systolic blood pressure (during the 14-year follow-up survey of residents 30–49 years old of Framingham, Mass.).

SOURCE: W.B. Kannel, T. Gordon, M. J. Schwartz, *Am J Cardiol* 27:335 (1974), with permission.

ical publication in 1971, in which two investigators, Evans and Rose, wrote: "In an operational sense, hypertension should be defined in terms of a blood pressure level above which investigation and treatment do more good than harm. Probably this critical level may vary with age and sex."

Youth carries no built-in guarantee that a person won't develop hypertension, either; for example, a survey of slightly more than 3,000 people aged 15 to 29 years in the biracial community of Evans County, Georgia, were examined between 1960 and 1962 and again between 1967 and 1969. This study demonstrated that a significant proportion of young people are hypertensive (defined as a blood pressure of 140/90 mm Hg or higher). Here are the specifics:

White males	19 percent
White females	12 percent
Black males	34 percent
Black females	31.6 percent

Regardless of what the studies will ultimately show about the role of heredity, race, sex, and age, one fact remains: There is nothing anyone can do to alter any of these variables. Consequently, it makes sense to focus on the factors that you do control—namely, your emotions, drugs, diet, exercise, and smoking habits.

Can Stress Cause High Blood Pressure?

Is the fast pace of our highly industrialized society a major cause of hypertension? Many doctors say so, and several studies support their view. Even an isolated disaster or a life-threatening event can precipitate hypertension. A striking example occurred thirty years ago in a small Texas town in which there was an enormous explosion. Of those who were either directly involved in the blast or situated nearby, a full 57 percent developed high blood pressure. Doctors nicknamed this "blast hypertension," since blood pressure fell to normal in most of the subjects once the stress of the experience subsided.

Similarly, another survey showed that people in high-tension occupations like air-traffic control had higher blood pressure than air force personnel with desk jobs. And, finally, as early as World War II, a British medical investigator found that the front-line soldiers had higher blood pressure than those who were not in the field.

Presumably, continued stress ultimately stimulates the autonomic nervous system to produce a permanent state of constriction of the arteries. Under normal circumstances, the body automatically responds to an occasional stress such as the threat of collision; various parts of the body are immediately called into coordinated play in order to prevent the accident. Once the danger has passed, all "systems" return to normal: you stop perspiring, ease your grip on the wheel, and so on. However, when you maintain a certain level of stress all day—because of a job, marriage, or other conditions—your body may ultimately adapt by simply "resetting" all the gears, and sustained hypertension follows.

Debate about the exact role of stress in hypertension continues, but few would argue that it does not play some role in the disease.

Can Medications Cause Hypertension?

Yes. In fact, even some very commonly prescribed pills such as oral contraceptives have been known to set off hypertension. In most women, however, blood pressure returns to normal when the pills are discontinued. The exact incidence of high blood pressure resulting from the Pill remains unknown, but it is considered an important, if uncommon, side effect. Other medications such as steroids and certain nasal decongestants may cause an increase in blood pressure, too.

Does Diet Affect Blood Pressure?

Again, the answer is *yes*. Obese patients having mild elevations in blood pressure frequently return to normal once they reduce. (Interestingly enough, consumption of a considerable amount of licorice can also elevate blood pressure.)

Alcohol. To date, little is known about the effects of mild alcohol consumption on blood pressure.

Salt. Quite a bit of information is available on the role of salt in hypertension. Doctors know that among populations whose salt intake is very low, high blood pressure is virtually nonexistent. Studies using rats that are genetically predisposed to hypertension show that they develop high blood pressure and die at an early age when placed on a high-salt diet. This same group of rats will live a full life without high blood pressure if their diets are low in salt.

Doctors are particularly worried about the sodium content of baby foods, so much so that within the last few years various consumer groups have pressured manufacturers to remove as much salt from these foods as possible. Unfortunately, even mothers who avoid these products and feed their babies from the table (perhaps because they find this cheaper or more convenient) may actually be doing their children a disservice. Certainly, many babies can eat smaller ground-up portions of most of the foods adults prepare for themselves *if* a lot of salt hasn't been added during the cooking process. Also, some foods simply are full of salt. Cow's milk, for instance, contains four times the amount of sodium that human milk does.

Just how much salt intake is required on a daily basis? Table salt—sodium chloride—is not an essential dietary additive. Most foods contain enough natural salt to fulfill your body's daily requirements for sodium. Yet Americans ingest anywhere from two to five times more salt than they need each day.

Presumably, extra salt in the body elevates blood pressure by a variety of mechanisms, one of which appears to be fluid retention. This results in increased pressure in the arteries. In a survey conducted by the National Heart and Lung Institute several years ago, it was found that persons with high blood pressure consumed four times as much salt and drank twice as much water over a seven-day period as a control group.

Water. Finally, even the chemical composition of drinking water has been cited as a cause of hypertension, but the specific effects of the various minerals on blood pressure are still unknown.

How Does Exercise Affect Blood Pressure?

Remember, as amazing as your heart is, it is not a magical organ, but a mass of muscle. Routine exercise goes a long way to maintain and improve overall cardiopulmonary fitness, because exercise not only tones muscles, but can also improve the interaction among the skeletal muscles, the heart, and the lungs, thereby enhancing the body's ability to work.

Most doctors feel that regular participation in some form of isotonic exercise (dynamic muscular activity such as running and swimming) will help you maintain cardiovascular health. Some studies have shown that regular exercise programs such as running and jogging may produce a drop in diastolic blood pressure. So, even if having high blood pressure is the only exception to your otherwise healthy condition, your doctor may advocate an exercise program for you. Certainly exercise, coupled with a weight-reducing plan (if it's needed), may be as effective and palatable for some patients as a lifetime of drug therapy. It is definitely cheaper, and your family can join in the fun to improve their over–all fitness and keep their hearts healthy, too.

Does Smoking Cause High Blood Pressure?

Here, the facts are surprising. Even in the Framingham survey, the smokers actually tended to have lower blood pressures. However, lest anyone interpret it as a green light on smoking, bear this in mind: although smoking may not play a role as a causative factor in hypertension, it is a clearly established risk factor for the development of coronary heart disease.

If this isn't reason enough to quit, remember: The American Cancer Society estimated that approximately 92,000 deaths occurred in 1978 as a result of lung cancer. (For more specific discussion of this subject, see Chapter 3.)

Hypertension is one of the three major risk factors in the development of coronary heart disease. Consider steps you can take to control it on your own:

> maintain normal weight
>
> reduce your salt intake
>
> get regular daily exercise
>
> control daily stress as much as
>   possible with breaks or vacations
>
> cut down on or eliminate smoking

You may be in very good health and doing all of these things right now and still develop high blood pressure, but don't be discouraged. This may be due to other factors not yet entirely understood. However, if you adhere to the principles discussed here, you may prevent your blood pressure from increasing even more. In addition, you may reduce the amount of drug therapy necessary for treatment.

A Medical Mosaic: Hypertension

How did hypertension rise from the medical ranks of private to that of four-star general, and become recognized as a full-fledged disease? In large part, one physician deserves the credit. In 1948, Dr. Irvine A. Page, now Consultant Emeritus of the renowned Research Foundation of the Cleveland Clinic Foundation, dared to challenge some outmoded theories.

Initially trained as a chemist, Dr. Page was among the first to realize that regulation of blood pressure is similar to orchestrating a symphony. Many different components are involved, and if something goes wrong with even one element, the entire system is disrupted. Because he strongly believed that hypertension stemmed from several factors, Dr. Page proposed what he called "the mosaic theory" of hypertension, and the name stuck. Scientists still agree with him that many mechanisms are involved in producing hypertension. (See Figure.)

According to Dr. Page's theory, multiple factors affect the regulation of blood pressure, but three major kinds of mechanisms stand out: chemical (such as excess cortisol and thyroid hormones), anatomic (such as the condition of organs) and neural (centers in the brain that control heartbeat and blood pressure may be off—also, stress and other emotional factors may be involved).

In addition to these factors, the mosaic theory also points out that blood volume

Figure 2.9: The Mosaic Theory of Hypertension

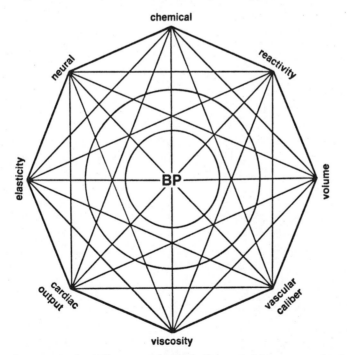

High blood pressure is a disease of regulation, and numerous factors are involved in this process. If the system is "off," blood pressure can increase. (BP=blood pressure.)

and blood viscosity, or thickness, may be involved, as well as cardiac output, i.e., the amount of blood the heart pumps in a given period of time. Peripheral resistance, another factor, represents the size of the arterioles, the network of blood vessels that delivers blood to all of the body's tissues. Are they constricted (narrowed) or dilated (open)? Just think of the nozzle on a fireman's hose to get the picture!

3

Cigarette Smoking Harms the Healthy Heart

If you smoke cigarettes, stop.
If you don't smoke, don't start.

There is no other way to say it. The evidence identifying cigarette smoking as a contributing factor to the development of coronary heart disease and lung cancer would fill volumes. The admonition cited above, which was coined by the American Cancer Society, succinctly defines the best and only way to deal with the problem of cigarette smoking. The approach is not new, but it gained considerable impetus when the official campaign against smoking was launched in 1964, and was reiterated by Joseph A. Califano, the former Secretary of HEW, in 1978. This chapter explains in some detail just how smoking harms the healthy heart.

The first surgeon general's report on smoking in 1964 stated, among other things, that the average cigarette smoker in the United States had a 70 percent greater chance of developing coronary heart disease than a nonsmoker. Since then, hundreds of studies have been carried out in order to learn more about the effect of smoking on health. In 1979, fifteen years after the initial report, a new, even more comprehensive report on smoking and health by the surgeon general was published by the U.S. Department of Health, Education and Welfare. A compendium of twenty-two scientific papers on smoking and health, commissioned by the surgeon general and reviewed by physicians and scientists who are experts in their fields, upheld the conclusions of the original report and included detailed discussions of such topics as the effects of smoking on women and children. Among its more specific findings were:

- Pregnant women who smoke cigarettes increase the risk of their giving birth to premature babies, and there is a growing amount of evi-

63

dence to show that children born to mothers who smoke cigarettes may be deficient in their physical, emotional and intellectual development.

- The number of teenage girls aged 12 to 14 who smoke cigarettes has increased eightfold since 1968.

- As the level of cigarette smoking increases, disease and death rates climb for women, just as they do for men; for example, since 1955 lung cancer has increased fivefold among women.

- Cigarette smokers who work in the asbestos, coal, rubber, textile, uranium, and various chemical industries are even more likely to develop lung cancer or heart disease than smokers in other occupations or nonsmokers on their own.

In summing up, the 1979 report stated that "cigarette smoking is the single most important preventable environmental factor contributing to illness, disability, and death in the United States."

SMOKING AND YOUR HEART

Over the years, many studies have been carried out to show the harmful effects of smoking on the heart. The Kingert study, for example, involved one million men and women, 40 to 84 years old. It showed that death from coronary heart disease increased for each sex and age group with the amount of cigarette smoking—the younger the age group, the higher the relative risk The youngest men who smoked two or more packs of cigarettes a day were at highest risk. In addition, other studies have demonstrated that the association of risk of coronary heart disease with cigarette smoking is independent of other risk factors such as an elevated level of cholesterol in the blood or high blood pressure. The risk of cigarette smokers dying from coronary heart disease is estimated to be at least double that of nonsmokers, and the risk of stroke is approximately five times greater. Depending on the presence of other risk factors, the risk of having a heart attack could rise to ten or more times above that of the nonsmoker.

In 1977, a committee of the American Heart Association noted that each year there were 325,000 premature deaths attributable to cigarette smoking; of these, 37 percent were from coronary heart disease, while 19 percent were caused by lung cancer. A recent surgeon general's report also devotes considerable space to the relationship between smoking and cardiovascular disease. In particular, the report stated that:

- Smoking is one of three major independent risk factors for heart attack; moreover, the effect is dose-related, synergistic with other risk factors for heart attack, and stronger at younger ages.

- Cigarette smokers are more apt to develop severe and extensive atherosclerosis of the aorta and coronary arteries than nonsmokers. The effect is dose-related.

- Smoking lowers the threshold for the onset of angina pectoris in patients with angina.

- Women who smoke and take oral contraceptives are at a significantly increased risk for both fatal and nonfatal myocardial infarction and thromboembolism.

- Cessation of smoking does reduce the risk of mortality from coronary heart disease, and after ten years off cigarettes, this risk approaches that of the nonsmoker.

How Does Smoking Damage Your Heart?

In many ways. First, the two major elements in cigarettes and cigarette smoke—nicotine and carbon monoxide—have deleterious effects on blood vessels. For example, it has been established through autopsies that cigarette smokers have considerably more atherosclerotic disease of the coronary and other arteries than nonsmokers, and these degenerative arterial changes in a smoker's heart are so frequent that the condition is referred to as "smoker's heart." These changes may result both from the carbon monoxide that is inhaled and the nicotine in cigarette tobacco. Remember, carbon monoxide is a poisonous gas. Among other things, carbon monoxide decreases oxygen delivery to heart muscle, which can result in dysfunction or damage to heart muscle cells.

Nicotine also has adverse effects on the cardiovascular system. Within ten or fifteen minutes after you begin to smoke a cigarette, and sometimes even sooner, your pulse rate quickens and blood pressure rises. None of the filters currently available can entirely remove these destructive elements, especially carbon monoxide: The level of tar and nicotine may be reduced, but this certainly does not make cigarette smoking "safe."

The postmortem studies mentioned previously showed that people who had smoked two or more packs of cigarettes a day had four times as much atheroma, a narrowing of the arteries with marked degenerative changes, as those who smoked infrequently. According to one study, fibrous thickening of the wall of the coronary arteries was present to an advanced degree in approximately one-fourth of those who had smoked two or more packs a day, compared to less than *1 percent* of those who had *never smoked*. The myocardial arterioles showed the most severe effects of cigarette smoking. Advanced thickening was found in 90 percent of smokers who smoked two or more packs a day, while the prevalence was slightly less than half this percentage among those who had smoked one to two packs a day. Among those who had never smoked, there was none. Although the specific cause of this condition is unknown, nicotine is strongly suspected to be the culprit. (See Figure 3.1.)

Has Cigarette Smoking Declined Since the 1964 Surgeon General's Report?

To the contrary. Although the number of adults who smoke cigarettes dropped from approximately 41.7 percent in 1965 to about 32.2 percent in 1978, the 1979 report states that the total number of cigarette smokers aged 17 and over climbed from an estimated 53.3 million in 1965 to approximately

Figure 3.1: How Smoking Can Increase Your Chance of Having a Heart Attack

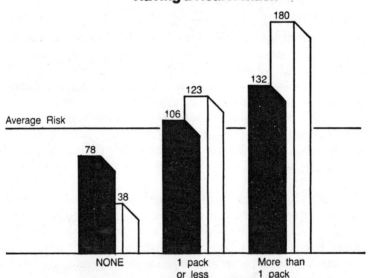

A man who smokes more than a pack of cigarettes a day has nearly *twice* the risk of heart attack and nearly *five* times the risk of stroke as a nonsmoker.

SOURCE: The Framingham Heart Study (men aged 30–62).

54.1 million in 1978. Although this change is small, it represents an 11.1 percent increase in the absolute number of adult female smokers (the absolute number of adult male smokers decreased by 8.5 percent). Although the number of teenage boys who smoke has remained virtually constant, the number of teenage girls who smoke has climbed at a steady rate. It is now estimated that approximately one-fourth of all teenage girls smoke, whereas roughly one-third of all teenage boys smoke. Finally, the gross consumption of cigarettes totaled 608 billion in 1976. (The figure represents an average of more than 11.5 cigarettes a day for every man, woman, and child over 18 years of age in the United States.) Cigarette consumption is also climbing at a steady rate of 2 to 3 percent a year.

More on Harmful Effects

It has been estimated by the American Cancer Society that at least 80 percent of all lung cancer is caused by cigarette smoking, which means that this disease is, to a large extent, preventable. Yet each year approximately 102,000 new cases of lung cancer are diagnosed, and 92,000 die of it annually (280 people a day). The death rate from lung cancer is climbing steadily among women, and it has increased more than twenty-five times in forty-five years for men. Worst of all, the prognosis for this particular type of cancer is very poor: the five-year survival rate is 8 percent for men and 12 percent for women.

Does Quitting Really Help?

Yes. Even among heavy smokers the risk of developing coronary heart disease decreases 25 percent in the first year of abstinence. In addition, most ex-smokers report immediate benefits: disappearance of morning cough and more stamina. At one asbestos plant in Waukegan, Illinois, all employees were recently required to stop smoking on the premises after studies showed that asbestos workers who smoked ran a 92 percent greater chance of developing lung cancer than those who did not.

How to Go About Quitting Smoking

No one will tell you that stopping is easy, because it isn't. Fortunately, however, there are many books, leaflets, pamphlets, and programs that can help you. For information write to:

American Cancer Society (ACS)
777 Third Avenue
New York, New York 10017
(212-371-2900)

Similarly, the American Heart Association offers a wide variety of films, leaflets, and pamphlets urging everyone who smokes to stop. If you are particularly concerned about weight gain while trying to give up smoking, the American Heart Association publishes a pamphlet that discusses this problem, entitled *Weight Control Guide and Smoking Cessation Program.*

Besides these organizations, you can contact SmokEnders®, the most effective group to date in helping people quit smoking. It was founded in 1969 by Jacquelyn Rogers, a compulsive smoker for twenty-two years. She and her husband, a dentist, devised a means to help her quit smoking. Since then, they have been teaching this method to others. Among the graduates are former Secretary of HEW Joseph A. Califano, singer Barry Manilow, and actress Rosemary Harris. Many organizations have been impressed enough to have hired SmokEnders instructors to help their employees quit smoking. Its "blue-chip" clients have included AT&T, General Electric, Johnson & Johnson, General Foods, Pepsico, Inc., Xerox Corporation, New York Stock Exchange, Nestlè Company, and many major banks and insurance companies.

SmokEnders has chapters all over the United States, as well as abroad. The instructors are all graduates of the program. There is a fee for the program, which consists of eight weekly meetings. Cost varies, but $100 is average. The program can also be repeated at a 50 percent discount. For information, call toll free: 800-227-2334. For more information about SmokEnders, contact the national headquarters:

SmokEnders®
37 North Third Street
Easton, Pa. 18042
(800-523-6155)

Public Health Campaigns

Despite all evidence, the tobacco industries continue to lobby to protect sales. In April 1978 Joseph A. Califano, former Secretary of HEW, pointedly asked tobacco company executives: "Is there anyone, including tobacco company lobbyists and executives, who would encourage their own children to smoke cigarettes?"

Both the American Cancer Society and the American Heart Association are campaigning to eliminate smoking. The AHA has called for the Federal Government to ban all cigarette advertising and to halt its $44.4 million annual subsidy to tobacco growers. It is also campaigning for laws that make it illegal to sell tobacco to people under 18 years of age; restriction of cigarette smoking in enclosed public places and in public areas where people work and play; and a ban on the sale of cigarettes in places where children can purchase them.

Whether or not these organizations will succeed in lowering cigarette consumption remains to be seen. In the interim, remember:

If you smoke cigarettes, stop.
If you don't smoke, don't start.

4
Living with Risk Factors Beyond Your Control

Although few physicians would argue that cigarette smoking, high blood pressure, or a diet high in animal fats do not contribute to the development of coronary heart disease, at least we can eliminate or modify these risk factors. Unfortunately, however, there are other variables over which we still have very little control. Diabetes, a positive family history of heart disease, and a person's age, sex, and race are all known to affect the risk of heart attack.

Diabetes, for example, is a disease that can develop in anyone at any time. Once you have it, there is no definitive cure, although a prudent diet and drugs can help normalize diabetic patients. There is also nothing you can do about your family's medical history—if one or more of your relatives died of heart disease, you cannot alter the facts.

You can, however, try to control some of the other factors in your "coronary risk profile." But before we outline the steps you can take, it is important to understand what diabetes is all about.

WHAT IS DIABETES?

Essentially, *diabetes mellitus* is a disorder of *metabolism*, the body's regulating process in which foods are broken down into their constituent chemicals and rebuilt into new substances or broken down and transformed into other chemicals that may be eliminated from the body or reused.

In diabetes, a key part of the metabolic process—the body's ability to utilize carbohydrates—is impaired. Sugars accumulate in the blood in excessive quantities and ultimately are excreted in the urine. The hormone *insulin*, which is produced by the pancreas, is instrumental in the metabolism of sugars. When the amount of insulin produced is insufficient—as in diabetes—the body is unable to metabolize carbohydrates adequately. The excessive accu-

70

mulation of sugar in the blood causes *polyuria* (increased urine volume), resulting in dehydration and a continual sensation of thirst, since abnormally large quantities of water are lost from the body.

There are two types of diabetes: *juvenile* and *adult-* or *maturity-onset.* These terms are somewhat misleading because juvenile diabetes, although it *generally* becomes evident during childhood or puberty, can also first appear in adulthood. Similarly, the adult-onset type of diabetes may appear in adolescents. Adult-onset diabetes is a milder form than the juvenile type.

Who Gets Diabetes?

Diabetes can develop in men, women, or children, but it is more common in women than men, and the incidence is greater among those over 40 years of age. Today it is estimated that up to 10 million Americans have diabetes mellitus, although not all victims are aware of it. The disease tends to be hereditary; if one of your relatives has, or had, diabetes, you are more likely to develop it than someone with a negative family history of diabetes.

What Are the Warning Signs?

There are numerous symptoms associated with diabetes:

Chronic thirst	Skin infections (boils, carbuncles)
Frequent urination	Visual disturbances
Chronic hunger	Vaginal itching
Weakness, malaise	Weight loss

Weight loss is particularly noteworthy when it occurs despite a good appetite and adequate food intake.

How Is Diabetes Detected?

To begin, a routine urinalysis is done. Even if sugar is not present in the urine, however, a physician may decide to order more specific tests, particularly if you have some symptoms suggestive of diabetes. In that case, a "fasting blood sugar" test may be done. For this test, the patient is required to fast, avoiding the intake of all food and beverages (except water), overnight. In the morning, a blood sample is obtained, and the concentration of sugar in it is determined. Again, however, a normal "fasting blood sugar" does not exclude the possibility of diabetes, since it's possible for blood sugar to be normal after fasting but elevated after eating.

A more specific index than the fasting blood sugar test is the "postprandial" (after eating) blood sugar test. After a patient has eaten a high-carbohydrate meal, a blood sample is drawn each hour for three hours. A high blood sugar usually means diabetes is present. A borderline, or a slightly elevated, blood sugar level warrants further investigation. In borderline cases, a glucose tolerance test is ordered. This is a very specific test. First, fasting blood and urine sugar levels are obtained; then, the patient is given a dose of sugar (in water) to take, and blood and urine samples are taken thirty minutes, one hour, two hours, and three hours later.

What Does Diabetes Have to Do with Coronary Artery Disease?

It has been established that in over half of all diabetics between the ages of 40 and 59, cardiac disease is the primary cause of death. In the population at large, coronary artery disease occurs more frequently among diabetics than among nondiabetics and is fatal earlier. Diabetes is considered an important risk factor for coronary artery disease and atherosclerosis of all arteries in the body. The reason for this is not known, but the metabolic defect in this disease clearly contributes to the premature degenerative process of the arteries, which, in turn, is responsible for many of the complications that result from diabetes. Worst of all, although a premenopausal female is less likely to develop coronary heart disease than a male of a comparative age, this advantage is lost to the female diabetic. Also, once a heart attack occurs in a diabetic, the prognosis is poorer than in the nondiabetic with coronary heart disease.

Unfortunately, many diabetics have other risk factors present. For example, they may also have high blood pressure, elevated levels of cholesterol and triglycerides, and be cigarette smokers. All of these factors, however, can be completely controlled if the patient makes an effort. Since obesity is often found among adult diabetics, dietary control alone is often sufficient to maintain normal blood sugar levels. Obviously then, risk of cardiovascular disease varies considerably among diabetics, depending on the presence of other risk factors and the patient's effort to control them.

In general, the Framingham Heart Study showed that individuals with impaired carbohydrate tolerance had at least a doubled risk of coronary heart disease, congestive heart failure, and atherothrombotic brain infarction (stroke), compared to those without this abnormality (See Figure 4.1.)

What You Can Do About Diabetes

The discovery of insulin in 1921 in Canada by Frederick G. Banting and Charles H. Best revolutionized the treatment for diabetes. Today it is estimated that approximately 1.25 million diabetics require insulin; 1.25 million

Figure 4.1: Data from the Framingham Heart Study, 18-Year Follow-Up

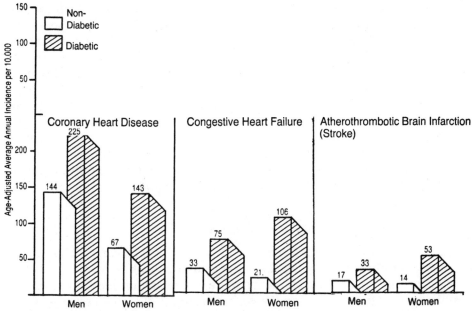

These charts show the risk of cardiovascular morbidity according to diabetic status in men and women aged 45–74.

SOURCE: W. B. Kannel, *Symposium on Cardiovascular Epidemiology* VI, 5 (October, 1976), with permission.

are controlled by drugs, and 3.5 million respond to dietary management alone. The remaining four million diabetics are uncontrolled, but many of these patients would probably fare better if they adhered to their prescribed diets.

If you have diabetes, a wide range of medical and social services are available. You can write to the American Diabetes Association (2 Park Avenue, New York, New York 10016), or to the Juvenile Diabetes Association (23 East 26 Street, New York, New York 10010) for information. These organizations can guide you to the best treatment centers for diabetes, as well as help you obtain a Medic-Alert Tag. The American Diabetes Association maintains affiliates in all states and has over sixty-seven branch offices. Numerous free pamphlets are also available, each providing various kinds of counseling. A sample of these includes: *Some Facts About Diabetes, Travel Tips for Diabetics, What You Need to Know About Diabetes, Career Choices for Diabetics, Employment*

Opportunities and Protections for Diabetics, School Children with Diabetes, Helping Your Child Live with Diabetes.

In addition, the ADA also publishes a bimonthly magazine, *Diabetes Forecast*, at subscription rates of $15 for one year and $30 for two years. The magazine publishes articles ranging from features on cooking, special camp programs for children, and pregnancy and diabetes, to advice on employment and insurance. Finally, many good cookbooks and other helpful guides for the diabetic are available.

Remember, if you follow your doctor's advice and keep your diabetes and any other "controllable" risk factors in check, the chances of your developing a cardiovascular problem may decrease. Mary Tyler Moore—actress, dancer, and businesswoman—and Jim "Catfish" Hunter, a retired pitcher for the New York Yankees—are diabetics whose careers show that you can live and enjoy life to the fullest, providing you take good care of yourself!

A Postive Family History Is a Risk Factor Too

As the old saying goes: "Friends you pick, relatives you can't." Thus, like diabetes, a family history of heart disease is another risk factor totally beyond your control. Consequently, it is even more important for those with a positive family history to eliminate and/or control as many of the other risk factors as possible. Although there is considerable scientific evidence to show that the incidence of coronary artery disease is related to family history, it is unclear to what extent this is due to genetic factors, since families also share similar social and dietary patterns. Nevertheless, there is clear evidence that the risk of coronary heart disease increases in close relatives of people who have had a heart attack early in life (prior to 50 years of age).

The important thing is to *know* your family history. How did your grandparents or your aunts and uncles die? If you've heard that your grandfather had "heart trouble," or your grandmother had a stroke or a "touch of" diabetes, the details of their illnesses could be significant. How old were they when they died? Have you lost a close relative due to "sudden death"? Has any relative had a heart attack and survived? What about high blood pressure? Is any relative currently taking medication for it—or did any deceased relative have high blood pressure? You should be thoroughly familiar with your family history—if it's negative for coronary heart disease, all the better for you—and if it's positive, you should make every possible effort to keep all other risk factors under control.

Throughout this book, we will point out ways for you to help keep risk factors under control, especially the "Big Three." Fortunately, all three can be controlled very well, providing you eliminate cigarette smoking, take medication as your physician prescribes it for you if you need it to control high blood pressure, and control your intake of saturated fats if your doctor recommends this to reduce your serum cholesterol level.

Age, Sex, and Race Also Affect Your Coronary Risk Profile

Many physicians feel coronary atherosclerosis is relatively common in men 20 years of age and older. Indeed, atherosclerosis is often regarded as part of the normal aging process; still, most experts agree that the high incidence of heart attacks in this country is not normal. It is one thing to discover during an autopsy that a 78-year-old man who died in his sleep had severe coronary artery disease, and quite another to learn on autopsy that a young man in his twenties also had extensive coronary artery disease.

Age. Recent statistics reveal that the most significant increase in the cardiovascular disease mortality rate is occurring among men aged 30 to 49. In general, however, most Americans who die from some form of heart disease are 65 years of age or older. To some, that may not seem so devastating; after all, 65 is considered "over the hill" by many. But with well over half the deaths that are attributable to heart disease occurring in that older age group, it is important to point out that similar trends are *not* reported in numerous other countries. It is equally important to emphasize that many individuals remain highly active and productive well into their seventies and eighties.

Sex. Your sex also influences the likelihood of developing coronary heart disease. It is known, for example, that before the age of 45 men are ten times more apt to develop cardiovascular disease than women are. By the age of 60 the ratio is still two or three to one. The incidence of cardiovascular disease among women, however, climbs dramatically after menopause.

Race. Race has been evaluated in terms of its role in the development of coronary heart disease. Statistics show that, proportionately, the rates of CHD are just about as high among black women as among white men, but why this is so is unknown.

Although diabetes, a positive family history of heart disease, and a person's sex, age, and race are beyond our control, they are factors that every physician takes into consideration in formulating a coronary risk profile for a patient

5
Exercise to Your Heart's Delight

Huff! Puff! Huff! Puff! The wicked wolf, perhaps, warming up to blow the house down? Quite the contrary. Today, huffing, puffing, grunting, and panting is the sound of America; the noise reverberates from racquetball courts in San Francisco to Sunday's congested bicycle paths in New York's Central Park. To date, a record 87 million American adults now claim to participate in some form of athletic activity. For some, interest in sports waxes and wanes—for them, it's just another passing flirtation with the latest trend. But a considerable number seems addicted—quite willing, in fact, to spout off with evangelistic fervor about the joys of running, jogging, bicycling, or whatever.

The urge to exercise is sweeping the country at such an extraordinary rate that even traditional "blue-chip" corporations have joined the crusade. For example, current estimates reveal that more than 300 well-known corporate giants, such as Pepsico, Inc., the Xerox Corporation, General Foods, General Motors, Chase Manhattan Bank, and McGraw-Hill, to name a few, have arranged for their executives to exchange their two-martini lunches for an hour on a squash court. Now, "corporate remodeling" doesn't necessarily mean new furniture for the executive suite. Rather, it signifies the installation of lockers, showers, exercise equipment, a running track and, in some cases, even an Olympic-size swimming pool—in short, everything the managers need to stay in shape.

Everywhere, sedentary America is getting on its feet again, and top physicians as well as sports suppliers concur: We're in the midst of an exercise explosion, and it looks like it's here to stay. Throughout the country, exercise spas and health clubs are cropping up all over; with an estimated 30 million tennis freaks now swarming the courts (you can't even get "wait-listed" to play in some areas), and, in New York, it's sometimes difficult to say which

76

are more numerous: the joggers going around Central Park's reservoir or the disco dancers at Regine's.

What's happening? Doctors have established that exercise improves cardiovascular fitness and possibly reduces the likelihood of heart attack; furthermore, it is beneficial in many other ways. In this chapter, we discuss exercise: what types help your heart, how and when to begin your program, and when to stop.

Many physicians currently advocate increased physical activity as one of the most effective ways to maintain cardiovascular health in individuals without disease, and as a form of therapy for certain patients with cardiac diseases. Nowadays, the subject of exercise arouses great interest: zealots extol it as a virtual health panacea and critics condemn it as a self-destructive form of behavior. Although knowledge of the benefits and limitations of exercise is incomplete, certain facts have been established which provide a rational basis for its evaluation. For example, it is now clear that increased physical activity does provide certain benefits to healthy individuals and selected patients with cardiac disease but that in some people, particularly in the latter group, it is neither beneficial nor safe. In order to have a better understanding of the role of exercise in health and cardiac disease, it is worthwhile to discuss the physiologic effects of exercise training, the requirements to produce these effects, the manner in which they can influence cardiac health, and the selection of individuals for exercise programs. It is also helpful to view exercise much as you view a potent drug—when properly prescribed to appropriate individuals, it has the potential to provide considerable benefit, but when self-administered it can be harmful, and even lethal. This admonition particularly applies to patients with cardiac disease and even to apparently healthy individuals who have been sedentary and are at high risk to have undetected cardiac disease.

THE CASE FOR EXERCISE

"Running for your life" used to imply that you were in trouble with the law and couldn't escape its clutches fast enough. Today, that phrase has an altogether different meaning. More Americans each year are joining the wave of sports enthusiasts who don their track shoes every morning or evening and sprint around their neighborhoods or around a running track for a few miles. If the movement has a Pied Piper, it is Dr. Kenneth H. Cooper, who is Director of the Aerobic Activities Center in Dallas, Texas. His book *Aerobics* has sold well over one million copies, and it is in part responsible for the five million people who now perform aerobic exercises regularly.

However, while Dr. Cooper has helped publicize the value of physical fitness in maintaining health, he is far from alone in his studies of the effects of exercise on the cardiovascular system. Findings from the Framingham Study also showed that exercise has an ameliorating effect on the clinical course of coronary heart disease. In general, over a ten-year period, fatal heart attacks occurred less frequently in those people with more active life-styles than in the group of people with sedentary jobs. Similarly, in a massive rievew of death certificates of two million middle-aged men from England and Wales, one investigator found an inverse relationship between the mortality from coronary heart disease and the level of activity required by the last job held by the individual.

Finally, two recent studies document that hard physical work or strenuous exercise, such as jogging or running, are particularly beneficial for your cardiovascular system, while less demanding activities, such as golf, may be of little value in enhancing cardiovascular fitness.

In a twenty-two-year study of 3,600 longshoremen in San Francisco, investigators found that those men between the ages of 35 and 54 who worked in the most strenuous jobs had the lowest risk of fatal heart attack. In fact, those who were less active ran a three times higher risk of having a fatal heart attack than their harder-working peers. Based on this study, the researchers concluded that a lack of hard physical work was actually equal to high blood pressure or cigarette smoking in measuring risk of a fatal heart attack. The longshoremen who worked at the less active jobs who also smoked cigarettes and had high blood pressure, had as much as twentyfold increase in risk of having a fatal attack.

In another study of 17,000 Harvard alumni between 35 and 75, fewer heart attacks occurred among those who regularly participated (at least three hours a week) in strenuous sports activities such as swimming, running, and jogging. Overall, these men used up an average of 2,000 calories or more each week as a result of their activities. The results of this large survey showed that strenuous activity had a protective effect on the heart, even when other risk factors, such as obesity or high blood pressure, were present.

With sports enthusiasts shelling out approximately $65 million annually for equipment ranging from exercise bicycles to virtually useless massager belts, it hardly seems necessary to promote physical fitness. Yet, estimates indicate that some 50 million Americans are physically inactive; that is, they do not regularly participate in any sport for the purpose of exercise. If you're one of them, this chapter is for you.

PHYSIOLOGICAL EFFECTS OF EXERCISE

Long-term aerobic (isotonic) exercise produces important changes in the body's response to physical activity, in contrast to isometric or strength-building forms of activity. Aerobic exercise consists of continuous, rhythmic activity of large muscle groups moving the body through space; for example, walking, cycling, jogging, and swimming, for extended periods of time. Isometric activity, in contrast, consists of static muscle contraction against a high resistance for a brief interval (e.g. weight lifting, pushing against a fixed resistance, etc.). Aerobic exercise, as the term implies, involves the increased transport and utilization of oxygen (the body's essential fuel) by the body's cardiovascular, pulmonary, and musculoskeletal systems. Through regular exercise, these systems actually develop a greater capacity for oxygen metabolism. The results are increased endurance and an ability to perform physical activity with less subjective and physiologic stress. No such beneficial effects on cardiopulmonary fitness result from isometric exercise.

In the healthy individual who pursues a program of habitual aerobic exercise, the following changes occur. First, the exercising muscles develop a greater capacity to remove and use oxygen from the blood that supplies them. This alteration is related to an increase in the energy-producing components (mitochondria) of the muscle cells and certain enzymes. The result is an increased work capacity of these muscles. The heart muscle in the normal individual increases in mass (hypertrophies), as does any muscle when subjected to increased work. Thus, the heart is able to pump larger volumes of blood to the body's organs with each beat. The skeletal muscles receive more oxygen and therefore gain a greater capacity for work. The improved function of the heart and the increased ability of the skeletal muscles to extract oxygen from the blood reduce the frequency of cardiac contraction (heart beats/minute) necessary to support skeletal muscle activity at levels below maximum effort. Thus, the heart rate is lower at rest and at submaximal levels of activity in the "trained" individual compared to the sedentary person. (See Figure 5.1.)

Certain hormonal changes also appear to contribute to this reduction in cardiac stress associated with exercise training. The blood levels of the cardiac-stimulating or excitatory hormones, epinephrine (adrenaline) and norepinephrine (noradrenaline), are lower after exercise training. It should be understood that although cardiac mechanical activity is lower during submaximal activity after exercise training, the pumping function of the heart is improved and it can deliver more blood per beat and has a higher maximum output. Therefore, maximum exercise capacity rises after training.

In addition to the ability to perform more work with less subjective stress, which contributes to a feeling of enhanced energy and reduced fatigue during a normal day's activities, other changes of *potential* benefit are associated with exercise training. These include alterations in body metabolism, in the blood, and in psychological status that may be advantageous in reducing the risk of coronary heart disease. On a stable diet, exercise will induce modest but definite reduction in body fat and weight, and in the concentration of tri-

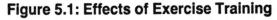

Figure 5.1: Effects of Exercise Training

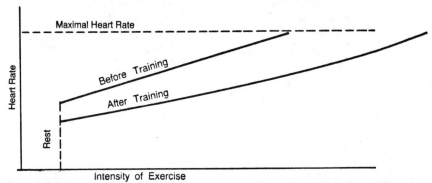

Reduction in heart rate response to all levels of submaximal exercise after training compared to heart rate measured before training.

---

glycerides (a form of fat) in the blood. Blood pressure is lowered in some individuals. Although blood cholesterol is not lowered, distribution into high-density lipoprotein (HDL) cholesterol and low density lipoprotein (LDL) cholesterol appears to be favorably affected. Thus, HDL cholesterol, which is associated with reduced risk of coronary heart disease, is increased, and LDL cholesterol, which increases risk, is lowered. The tendency of the blood to clot within arteries is diminished, possibly decreasing the potential for coronary thrombosis and myocardial infarction. Improved emotional outlook is experienced by many adherents of exercise programs, who report less tension, depression, hypochondriasis, and insomnia. Indeed, some individuals can become "addicted" to exercise in the sense that they experience negative side effects when unable to engage in physical activity for extended periods.

It should be noted that there is *no* evidence in humans, either healthy or with coronary artery disease, that exercise produces changes in the coronary vessels. Studies have shown no signs of increased auxiliary (collateral) coronary arteries or enlargement of the native coronary circulation. Atherosclerotic narrowings of the coronary arteries have not been shown to regress after exercise (or dietary programs), and such alterations would not be anticipated in light of the chronic, scarred, fibrotic and calcified composition of the atherosclerotic deposits which are hard and firmly organized within the blood vessel wall. The potential benefits of exercise in healthy people and in patients with coronary artery disease accrue primarily from the physiologic alterations enumerated previously. Their specific value to patients is considered separately below.

There is evidence that individuals who are physically active throughout their lives may have a lower death rate from coronary heart disease than sedentary individuals, but considerably more research is necessary on this question; it may be that inherently healthy individuals are the ones who engage in physical activity, rather than that the activity confers a protective effect. Another interesting finding was noted in the Health Insurance Plan of New York City: Survival from a first myocardial infarction was higher in previously active individuals than in sedentary patients.

Figure 5.2: O_2 Consumption and Heart Rate During Exercise

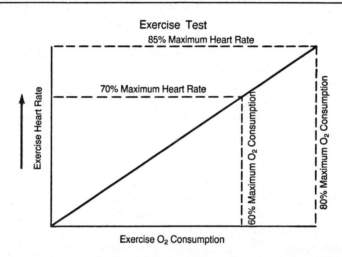

Relationship between an individual's oxygen consumption and heart rate during exercise. Note that 60% of maximum oxygen consumption matches 75% of maximum heart rate and 80% of maximum oxygen consumption matches 85% of maximum heart rate. The benefits of exercise training usually require exercise intensity associated with 60–80% of maximum capacity, as measured by oxygen consumption.

Requirements for Production of a "Training Effect"

To produce the beneficial effects of exercise, several criteria must be fulfilled. These relate to type of exercise, intensity, frequency, and duration.

As indicated previously, exercise must be of the aerobic type. There are many forms of aerobic activity, so a person should be able to select one that he will enjoy and can adhere to (Table 5.1). It should be performed to an intensity that is 60 to 80 percent of the individual's maximum capacity, which refers to percent of maximum oxygen utilization measured during an exercise test. This usually corresponds to about 70 to 85 percent of heart rate at maximum exertion as determined during an exercise test. (See Figure 5.2.)

Measurement of oxygen consumption during exercise testing requires complete apparatus that is not available in most exercise laboratories, but the relationship between oxygen consumption and the heart allows reasonable estimation of appropriate training levels. A *crude* means of estimating one's maximum heart rate and calculating target heart rates for exercise is provided by the formula: 220 − age = maximum exercise heart rate. Thus, for a 40-year-old person, estimated maximum heart rate is 220 − 40 = 180 beats/minute; 70% of 180 = 126 beats/minute for an exercise target heart rate. It is emphasized that the formula 220 − age provides a very rough approximation of maximum heart rate in the individual and can err considerably below or above the true value. Maximum heart rate determined during an exercise test is the truest and safest means of obtaining this information. However, in healthy individuals who desire programs of mild activity, the mathematical approximation of maximum heart rate may be acceptable.

Exercise must be performed a minimum of three times weekly, preferably on alternate days, to allow rest and recovery. Daily high-intensity activity is preferred by athletes and other highly-conditioned persons who have safely progressed to these levels. The duration of exercise should be a minimum of twenty minutes. If lower levels of activity such as walking are pursued, it is preferable to perform for minimum intervals of thirty to forty minutes. Each exercise period should be preceded and followed by a brief (five minutes) warm-up and cool-down period. The former usually includes stretching exercises and a gradual build-up of the type of activity to be pursued, and the latter consists of a gradual slow-down rather than abrupt cessation of activity. Adherence to the foregoing principles will result in demonstrable physiological changes in six to eight weeks or less. It has been found that the resting pulse rate falls about one beat/minute for each week of an exercise program of the type outlined here.

It is important to sound a cautionary note concerning healthy but previously sedentary adults over age 35 who embark upon a program of augmented physical activity. If this is to involve more than mild activity (walking, low-level cycling), a physician's clearance and guidance should be obtained. The

Table 5.1. Aerobic Types of Activity

1. Walking	4. Swimming	7. Rope skipping
2. Jogging	5. Skating	8. Aerobic dance
3. Cycling	6. Rowing	9. Cross country skiing

physician will perform an evaluation and may order an exercise test or other studies, depending upon the individual. No patient with cardiac disease should pursue increased activity without first consulting a physician. Untoward events during exercise have most often occurred when individuals have engaged in self-prescribed physical activity or have exceeded the limits indicated to them by their physicians. These simple precautionary measures will enhance the safety, benefits, and pleasure of exercise.

The benefits of aerobic exercise correlate directly with the level of intensity that can be safely sustained, but a major problem in this regard is always compliance. As you probably realize, sticking to an exercise regimen—especially a rigorous one—is difficult. A number of people do adhere to strict jogging regimens, for example, but these people still represent a minority of the population. In fact, there is a very large drop-out rate from exercise programs involving high levels of activity. Usually, boredom and/or a number of muscle and joint problems account for the drop-out rate. Clearly, the ideal form of exercise is one that is relatively easy to carry out, requires nothing in the way of expense (for equipment, etc.), and is enjoyable. Walking fulfills all of these criteria. In fact, we believe it is the ideal mode of activity: it provides the benefits of exercise to the largest number of people over the longest period of time. It can also be carried out as a family activity, presents the fewest limitations in terms of age and state of health, and is least likely to result in adverse effects. Furthermore, walking is a form of exercise that can be done daily—alternate days off to relax the muscles are not required.

To avoid boredom, one can vary the routes; often, an hour or so of walking provides the individual with a peaceful and pleasurable interlude. Finally, the likelihood of compliance by parents sets a good example for children, who also learn to establish a routine pattern of activity—and walking is also a very safe form of exercise. In fact, for cardiac patients, it is an excellent form of exercise, although even walking should not be undertaken without the consent of your physician if you have some form of heart disease.

How Walking May Benefit the Heart. Recent studies have shown that walking produces a cardiovascular "training effect"; that is, after several weeks of a daily, brisk walk for 30–40 minutes for 5–7 days a week, the heart rate associated with the initial speed of walking will be lower than at the time of the initiation of the walking program. These findings demonstrate that the body has adapted to the exercise and has become more efficient at it, and that the heart does not have to beat as fast to sustain a given pace of walking. These beneficial effects were recently demonstrated in a group of coronary heart disease patients at the University of California, Davis, by one of us (EAA), Dr. Rudolph Dressendorfer, and Ms. Joan Smith.

Walking is also effective in reducing weight; a study carried out in the mid-1970s showed that one hour of daily walking by obese women for one year, *without* changes, resulted in weight losses of as much as 40 pounds during that period. More studies are needed to explore in detail the physiological effects of walking, but it is clear that it does produce many of the benefits of aerobic exercise.

Still, walking is a low-intensity activity; as such, it must be performed for a relatively long period per session, at frequent intervals, to produce the desirable physiologic effects. Strolling with frequent stops is not nearly as effective. Walking as a form of aerobic exercise requires a brisk pace for 30–40 minutes per session at least three times a week (heart rates in sedentary individuals can reach 130 beats/minute) to produce a heart rate of 100–120 beats/minute (depending on the person's age, general health, etc.).

As with all exercise programs, walking should be started at a slow pace for a relatively short period of time (10–15 minutes), and one should build up gradually in exertion over the first two weeks. This approach should obviate any joint or muscle aches.

How to Start Your Exercise Program

1. First, give your program some serious thought. Remember, your objective is to select an activity that you will enjoy and, therefore, that you will want to engage in for the rest of your life. Don't consider running or jogging, for example, just because they are "in" at the moment. Finding a partner to run with who runs at the same speed you do is somewhat difficult; so if you don't particularly enjoy doing things alone, you could lose interest quickly.

Similarly, if you are quickly put off by joining clubs, buying equipment, and so on, you may find that to play squash, which at first glance might seem appealing, has requirements that are really more trouble than the game itself is worth to you. Once you do settle on an activity, however, plan enough time.

2. To reap maximum benefits, you must faithfully follow your exercise program. It should be demanding and challenge the cardiovascular system, but it should not exhaust you or leave you on the verge of collapse.

3. Finally, keep in mind that an exercise program is individual. Don't concern yourself if a neighbor ten years older who has been running for a shorter period of time can now run longer than you can. For everyone who starts to exercise to improve cardiovascular fitness, the objective is the same: to build up physical tolerance and endurance. But, remember, these vary according to the individual. For example, after you have been running for a while, your cardiovascular system may no longer be challenged by a particular walking or jogging speed, and you might have to increase your pace in order to hit your "target zone"—the point at which you are exercising hard enough to achieve cardiovascular fitness, but not so much as to strain yourself. Pages 92–93 illustrate appropriate "warm-up" exercises for you.

How to Find Your Target Zone—The Pace That's Best for You

It is best for a sedentary person to visit his physician for a physical examination before beginning an exercise program. If you are over 35 and male, your doctor may want you to have an exercise "stress test." Your doctor should also help you select the activities and the pace that are best for you.

If you have an established cardiac condition or another known disease, such as arthritis, you should see your physician before you undertake any strenuous activity program. Females and males under 35 who have always been in good health can probably forego an extensive checkup prior to starting an exercise program if they follow instructions, take it slowly at first, and consult their physician if any signs or symptoms develop.

In order to achieve cardiovascular fitness, you need to exercise enough to hit your target zone—the pace that is best for you. (See Figure 5.3) Remember, the *maximum* heart rate for a particular individual can only be determined by an individual exercise test. In patients with cardiac or other limiting conditions, accuracy in determining the target heart rate is *essential*, and exercise

Figure 5.3: Maximal Attainable Heart Rate and Target Zone

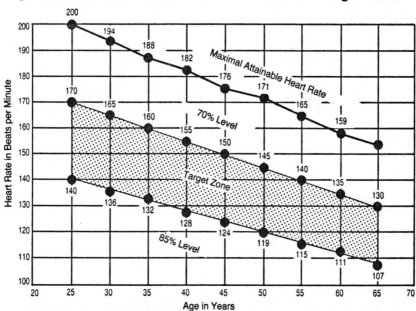

The numerical values shown here are "average" values for the given age. However, the target zone for approximately one-third of the population may differ from these values.

SOURCE: From *Beyond Diet . . . Exercise Your Way to Fitness and Heart Health*, Lenore Zohman, M.D., Best Foods, CPC International, Englewood Cliffs, N.J., with permission.

should only be undertaken after consultation with a physician. An exercise test is needed to ascertain whether a particular exercise program is safe and at what intensity it should be pursued. Spend five to ten minutes warming up to loosen your muscles and joints and stave off stiffness, soreness, and possible injuries. Once you start to exercise, hit your heart rate target zone and *stay* within that range for twenty to thirty minutes. Finally, your exercising should taper off with "cool-down" exercises over a five-minute period. (See Figure 5.4.)It is inadvisable to discontinue strenuous exercise abruptly since this does not permit the blood to circulate back to vital organs, such as the brain; light-headedness or other symptoms can result from abrupt termination.

How to Take Your Pulse

You can measure your pulse by locating it at the carotid artery in your neck, or at arteries in your wrist, your groin, or in the bend of your elbow. (See Figure 5.5.)Measure your pulse rate after your warm-up exercises; at that time, it should be well below your target heart rate. Then, move into your more vigorous regimen, and check again within five minutes or so to see if you have hit your target rate. To take your pulse during exercise, simply stop for ten seconds while measuring it and multiply the number of beats you feel by six. (Do not attempt to measure your pulse for a full minute, or even fifteen seconds,

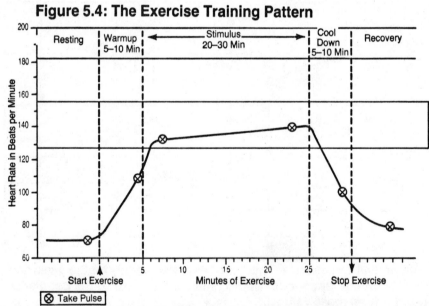

Figure 5.4: The Exercise Training Pattern

SOURCE: From *Beyond Diet . . . Exercise Your Way to Fitness and Heart Health*, Lenore Zohman, M.D., Best Foods, CPC International, Englewood Cliffs, N.J., with permission.

Figure 5.5: How to Measure Your Pulse

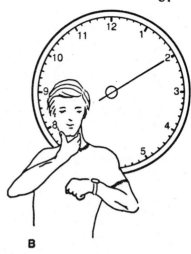

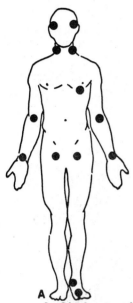

A: Circles mark the sites on the body where your pulse rate can be measured.

B: Measure your pulse for ten seconds and multiply by six to establish your pulse rate.

SOURCE: From *Beyond Diet . . . Exercise Your Way to Fitness and Heart Health*, Lenore Zohman, M.D. Best Foods, CPC International Englewood Cliffs, N.J., with permission.

---

because your heart rate drops very rapidly after exercise.) If you haven't reached your target rate, step up your activity; if you exceed your target rate, slow down. Also, measure your pulse immediately after you stop exercising.

In order to derive the most benefit, exercise three or four times a week. The days "off" allow you to recover from vigorous exercise and this helps to prevent exhaustion, especially if you have been sedentary. Don't exercise just Saturday and Sunday and skip the rest of the week. This is the "weekend athlete" syndrome, and the positive effects of exercise are somewhat lost when more than a day or two intervenes between activities. Also, the hazards of occasional bursts of activity, especially if they are vigorous, can be considerable.

How Are You Doing?

After a few weeks, your cardiovascular fitness begins to improve. During this period, you may experience some soreness or other aches as outlined, but these can generally be relieved by the remedies listed. If symptoms persist, see your doctor.

After six weeks or so, you will probably have to increase the level of your activity in order to hit your target heart rate. For example, as your body becomes conditioned, you may discover that you don't hit your target rate even after five minutes or so into the activity. In that case, increase your pace. Regardless of what your target heart rate is, you should stay within it for at least twenty minutes or so for exercises to be effective.

Put Your Daily Routine to Work for You

If you feel that you simply don't have time for a beneficial routine, try to reprogram your normal activities. For example, a housewife who feels pressed for time may believe it is all but impossible to find a half hour in the day in which to exercise. However, studies show that the average housewife walks more than fifteen miles a day in the course of performing her regular chores. Now, rather than walking up and down the stairs all day, she could build up a routine in which she runs up and down them, putting this back-to-back with more strenuous chores: cleaning windows vigorously, scrubbing floors, and the like. If you must do this sort of work, do it in such a way as to derive some direct personal benefits from it. If you have to walk the dog, don't walk, run. If you must keep several outside appointments, don't drive to all of them; instead, leave a bit earlier and press yourself into walking briskly to your destinations. Use stairs instead of elevators.

On the other hand, if you feel you would do better using an exercise bicycle or a rowing machine, but you haven't the space or the funds to purchase equipment, check with friends. You could pool resources; for example, several people could form an exercise club together. One may contribute space in a garage or cellar, and whatever else is needed can be bought collectively. Sometimes, buying many pieces of sports equipment at once entitles you to a discount. Or, each of you can contribute one piece of equipment to your at-home gym. Occasionally, secondhand equipment is available at good prices, so try the want ads too. But remember, whatever exercise program you choose and however you organize it, stick with it. In the long run, you'll feel a lot better for it!

On the following (pages 89-93), we have provided you with some guidelines to help you monitor your own exercise program. For example, page 89 lists symptoms associated with exercise that may mean you should consult your physician; page 90 provides you with a preliminary medical checklist, page 91 lists aches and pains you can manage yourself and pages 92-93 show you several easy, warm-up exercises.

Guidelines: When to See Your Physician

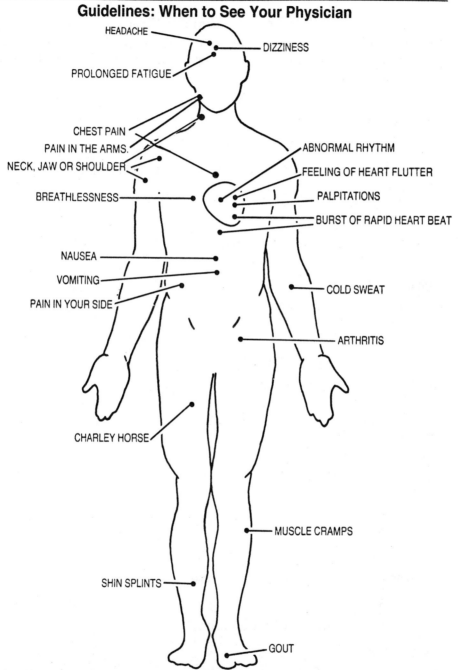

HEADACHE
DIZZINESS
PROLONGED FATIGUE
CHEST PAIN
PAIN IN THE ARMS
NECK, JAW OR SHOULDER
ABNORMAL RHYTHM
FEELING OF HEART FLUTTER
BREATHLESSNESS
PALPITATIONS
BURST OF RAPID HEART BEAT
NAUSEA
VOMITING
PAIN IN YOUR SIDE
COLD SWEAT
ARTHRITIS
CHARLEY HORSE
MUSCLE CRAMPS
SHIN SPLINTS
GOUT

If any of these symptoms are associated with exercise, discontinue your exercise program and consult your physician.

SOURCE: L. Zohman, M.D. Adapted from *Beyond Diet . . . Exercise Your Way to Fitness and Heart Health*. Best Foods, CPC International, Englewood Cliffs, N.J., with permission.

A Preliminary Medical Checklist

Review this list before you begin any exercise program. If any of these risk factors or chronic problems apply to you, you should consult your doctor before beginning an exercise program.

Risk Factors

A positive family history of heart disease

Age (Adults over 35 should consult their physician before initiating any exercise program.)

Cigarette smoking

Diabetes

Elevated serum cholesterol

High blood pressure

Overweight (by more than fifteen pounds)

Chronic Conditions or Illnesses

Arthritis (any form including bursitis, rheumatism, etc.)

Asthma

Chronic bronchitis

Emphysema

Gout

Headaches (frequent and/or undiagnosed)

Leg cramps when you walk

Orthostatic hypertension

Pain in any joints when arising in the morning

Palpitations

Shortness of breath when walking, climbing stairs, running, etc.

Unexplained dizziness

Aches and Pains You Can Manage Yourself

Problem	Description	Remedy
Blisters	Swellings that contain watery fluid.	Caused by irritation to the skin (eg., your shoe rubbing against your heel). Before skin actually "blisters," put vaseline on it and cover with a gauze pad. If a blister develops, wash it with soap and lukewarm water and cover with a gauze pad. Don't puncture the blister. If it becomes infected, see your doctor.
Charley Horse	Ache, pain, or stiffness in muscle results from strain; sometimes a ligament is torn.	Take aspirin and a hot bath, and discontinue the part of your exercise program that strains the muscle. For immediate relief, massage.
Pain in Calf Muscles	Consistent pain.	Be sure you are wearing proper track shoes; try to avoid running or jogging on pavement. If cramps continue for a few weeks, see your doctor.
Shin Splints	A "wastebasket" term to describe muscle strains on the back and front part of the lower leg.	Be sure track shoes fit properly. Avoid running or jogging on concrete. Be sure you aren't running with your feet turned out.
Prolonged breathlessness (10 minutes or so after exercising) Prolonged fatigue (Several hours after exercise) Nausea, Vomiting		Exercise is too vigorous for you—slow down. Stay at lower end of your target range.

Cardiovascular Warm-up Exercises from the University of California, Davis, Department of Physical Education and the Division of Cardiovascular Medicine, School of Medicine

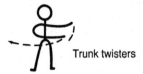
Trunk twisters

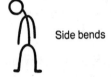
Side bends

Arm circles a) forward
b) backward

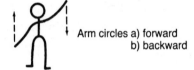
Full trunk circles (both directions)
bend over, sweep arms down in front of
you, swing arms up and around over
your head

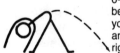
6-inch toe-touch
bend over, reach out and to the left of
your left foot; stand up; bend over again
and reach out and to the right of your
right foot (6 inches on each side)

Side lunge: lunge to both sides

Shoulder square with shrug and circles
interlock your hands and put arms over
your head, palms facing the ceiling;
shrug your shoulders up and down

The wringer
lay flat on the floor; lift your right leg
over your left and try to touch toe to
floor; you should turn your head to the
right simultaneously; reverse (cross left
leg over right and turn your head to the
left)

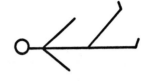

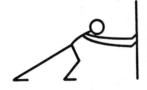

The rocker
bend knees, hands should clasp knees;
rock forward and backward

Sit-ups
raise head and back only ; look at toes
(you can also do this exercise with your
knees bent)

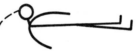

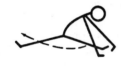

Sitting toe reaches
sit in the straddle position, swing arms
to left to touch the left toe; repeat to the
right

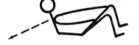

Calf stretch
place both arms straight out with palms
against a wall; bend left leg back and
stretch; repeat with right leg

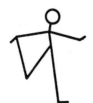

Ankle hold
with left arm against a wall, pull up right
ankle with right hand, hold; drop ankle
to floor. Repeat with left ankle, using
right arm for support against wall.

6

Obesity:
Every Extra Pound Makes Your
Heart Work Harder

Fat men are more likely to die suddenly than the slender.

—Hippocrates

What do your heart and circulatory system have in common with auto design and gas mileage? "Nothing," you say. You might reconsider after reading an advertisement published by General Motors Corporation's customer information service. Entitled *How Weight Affects Gas Mileage*, its opening statement proclaims: "The savings can be doubled if weight is removed in the design stage." We read on, and learned that, essentially, it boils down to simple multiplication: if the exterior dimensions of an automobile are trimmed in the design stage, the bumpers don't have to be so long, the frame doesn't have to be as big, and so on. This eliminates weight; then the savings begin to multiply. For example, if you took 100 pounds of golf clubs out of your car trunk, you might, depending on the car, save about five gallons of gas in 10,000 miles. However, if you take that same 100 pounds out of the car in the design stage, then you can effect savings all the way around—smaller engine, transmission, axles, tires, and so on. In general, if you run the car properly—light foot on the gas, the "mechanics" kept in good condition—you'll conserve energy and get more miles per gallon.

Well, that's how it is with your cardiovascular system. If the "exterior dimensions" are trim, then the savings are multiplied. For example, an obese person needs more blood vessels—miles and miles more in some cases—to nourish millions of "extra" cells. Thus, obesity requires that the heart pump more blood and pump it farther, and because the obese person isn't in good physical condition, the heart has to work harder to pump the blood through the arteries and veins. Just as a defective spark plug can diminish MPG, so

94

obesity can increase the wear and tear on your heart. The result is, the heart can "give out" sooner than it would if the "exterior dimensions" were lighter. In other words, this chronic overwork can result in impaired function of the heart, increased vulnerability to a variety of heart diseases and reduced longevity.

In this chapter, we will describe some of the most effective contemporary weight reduction programs, and provide a list of clinics for children to help you help them stay trim and healthy.

HOW OBESITY AFFECTS YOUR HEART

Even Hippocrates recognized the price of obesity. Although moderate obesity—in the absence of *all* other risk factors—may be associated only with a slight increase in the risk of developing coronary heart disease, most physicians agree that obesity predisposes you to the development of other risk factors, such as diabetes, high blood pressure, and, possibly, elevated serum cholesterol. In addition, obesity increases the work load of the heart. Finally, obese people are less likely to exercise than the nonobese; thus, a sedentary life-style sets in. Add it all up, and you have a situation that endangers your heart.

Unfortunately, obesity is one of the most common health problems in this country today. Despite the million-dollar mass media blitz that continually drives home the message "THIN IS IN," the fact remains that more than 40 percent of American women aged 40 to 49 are obese (obesity is defined as 20 percent or more above ideal weight) and 30 percent of adult men are obese. In this country, the prevalence of obesity has doubled since the turn of the century; worst of all, the trend has affected adolescents, and it is currently estimated that at least 25 percent of the nation's children are obese.

Particularly in young children and adolescents, obesity poses a challenge, for several reasons. It is difficult, if not impossible, for example, to motivate them by a threat of impending disease, since the medical consequences of obesity are usually long-range. Yet a growing number of clinicians are beginning to think that, in many cases, the development of coronary heart disease may be partially traced to social and dietary patterns established in childhood. Over 60 percent of the children who are obese by the age of four become overweight adults; more than 80 percent of all obese children remain overweight as adults; and, if these youngsters don't lose weight by adolescence, the odds against their ever doing so rise to twenty-eight to one.

Theories abound as to the exact causes of obesity. There is evidence which indicates that genetic factors play a role. Certain biochemical and anatomical dysfunctions may be involved. The adipose, or fat, cells present in the body have recently been evaluated for their significance in the onset of obesity.

Finally, psychological factors may come into play. Regardless of the cause of obesity, steps can be taken to correct the condition. There are also provisions you can make to prevent obesity from developing in children—and that's another step in caring for your heart and theirs, and in helping to keep all your hearts healthy.

Prevention of Obesity in Children

Obesity is difficult to define in children under two years of age, but the child's height and weight should be recorded routinely and compared to standardized charts. As long as your child is developing normally, you need only keep him or her on the right track. Here are a few suggestions: (1) provide fresh fruits and vegetables for snacks instead of junk foods; (2) fruits and vegetables can be pureed in a blender for feeding infants; and (3) avoid products with additives such as MSG (monosodium glutamate), extra sweeteners, or saccharin.

During childhood and adolescence, the same general rules apply. In addition, avoid soft drinks—fruit juices are better. Fortunately, studies have shown that the inborn "sweet tooth" is a myth—you and your children don't have an innate drive to eat candies and cakes.

To help your children eat properly and avoid obesity, get them involved in preparing their own meals. Let them shop with you and teach them to read food labels. Let them plan and cook meals as their age permits. If this is presented as a privilege, not a chore, you'll get much better response. Simply establish basic rules: for example, they can select one of their "favorite" dishes for dinner—even spaghetti—but show them how to serve pasta as an integral part of a balanced, nutritious meal. Don't, however, use food in any "punishment" or "reward" system. And don't forget to encourage regular exercise.

Help When Weight Creeps Up

For many people, the experience of losing weight resembles that of Mark Twain in giving up smoking. He found it very easy, having done it hundreds of times. Losing weight is difficult enough, as many of us know, but the real problem lies in keeping it off. What's the solution? Unfortunately, although obesity is recognized to be a disease, there is no cure. But there *are* steps you can take to help yourself. In most cases, however, the bottom line is simple and clear-cut: eat less and exercise more. The trick is to avoid the "yo-yo" syndrome—letting your weight slide up and down the scales in rhythmical patterns.

There are safe approaches to weight reduction, and some not so safe. Virtually every obese person we know has tried one or all at some point: The Atkins

Diet, The Stillman Diet, The Scarsdale Diet, The Grapefruit Diet, The Drinking Man's Diet, The No-Aging Diet, and so on. For most, the initial weight loss is incentive enough to keep control for a while, but ultimately the weight creeps up again.

Weight control varies from person to person. People who have been of average weight all their lives and begin to put on a few extra pounds at 45 or so differ from those who have a chronic weight problem. For the former, a reasonable low-calorie diet does the trick, and many people who gain five or ten pounds can lose it and keep it off successfully. Similarly, a normal woman who retains a few extra pounds after childbirth is generally able to reduce to her average weight again. Those who "yo-yo," however, clearly have special dietary problems. For them, it's a lifelong "battle of the bulge"; consequently, the obvious solution is a lifelong program. A temporary, remedial low-calorie plan is no solution simply because it has no long-term effect. In our opinion, there are four fairly effective methods of weight reduction. These plans are not only aimed at helping you lose weight (any low-calorie plan can do that), but they have also been developed to help keep your weight permanently under control. To be forthright, we cannot tell you that getting weight off and keeping it off is easy—it is not. Long-term follow-up statistics of weight reduction programs show that only one in twenty persons is even capable of losing twenty pounds, and less than one in a hundred has kept the weight off for more than a year.

Nevertheless, there are victors. Before you undertake any diet, however, see your physician. Our recommendations follow.

TOPS Club, Inc.
4575 South Fifth Street
P.O. Box 07489
Milwaukee, Wisconsin 53207
(414-482-4620)

TOPS (Take Off Pounds Sensibly) and KOPS (Keep Off Pounds Sensibly) were established in 1948 by Ms. Esther Manz. There are 12,500 chapters in the United States, Canada, and twenty-four foreign countries, with more than 330,000 members. Membership fees are $12.00 for the first two years, and $10.00 per year thereafter. There isn't any specific diet plan; rather, members consult a physican for an appropriate diet and determine a weight goal. Weekly weigh-ins are held privately. Meetings vary—some groups invite guest lecturers, others simply meet and talk over common problems.

Weight Watchers International, Inc.
800 Community Drive
Manhasset, New York 11030
(516-627-9200)

Weight Watchers has had considerable success. They teach the key elements of long-range weight control, each of which is mandatory for continuing success: how to eat balanced meals, how *much* to eat, *when* to eat (and when *not* to eat). In addition, Weight Watchers helps you to "retrain" your eating habits.

Finally, Weight Watchers has a line of frozen foods and special restaurants. Fortunately, since the latter cover a wide choice of foods, eating out remains interesting.

Weight Watchers is listed in local phone directories.

Overeaters Anonymous (OA)
World Service Office
2190 190 Street
Torrance, California 90504
(213-320-7941)

Established in 1960, the approach of this organization is similar to that of Alcoholics Anonymous (AA). Members attend meetings anonymously; no dues, but contributions are accepted. This group recognizes that obesity is a disease and that *compulsive* eating is a *progressive* illness. Like alcoholism, it can't be cured, but it can be arrested.

OA does not endorse any specific diet, although it has developed a simple low-carbohydrate, low-calorie diet. Members can attend OA meetings and follow their own dietary plans.

OA's overriding motto is "Just For Today." The overeater learns—day-by-day—that he or she need only worry about not overeating *today*. OA members are very supportive of each other; like AA members, they get through one day at a time. At each meeting, a "leader" starts things off, others tell their stories, and a discussion follows. At the close, the leader will announce that experienced members are available to "sponsor" any new member.

For compulsive overeaters, OA is *definitely* worth a visit. You certainly haven't got anything to lose—but pounds—and this time, the loss may be permanent. In New York City, midday meetings may be attended by thirty people or more: lawyers, business executives, salesclerks, even models.

For information, check your phone directory or write to the address above.

The Diet Workshop
111 Washington Street, Suite 300
Brookline, Massachusetts 02146
(617-739-2222)

Founded in 1965 by Ms. Lois Lindauer, the Diet Workshop currently has affiliates in 29 states, the District of Columbia, and Canada.

Additional information may be obtained by writing to the address above.

Behavior Modification

This method can be used to manage numerous problems, from fingernail-biting to obesity. In coping with obesity, your counselor for this program will carefully analyze your eating patterns. In order to establish your behavioral record, you are permitted to eat what you want, when you want, for a week or ten days, but you *must* keep an exact record of what you ate, when you ate it, and how you felt at the time you ate. Your feelings help the counselor determine the stimuli that may have initiated the "eating episode."

Most behavior modification programs set three objectives: (1) to alter the situation in which the stimulus occurred; (2) to help you control the act of eating itself; and (3) to reinforce positive behavior. Children can also be taught behavior modification.

This program usually offers counseling, advice on nutrition, and so on. To find an expert, ask your physician, check with your local branch of the Health Department, or call either your community hospital or a medical school. A university or college department of psychology may also be able to help you.

Fasting

This is the most drastic of all methods of dieting. Few physicians will place a patient on this diet (which generally consists of water, vitamins, and a protein supplement) unless the patient is considerably overweight—at least fifty pounds. It is *definitely* not designed for a loss of ten to twenty-five pounds. Also, fasting should not be undertaken without careful medical supervision. Several reports have linked the use of liquid protein supplement with sudden death.

Occasionally, a physician will recommend that an extremely obese patient fast, providing careful evaluation and tests are made every week. If you are interested in fasting, contact your physician or a university-affiliated hospital. This diet can be fraught with medical complications; thus, medical supervision is mandatory.

Fasting Program Supplement

A relatively new fasting program supplement is available in a number of cities, but *only* under medical supervision by a physician. (Most physicians will not consider this diet for you unless you are 20% over ideal weight.) After a careful medical evaluation, patients accepted for the dietary regimen are given packets of powder (five to be taken per day) that contain 60 calories each (a total of 300 calories per day). The powder comes in chocolate, vanilla, orange and cherry flavors, and may be mixed in water, plain tea, black coffee or diet sodas. Potassium supplements and vitamins are also recommended by physicians. For more information, see your physician, or write to The Delmark Company, Minneapolis, Minn. 55416. (Ask for information about Optifast.®) Similarly, the Cambridge diet,™ although available over-the-counter, should not be undertaken until you see your physician.

Other Methods

We have purposely ignored diet pills since we feel these have no place in the management of obesity. Similarly, intestinal bypass surgery is indicated in very few cases. Having your jaw wired shut is a radical approach to a problem that will, in all likelihood, be with you for life.

Overweight people must accept dieting as a way of life—not as a punishment. For example, an 1887 cartoon in *Harper's Weekly* shows a patient (dissatisfied with dietary restrictions) telling his physician: "Say, Doc, I'm blamed if I'm going to starve to death, just for the sake of living a little longer." Obviously, there's little point to that. Therefore, your primary objective is to find a weight reduction program that is tolerable, and to follow a maintenance plan that lets you eat sensibly and enjoyably afterward.

A Guide to Weight Control Clinics

Several specialized obesity clinics are operating in the United States. Programs vary, ranging from strict plans to behavior modification techniques, all under medical supervision. Besides these facilities, your local YMCA or YWCA may offer some type of weight-reducing program.

Dietary Rehabilitation Center
804 West Trinity Avenue
Durham, North Carolina 27710
(919-684-6331)
Established: 1972. Consult the center for additional information.

Heart Health for Diet and Weight Control
Stanford Heart Disease Prevention Program
Stanford University School of Medicine
Stanford, California 94305
(415-497-6051)
Established: 1977; fees: contact program; primary treatment modality: educational.

Vanderbilt Weight Management Program
Department of Psychology
Vanderbilt University
Nashville, Tennessee 37240
(615-322-3524)
Established: 1976; fees: depends on program selected. Programs: (1) educational program, 8–16 week commitment, $90; (2) weight management specialist training, nine months commitment and one year's work in field; fees: contact Dr. Katahn; (3) intensive clinical program, six months commitment, $650; primary treatment modality: combined.

FOR ADULTS AND CHILDREN:

Clinic for Eating Disorders
Department of Psychiatry
University of Cincinnati
559231 Bethesda Avenue
Cincinnati, Ohio 45267
(513-872-5150)
Established: 1974; fees: $45 for initial interviews; $45 per session; no minimum commitment; primary treatment modality: behavioral.

The Outpatient Nutrition Center
New England Medical Center Hospital
171 Harrison Avenue
Box 783
Boston, Massachusetts 02111
(617-956-5273)
Established: 1918; fees: contact center; minimum commitment: individual; primary treatment modality: nutritional.

The Weight Control Unit of the Obesity Research Center
St. Luke's Roosevelt Hospital
Suite 3D
411 West 114 Street
New York, New York 10025
(212-870-1743)
Established: 1977; fees: contact center; minimum commitment: individual; primary treatment modality: combined.

7

How Alcohol Affects
Your Heart

In the last few years, alcoholism has joined the ranks of so-called bad habits that have finally revealed themselves to be diseases, and today physicians and consumers are growing increasingly aware of the pitfalls of excessive alcohol consumption. The problem for many, however, is: What constitutes too much alcohol? Is it the two-martini lunch, followed by a cocktail at 6 P.M., and then wine with dinner? Or could simply having a drink every day be considered "excessive"?

In the following section, we will discuss the effects of alcohol on the heart. Our objective is to show you how to promote cardiac health. Although we feel the moderate use of alcohol is permissible for many individuals, one must remain aware that alcohol is a chemical substance. It is toxic to most tissues and the use of it by some individuals may result in alcoholism. For those who have, or suspect they have, a drinking problem, we have included a useful guide to various medical and social facilities as well as a selected list of leaflets and pamphlets about alcohol and its effects.

IS DRINKING BAD FOR YOUR HEART?

In moderation, no. Most experts agree that two drinks a day, say, two glasses of wine with dinner, is within acceptable limits for most individuals. Recently, however, several medical reports have shown an association between limited alcohol intake and reduced rate of heart attack. These limited data should be viewed as inconclusive at this time.

One interesting finding that has emerged from the Honolulu Heart Study showed that men (in this study, all the men were of Japanese descent) who drank up to two ounces of pure alcohol per day had significantly fewer heart attacks than nondrinkers. In part, investigators have hypothesized that this

103

may be because consumption of alcohol produces a rise in the levels of high-density lipoproteins (HDLs) in the blood. As we discussed in Chapter 1, a high level of HDLs has also been associated with a decreased incidence of coronary heart disease. Lest this information send you running to the nearest bar, bear in mind that a high level of HDLs does not mean that you will not have a heart attack; also, there are other, more acceptable methods of raising high-density lipoproteins in the blood such as weight reduction and exercise. Finally, as the study directors themselves pointed out, this drinking was not associated with a lower overall mortality.

Excessive drinking is known to have adverse effects on the heart, as well as on other organs of the body such as the liver and the brain. Several studies show that the cumulative effects of continual heavy alcohol intake can produce metabolic and morphological abnormalities of the heart muscle that may precede clinical signs and symptoms. In some cases, these abnormalities progress to arrhythmias, thromboembolism, and/or congestive heart failure. These conditions can develop as a result of prolonged excessive drinking.

The medical term for the cardiac syndrome resulting from chronic excessive alcohol consumption is *alcoholic cardiomyopathy*. (*Cardio* means "heart," *mys* is Greek for "muscle," and *pathos* is Greek for "disease.") This syndrome can sometimes be reversed—unlike damage to the brain as a result of alcohol—but only by totally avoiding alcohol. To problem drinkers, however, abstinence from alcohol may seem impossible; luckily, it doesn't have to be. On June 10, 1935, Alcoholics Anonymous (AA) was founded by William G. Wilson, a New York City stockbroker, and Robert Smith, a surgeon from Akron, Ohio. More than any other organization or treatment plan, AA has helped alcoholics achieve and maintain sobriety. Because alcoholism is a growing problem in this country—especially among teenagers—we will discuss the significance of this disease, not only because its effects can damage the heart, but also because it is both preventable and controllable, providing the drinker understands what alcoholism is all about.

What Is Alcoholism?

Alcoholism is a chronic, progressive disease—not a "bad habit" that comes and goes at a drinker's whim. Similar to diabetes and hypertension, there is no "cure" for it, but recovery is possible.

Who Becomes an Alcoholic?

Anyone can. If their mothers are alcoholics, infants can be born addicted to alcohol. This condition is referred to as the *fetal alcohol syndrome*.

Contrary to popular opinion, the average alcoholic is not found in a stupor on skid row, nor is he or she sprawled in a flophouse. Instead, many alcoholics are high-school and college students, athletes, housewives, socialites, business people and even doctors. Alcoholism is not selective—it can afflict anyone, of any age, sex, or nationality.

Is Alcoholism a Common Problem?

Unfortunately, alcoholism is far more common than most people think. Many problem drinkers who strongly suspect that they are alcoholic are afraid to seek help because the "stigma" formerly associated with the disease persists. Often relatives deny that there is a problem, friends are reluctant to speak up, and many employers will ignore it as long as possible. Failure to acknowledge the existence of alcoholism results in millions of people not getting the help they need.

More specifically, government statistics indicate that alcoholism is the leading drug problem in this country; one in ten drinkers in the United States becomes an alcoholic; in other words, of the 100 million adults who drink, 10 million are alcoholics, at a cost to government and industry of $25 billion annually (1974 estimate). Even more alarming: approximately 500,000 teenagers are alcoholics and the number is rising. Years ago, male alcoholics outnumbered females four to one; today, the ratio is about even.

Despite these enormous numbers, many people still consider alcoholism "unusual." It's probable, however, that you know someone who is an alcoholic. Studies have shown that approximately 40 percent of the patient population in any hospital is made up of alcoholics, although few of the patients are hospitalized for that disease. In such cases, doctors are treating conditions which are often simply the results of alcoholism, such as chronic anemia, cardiomyopathy, and liver disease, rather than treating the primary disease.

How Do You Know If You Are an Alcoholic?

Again, like diabetes and hypertension, alcoholism ranges from mild to severe. Keep in mind, however, that it is a progressive disease. Left uninterrupted, it will ultimately overcome its victim.

No one can say "four drinks a day" or that "getting drunk every Saturday night" equals alcoholism. Some people with the disease don't begin drinking until after 6:00 P.M. or so every night. Others, surprisingly, go weeks without a drink (which leads them to believe that they can control their problem when they can't) and then go on a binge. They may get drunk on a "party weekend"—"like everyone else," they rationalize—and then go a few more weeks without drinking.

There are some questions that you can ask *yourself*, and we have listed them here. Even one *yes* warrants careful evaluation on your part, but it is not strongly diagnostic in itself. But if you catch yourself saying, "But everyone answers yes to some of those questions," be assured that that is not true.

If you need to seek help, we recommend that you make a call to AA first. Whoever answers the phone will give you information, support, and guidance—the last thing you will encounter with any member of this group is condescension. All of these people have experienced what you are going through, and they all want to help you. They aren't evangelists; you can attend any AA meeting free without participating. No one will ask your name or purpose.

If you go to your physician, he or she may be willing to counsel you over a period of time—in addition to AA—or may refer you to a psychologist or psychiatrist. Many excellent counselors—psychiatrists, psychologists, social workers—are not necessarily experts on alcoholism, which is a complex disease. Consequently, we advise you to consult someone who is known for skill in managing alcoholic patients.

Remember that you are not alone. It certainly must have been very difficult for Betty Ford, Joan Kennedy, Wilbur Mills, and Dick Van Dyke, among others, to admit their addictions publicly, but they each benefited from participating in recovery programs.

Check Yourself: Are You Drinking Too Much?

Have you ever suffered a lapse of memory (a "blackout") as a result of drinking?

Have you ever heard strange sounds or seen strange sights as a result of drinking?

Has drinking ever interfered with your job (you were late to work or left work early, etc. because you didn't feel so well)?

Has drinking ever made you physically ill, e.g., hangover, vomiting, or the morning-after "shakes"?

Do you find it difficult to leave an unfinished drink behind?

Do you often think about drinking?

Have you been drunk more than once in a year?

Have you ever been physically violent or experienced any sort of personality changes as a result of drinking?

Do you drink to relieve anxiety and/or depression?

Have you lost friends as a result of drinking or selected new "drinking friends"?

Do you drink to block out financial or marital problems?

Do you find that you drink to celebrate your successes and mourn your failures?

Do you find that you are anxious to continue drinking long after others have had enough?

Have you ever concealed your drinking—by hiding a bottle, sneaking a drink, or lying about the amount you've had to drink?

Have you ever taken a drink or two before going out, just in case you may not get the drinks you require during the evening?

Have you ever poured yourself a drink the morning of a hangover "for medicinal purposes," using "the hair of the dog that bit you" justification?

Have you ever telephoned long distance while drinking—and perhaps not fully recalled the content of the conversations the following day?

Have you noticed a change in your alcoholic tolerance—either an increase or a decrease—during the past few months?

Do you ever find it difficult to stop drinking once you have begun?

Do you ever eat lightly or not at all while drinking, so as not to interrupt your "high"?

Have you ever awakened following an evening of drinking and felt remorse, guilt, or embarrassment about your behavior the night before?

Do you find yourself making resolutions about your drinking that you are unable to keep?

Do you drink alone or have a few drinks in the morning in order to start the day?

Where Alcoholics and Their Families Can Go for Information and Help

Several organizations are known to have very effective programs, but many other good centers, as well as thousands of qualified counselors, are available. Your own physician may be able to recommend the best facility in your area; or check with your local medical association or the National Council on Alcoholism, 753 Third Ave., New York, N.Y. 10017 or write to Alcoholics Anonymous, P.O. Box 459, Grand Central Station, New York, N.Y. 10017.

8

New Light on an Old Risk Factor: Stress

Don't get excited, don't run, jump, or frisk.
Play everything cool, man—your heart is at risk.
Neglect your profession although you adore it
(With Type A behavior, oh brother, you're for it).
Ignore all your problems, stay constantly pensive,
Because if you don't, you'll end up hypertensive.
Stop eating butter; cholesterol rises.
And eggs are as bad, just as full of surprises.
Fats that are saturate are diabolic.
Triglycerides zoom and you soon wax embolic.
Toss out all your smokes or you're doubly stung:
Not just in the heart, boy, but smack in the lung.
Eschew all those sweets, you'll get hyperglycemic
(Or maybe it's *hypo*—there's grounds for polemic).
Lay off that rich diet, forget the martinis,
No pastries, potatoes, no blintzes or blinis.
They all make you fat, to your ticker's great dread . . .
Oh hell, let's forget it—you're better off dead.*

According to Dr. Hans Selye, President of the International Institute of Stress at the University of Montreal, Quebec, however, "Stress is the spice of life," and, indeed, it is. Most of us share this sentiment. We look forward to each day, ready to go, not knowing what pleasure or pain awaits us, but prepared to take the bad with the good. Since about ten years ago, virtually everyone, from research scientists to physicians, office workers, and housewives, has been clamoring to know just what price we pay for this "spice of life." Lately, it seems that our ailments, from routine headaches to free-floating

---

*Roger Starr, *Emergency Medicine* (September 1977), p. 31, with permission.

anxiety, depression, indigestion, ulcers, insomnia and, last but not least, heart attack, are being partially attributed to this entity called *stress*.

Exactly what is stress? Is it normal or is it another epidemic disease of the twentieth century? Does stress affect your heart? And, if so, how? In this chapter, we define stress, discuss its potential role in heart attack, and outline methods to help you cope with it.

WHAT IS STRESS?

Webster's Seventh New Collegiate Dictionary defines *stress* as "a physical, chemical, or emotional factor that causes bodily or mental tension and may be a factor in disease causation." Long ago, in fact, early historians knew that stress—be it good or bad—could cause, among other things, sudden death. Pliny the Elder wrote of a mother who, on seeing her son back from Cannae after she had already heard news of his death, promptly collapsed and died.

Centuries later, William Harvey, credited with the discovery of the circulation of the blood, wrote in his treatise *De Motu Cordis* about a man who, having been injured by someone upon whom he could not take revenge, "was so overcome with hatred and spite and passion, which he yet communicated to no one, that at last he fell into a strange distemper, suffering from extreme oppression and pain of the heart and breast." Shortly thereafter, he died.

In the seventeenth century, another noted English physician and surgeon, John Hunter, who knew he suffered from angina, once remarked: "My life is at the mercy of any rascal who shall put me in a passion." He died in 1793, reportedly during an intense debate at a hospital board meeting.

Then, in the nineteenth century, William Osler, an internationally known clinician, observed that many patients with coronary heart disease are "keen and ambitious, the indicator of whose engine is always set 'full speed ahead.' " In another segment of the same work he wrote that "Every affection of the mind that is attended with either pain or pleasure, hope or fear, is the cause of an agitation whose influence extends to the heart."

This interest in the role of stress in heart disease continued sporadically over the next hundred years or so. In 1945, one medical investigator reported that several mechanisms seemed to be involved in coronary occlusion, including "a compulsive striving for achievement and mastery which never seems to end." Most recently, Drs. M. Friedman and R. Rosenman wrote a book entitled *Type A Behavior and Your Heart*, which is about the association of certain personality traits with heart disease. The problem is, since stress is unavoidable, how can we know when we have exceeded the limit?

Strange as it may seem, we cannot survive without stress. Our bodies are designed to adapt to a wide range of challenges, both physical and emotional. Each adaptation—be it white blood cells rushing to an injured area to facilitate tissue repair, or a tension-relieving burst of tears—is a response to stress. Man's nervous system either adapts to a stress or challenge, or resists it—a dual response pattern classically referred to as "fight-or-flight." Either way, the nervous system interprets the signals and instantaneously transmits the message to the brain. A decision is quickly made, and the response "message" whizzes along the nerve pathways to trigger your reactions. For example, if you are swimming in the ocean and see a fin suddenly emerge from the water not too far away, a chain reaction occurs. You decide to resist, and a series of involuntary responses takes over your behavior: your blood pressure increases, you breathe faster, and your heart rate quickens. Then, you swim away from the impending threat of the fish as fast as possible.

Man has responded in this classic "fight-or-flight" pattern for centuries. Today, we cannot always respond to our daily stresses in such clearly defined black and white physical terms. More often than not, we have to settle for a "grin and bear it" approach. In other words, the energy that is released for "fight-or-flight" has to be channeled elsewhere. If your boss screams at you or an Internal Revenue agent subjects you to intensive questioning, all of your feelings of hostility and contempt are usually suppressed, since it would be most unwise to screech back at your boss or to argue assertively with an IRS agent. Unfortunately, these negative feelings—directed inward over a prolonged period—may be harmful to your health.

To learn more about the role of stress in disease, and cardiovascular disease in particular, numerous medical investigators have begun to explore in depth the influence of man's environment and personality upon the health of his heart. Four decades ago, a world-renowned pioneer in stress research, Dr. Hans Selye, originated the idea that both physiologic and emotional stresses produce a very distinct pattern of physical responses. Since then, many studies have been conducted to determine the precise effects of stress on the heart. One of the better known teams of investigators, Drs. Thomas H. Holmes and Richard H. Rahe, psychiatrists at the University of Washington Medical School, devised a simple questionnaire to evaluate specific life events (positive ones, like marriage, as well as negative ones, like the death of a spouse) that cause stress. Each event was assigned a numerical value, ranging from 11 to 100. If a person's test total exceeded 300 points within a single year, he or she was considered to be in a state of significant stress that could have psychological or physical consequences, or both.

Despite the common tendency to blame one's job for myriad symptoms or problems ranging from chronic fatigue to increased arguments with one's spouse or new difficulties with a child, Drs. Holmes and Rahe only listed 10 out of 43 job-related questions. The numerical value, or "life-crisis units," attributed to these questions fell below those assigned to more personal events; for example, divorce rated seventy-three, and a business readjustment only thirty-nine. It is worthwhile to note that, if job-related tensions *per se* were largely responsible for the coronary epidemic, we would have few top executives over the age of 55 running our corporations.

Using the scale devised by Drs. Holmes and Rahe, several investigators found that among 279 survivors of heart attacks in Helsinki, Finland, there was a rising rate of life change for the six months immediately before infarction (heart attack). In another large-scale study from Sweden, women who had had a myocardial infarction scored notably higher than the healthy reference population both on aggression and on a combined group of traits called "neurotic self-assertiveness." (This group includes feelings of guilt and defense of status.) Finally, in two separate studies, the Western Electric Study conducted in 1964 and a study involving Israeli civil service workers, certain factors such as interpersonal problems, depression, anxiety, and neuroticism were identified as precursors primarily of angina pectoris (chest pain associated with coronary artery disease), but not consistently with heart attack. Other studies suggest that obsessive personality traits and excessive control of emotions seem to be linked especially to heart attack.

Medical scientists are still uncertain about the mechanisms involved in the etiological role stress may play in the development of coronary heart disease, but reports that have appeared within the last five years continue to support the concept of a "coronary-prone" personality. In particular, the popular book by Drs. Friedman and Rosenman defines the classic "Type A," or coronary-prone personality as competitive, excessively hostile and driven, overcommitted to his or her job, intensely striving to achieve, and easily made impatient. Using these factors, Drs. Friedman and Rosenman designed a structured interview to measure the coronary-prone behavior pattern. At the outset, men who were to participate in the Western Collaborative Group Study were interviewed, and then the incidence of clinical coronary disease was assessed at four-, six-, and eight-year intervals. The men who had a "Type A" personality according to their initial interview had a 1.7 to 4.5 higher rate of new coronary heart disease than those who possessed "Type B" personalities.

Based on these and other reports, numerous medical and research institutions have sprung up to investigate stress and its role in disease. Today, approximately 5,000 different findings a year dealing with stress are reported; in fact, two medical publications are devoted to the subject of stress: *The Journal of Human Stress* and *Stress*. And of course, institutes such as Dr. Selye's International Institute of Stress are also devoted to the study of the effects of stress on health and disease. To help you cope with stress, we will discuss the major methods currently in use and suggest where you can go for additional help.

Are You a "Type A" (Coronary-Prone) or a "Type B" Personality?

The following questions are adapted from *Type A Behavior and Your Heart,* by Drs. M. Friedman and R. H. Rosenman, in which they outline behavior patterns characteristic of a coronary-prone personality, "Type A." "Type B" personalities seem to have a lower incidence of heart attacks. A preponderance of "Yes" answers will indicate that you have a "Type A" personality.

"Type A" Personality Traits
1. Do you explosively accentuate various key words in your speech?
2. Do you mutter the last few words of your sentence?
3. Do you walk, eat, and move rapidly?
4. Do you feel impatient at the rate events take place? (For example, a car ahead of you driving at a pace you consider too slow.)
5. Are you inclined to do two or more things at once? (For example, talk on the phone, prepare a list of things to do, and perhaps look over the morning newspaper.)
6. Do you almost always try to turn the conversation around to subjects that interest and intrigue you?
7. Do you feel guilty when you relax?
8. Do you schedule more and more things in less and less time? (A chronic sense of time urgency is a core component of "Type A" behavior pattern.)
9. When meeting a coronary-prone person, do you feel compelled to challenge him or her?
10. Do you have characteristic nervous gestures, such as clenching your fist, grinding your teeth, and so on?
11. Do you feel any success you have achieved is due to your ability to get things done faster than your fellow man?
12. Are you preoccupied with getting the things you consider worth *having?*

"Type B" Personality Traits
1. Are you free of *all* the habits listed for "Type A" personalities?
2. Do you rarely, if ever, suffer from a sense of time urgency?
3. Do you rarely, if ever, harbor free-floating hostility?
4   Do you rarely, if ever, display or discuss your achievements?
5. When you play, is it for fun and relaxation?
6. Can you relax without guilt, and work without aspiration?

How to Live Compatibly with Stress

First, it's important for you to realize that how you *perceive* a certain event has a lot to do with whether or not the stress associated with it might be harmful. For example, a 45-year-old man with a sick wife and five dependent children literally might collapse if he were fired from his job, whereas another man the same age, perhaps with a high-salaried wife and no offspring, might be relieved to be fired from a job that he did not particularly like. Another important aspect is that stress is derived from both joyous and sad occasions. The wedding of a daughter, for instance, can cause as much emotional wear and tear on you as the death of a close friend. To distinguish between "good" and "bad" stress, Dr. Selye coined the term *eustress* (*eu* is Greek for "good"). *Distress* describes negative stressful events.

Numerous organizations and societies help people learn how to cope with stress. In addition to these (many of which are hired by corporations to help employees), a variety of self-help methods are available. These include yoga, meditation, the Relaxation Response, biofeedback, exercise, behavior modification, and the pursuit of simple leisure activities. Many of these methods, such as yoga and meditation, have received a great deal of attention in the last few years in the Western world, but the ideas and techniques are actually centuries old. We will present only the essentials of each of these approaches to handling stress. Your local bookstore undoubtedly has numerous books available on these subjects.

The Stress Test

Review these events and total your score for the last year. If it exceeds 300 points, watch out—that's considered a state of significant stress.

Events	Scale of Impact
Death of spouse	100
Divorce	73
Marital separation	65
Jail term	63
Death of close family member	63
Personal injury or illness	53
Marriage	50
Fired at work	50

Marital reconciliation	45
Retirement	45
Change in health of family member	44
Pregnancy	40
Sex difficulties	39
Gain of new family member	39
Business readjustment	39
Change in financial state	38
Death of a close friend	37
Change to different type of work	36
Change in number of arguments with spouse	35
Mortgage over $10,000	31
Foreclosure of mortgage or loan	30
Change in responsibilities at work	29
Son or daughter leaving home	29
Trouble with in-laws	29
Outstanding personal achievement	28
Spouse begins or stops work	26
Begin or end school	26
Change in living conditions	25
Revision of personal habits	24
Trouble with boss	23
Change in work hours or conditions	20
Change in residence	20
Change in schools	20
Change in recreation	19
Change in church activities	18
Change in social activities	18
Mortgage or loan less than $10,000	17

Change in sleeping habits	16
Change in number of family get-togethers	15
Change in eating habits	15
Vacation	13
Christmas or Hanukkah	12
Minor violations of the law	11

T.H. Holmes and R.H. Rahe, "The Social Readjustment Rating Scale," *Journal of Psychosomatic Research* 11 (Pergamon Press, Ltd., 1967). Reprinted with permission.

Yoga

Yoga is concerned with the health and well-being of the whole individual. Yoga exercises (*asanas*) involve various sustained postures. Some, such as the locust, plough, and lotus positions, are better known than others and are frequently incorporated into other exercise plans.

Yoga also includes a series of breathing exercises designed to bring about relief of tension through deep relaxation.

Transcendental Meditation

People meditate in various ways which range from the self-made plan to more extensive programs. For some, meditation just involves a regular daily routine of sitting comfortably or reclining in solitude for fifteen or twenty minutes, listening to soothing music or maintaining silence while resisting all distracting thoughts. This can take place early in the morning and/or before retiring in the evening.

Transcendental Meditation (TM), on the other hand, is a specific but simple and easy-to-learn technique in which the individual is taught the seven steps of the transcendental meditation methodology.

The concept of meditation dates back thousands of years; Buddha, for example, believed that meditation could lead one to a state of peace. However, the idea that such an approach could help to relieve stress or lift one's spirits did not catch on in the United States until 1959, when an Indian man named Maharishi Mahesh Yogi introduced a meditation technique simpler than the traditional one. Since then, it has been estimated that more than one million Americans have joined the ranks of meditators, and the numbers swell each month.

Unfortunately, many people think TM is occult and that only religious "freaks" or social outcasts are involved in it. To the contrary, numerous doctors, lawyers, businessmen, teachers, and housewives practice TM, and many companies have hired TM instructors to train their employees in this technique. Much of the interest of corporations in TM stems from reports in medical and trade literature showing that the meditative state can create a highly relaxed condition, and that this can result in greater work productivity, better concentration on the job, less absenteeism due to emotional fatigue or illnesses precipitated by "nerves," and so on. To date, more than 150 studies on the physiological and psychological effects of TM have been published. The reports reveal varying degrees of success with TM. We feel it is important for you to understand what TM is, and what it is not, before you decide whether this method of reducing stress is for you.

Essentially, the individual sits in a comfortable chair and slowly repeats the *mantra*, a two-syllable sound that the mind can focus on. After a few minutes, the muscles begin to relax, and a feeling of calm takes over. Most people who learn the TM technique from a qualified instructor and practice it at home say that they feel refreshed, relaxed, and revivified after they have meditated.

To find out more about Transcendental Meditation, and the types of programs available in your area, you can contact one of the TM centers in your area.

Relaxation Response

Published in 1975, *The Relaxation Response* was written, with Miriam Z. Klipper, by Dr. Herbert Benson, Associate Professor of Medicine at Harvard and Director of the Hypertension Section at Boston's Beth Israel Hospital. In it, the author outlines "four basic elements" underlying the elicitation of the relaxation response. Basing his theories on many Eastern and Western writings, the author has determined that the relaxation response is an innate capability that has always existed and that has been indirectly reflected in many religious teachings. The four elements required for meditation effective enough to elicit the relaxation response are:

a quiet environment	a place where all internal and external distractions are avoided.
an object to dwell upon	gaze at a symbol; concentrate on a feeling; repeat a particular word or sound—the purpose of this is to eliminate other thoughts.
a passive attitude	eliminate all thoughts and distractions from your mind—this is essential to eliciting the relaxation response.
a comfortable position	assume a position (sitting, kneeling, etc.) that will enable you to stay still comfortably.

Dr. Benson recommends sitting with your eyes closed, then relaxing your muscles, beginning with your feet and working up to your face. Breathe through your nose, and continue for ten or twenty minutes. You are encouraged to do this once or twice daily, but not until two hours after eating.

Biofeedback

In the last few years, this technique has passed from the hands of the faddists into the laboratories of respected research and medical institutions. Today, biofeedback is being used to alleviate migraine headaches, high blood pressure, and assorted problems. Results vary, depending on the problem and the individual involved.

Essentially, biofeedback takes a "mind over matter" approach. It is used to help one identify certain feelings associated with, say, a migraine. The idea is to stave off those feelings that occur prior to the onset of a migraine by voluntarily relaxing and learning how to raise hand temperature (indicating that the blood vessels have dilated or relaxed). Specific relaxation exercises are taught; then, the patient is usually hooked up to an electromyograph (EMG), which monitors the electrical activity of muscle at various points. When the patient sees a certain pattern emerge, he is instructed on how to alter the pattern by means of various exercises. The idea is to "reprogram" certain responses. More research is required before we can fully know the uses and limitations of this technique. If you are interested in learning more about this method, see your physician first. He or she can probably refer you to the nearest medical facility utilizing this technique.

Exercise

For many, jogging or running, a calisthenics workout at the gym, or a regular dance class seems to provide sufficient relief from daily tensions. Fortunately, membership in a gym need not be a large expense—many offer group and/or family memberships, and your local YMCA or YWCA may also be giving instructions in dance, exercise, or yoga. Of course, a wide variety of sports can be pursued. Squash and tennis, for example, are surefire ways to work off stress, and swimming and golf—or just a peaceful walk in the park—can go far to help you feel better.

On the other hand, if you feel that it is only recently that your life has become particularly stressful, we offer the following tips:

- Beginning today, set aside fifteen minutes to enjoy by yourself. Do nothing, just relax.
- Identify as many sources of stress as possible, and try to devise means to work around them. For example, if you dread phone calls during dinner, leave the phone off the hook for an hour or so.
- If you feel you don't have enough "free" time, start to program

some for yourself right now. Pick one night a week for a play, movie, or a night at home talking, reading, or watching television, and don't let anyone deter you!

- If you work, build in one or two lunch hours a week that are yours "free." Don't have lunch with co-workers or run out and do five errands. Instead, spend the time in "new" surroundings such as your local library, a museum, the zoo, or an aquarium.

Behavior Modification

Like biofeedback, this technique is used to help people manage numerous disorders, ranging from drug abuse problems to overeating. Those who feel that they are caught up in a stressful life-style and could benefit from this methodology—learning how to alter "bad" habits and substitute better ones—should consult their physicians for an appropriate referral. (See Chapter 6.)

Leisure Activities

With so many people eager to escape the "nine-to-five" syndrome, the pursuit of leisure activities has grown appreciably during the last decade. In 1977, for example, Americans spent a record $160 billion on pleasurable activities, and today, more than 300 colleges and universities offer courses in leisure studies. Now, everything from hang gliding to scuba diving is being explored. Whatever activity you pursue, the purpose should be enjoyment. If it's bothersome in any way to you—avoid it. Leisure time should be used just for relaxation and fun!

Medical Help

If the stress and tensions of daily life leave you feeling continually anxious, depressed, or on the verge of cracking, by all means seek medical help. Do *not* make the mistake of turning to alcohol or drugs for relief. Once enslaved by chemicals, it is most difficult to break the cycle.

Begin by consulting your physician for a checkup, and discuss your problems candidly. Don't be a stoic; if you feel you need counseling, press for the name of a good psychiatrist, psychologist, or social worker. Many physicians will guide you to appropriate behavior modification clinics, biofeedback laboratories, and so on, *if you ask*. Fortunately, several current medical plans will cover these expenses; if yours does not, ask your physician or your local Mental Health Association to assist you in locating an appropriate counseling facility. Remember, virtually everyone needs help with one problem or another at some time, so don't hesitate to seek advice.

Regrettably, more and more Americans today are muttering such things as "he's killing himself," or "she's a 'workaholic,' " or "he's worried to death about that project." Whatever happened to "I'll do it in my spare time," or "I'm just killing time," or "I'll do it in my time off"? No doubt the intense pressure to succeed accounts for some of this change. We teach our children—beginning in kindergarten—how to compete effectively, in order to gain admission to the "best" high school, the "best" college, and so on. The emphasis always seems to be "onward and upward"—on both the corporate and social ladders. Even the book market today is flooded with titles such as *Looking Out for Number One, Pulling Your Own Strings, Success!, Power!, The Joy of Money,* and *The Managerial Woman.* We could probably benefit from a little less emphasis on the drive "to win" and a little more on learning simply how to enjoy life. Matthew the Apostle summed it up best when he wrote: "And which of you by worrying can add one unit . . . to the span of his life?"

Specialized Programs to Help You Cope with Stress

In addition to the Transcendental Meditation Centers, Life Extension Institutes also offer various services, ranging from instructions in other types of meditation techniques to biofeedback, all designed to help you cope with stress. Write to:

Life Extension Institute (LEI), Main Office
1185 Avenue of the Americas
New York, New York 10036
(212-575-8300)

The Center for Applied Behavioral Sciences
Menninger Foundation
Box 829
Topeka, Kansas 66601
(913-273-7500)

While these are held primarily for executives, through corporate contracts, some programs are available to individuals, too. To date, more than 12,000 companies, including IBM and Chase Manhattan Bank, have taken advantage of these seminars, which are conducted either at the Menninger Foundation in Topeka, Kansas, or at a site selected by the client.

PART II
Anatomy and Physiology of the Cardiovascular System

How does your heart work? The uninterrupted circulation of blood throughout your body continues day in and day out, thanks to the remarkable pumping action of the heart, but most of us would be hard put to explain how the heart actually accomplishes this action—and usually with such on-going rhythm.

Yet, every day, without fail, your heart beats approximately 100,000 times, with just a split second's rest between beats, moving 4,300 gallons of oxygen-rich blood through a 60,000 mile network of tiny blood vessels and major arteries. If all your blood vessels were joined end to end, they would reach from New York to California and back ten times. In this chapter, you can learn how your heart functions.

9
How Your Heart Functions

The amount of recycled blood pumped by the heart varies from person to person; however, the heart of an average-sized man pumps about three ounces of blood with each contraction or heartbeat. At rest, the man's heart pumps about five liters of blood per minute. But the heart can pump considerably more than that when necessary—up to four or five times as much during manual labor or exercise, for example. Then, a healthy heart may pump up to twenty to twenty-five liters of blood per minute. (One liter is a little more than a quart.) In the course of a year, the average adult heart pumps about 1.4 million gallons of blood, which amounts to 105 million gallons during a lifetime of seventy-five years—enough to fill over 10 million Volkswagen "Bug" gas tanks!

To understand how the heart accomplishes this, let's take a closer look at how your cardiovascular system works.

The Birth of Your Heart

Like every major organ in your body, your heart begins to develop and take shape virtually from the time of your conception. In fact, by the seventh week of pregnancy (often before some women realize they are pregnant), the heart has reached its definitive four-chambered fetal structure. The heart continues to develop normally along with the rest of the fetus's tissues and organs until birth.

Anatomy

Size and location. If you look at your fist, you'll have a good idea of the actual size of your heart. The average adult heart weighs about ten ounces. It lies above the diaphragm and beneath the sternum or the breastbone. Contrary to common belief, the heart is actually located in the center of the chest between the lungs, not just on the left side. However, because the left ventricle (the major pumping chamber) is larger than the right ventricle, the heart does extend to the left side of the chest, where you can feel it beating.

Structure. Although the heart is often drawn to look like a valentine, it really is a cone-shaped, hollow, muscular organ. The key word here is "muscular." It is through the contraction of the muscle, and the integrated functioning of its specialized parts, such as the muscular walls, the valves and the electrical cardiac conduction system, that the heart is able to perform its strenuous pumping action in a continuous, coordinated manner to fulfill the needs of the body's organs for oxygen-rich blood. (See Figure 9.1.)

Figure 9.1: Anatomy of the Heart

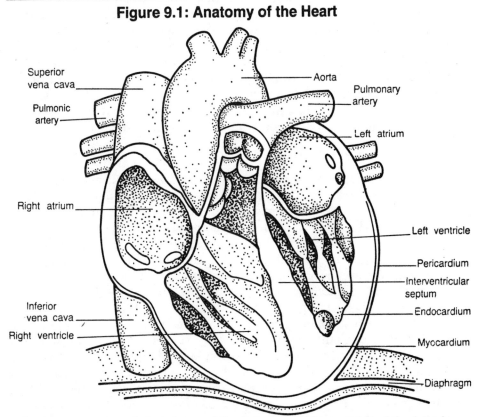

Basic anatomy and chambers of the heart; anterior aspect of the interior of the heart.

Tissue Layers of the Heart

Pericardium. The heart is enclosed in a tough fibrous sac called the *pericardium* (*peri* is Greek for "around," and *kardia* is Greek for "heart.")

Myocardium. The heart itself is composed of three distinct tissue layers: the myocardium, the endocardium, and the epicardium. The *myocardium* is the muscular portion of the heart, the thick middle layer. You've probably heard of the phrase "myocardial infarction" or "infarct" (MI), the medical name for heart attack. *Myocardial infarction* means that this layer of heart tissue—the myocardial tissue—has suffered an infarction. *Infarction* is a technical term meaning death of tissue due to lack of oxygen supply. Thus, the scientific term for *stroke* (when it is due to cerebral artery atherosclerosis) is *cerebral* or *brain infarction.* Death of myocardial cells may be due to lack of oxygen resulting from obstruction of circulation to the area. Thus, when blood flow is obstructed to myocardial or heart tissue for a prolonged period, *necrosis* or tissue death can occur, and a myocardial infarction (heart attack) may result. Later, we will explain in more detail how this happens and outline the steps you can take that may help to reduce the likelihood of its occurrence.

Endocardium and epicardium. The *endocardium* consists of a thin fibrous membrane of flat endothelial cells. Similar to the material that lines the blood vessels, the endothelial cells line the inside surfaces of the myocardium. The *epicardium* is the thin outside covering of the myocardium.

Heart Chambers and Valves

Your heart has four hollow chambers or cavities, each formed by muscular walls of varying thickness. The heart chambers are referred to as the left and right sides of the heart; however, most of the left side is actually *behind* the right side, which forms most of the front of the heart. (See Figure 9.1.)

Atria. Each side of half of the heart consists of a thin-walled chamber, the *atrium,* located just above a thick-walled chamber, the *ventricle.* The *atria* (plural of *atrium*) are the holding, or receiving, tanks of the heart. They receive a certain amount of blood from the venous system and the lungs, then contract rhythmically, ejecting the blood into the ventricles.

Ventricles. The *ventricles* are thicker than the atria because they must pump the blood out through the circulatory system. The left ventricular wall is three times as thick as that of the right ventricular wall, since it has to generate three times as much pressure to pump blood through the systemic circulatory system as the right ventricle generates to propel blood through the pulmonary circulatory system. Rhythmical contraction of the heart's muscular walls enables the blood to move through the atria and the ventricles in a continual pulsatile manner. (See Figure 9.2.) Ventricular muscle is arranged in spiral bands that provide the myocardial tissue with the strength and elasticity for this ongoing pumping activity.

Figure 9.2: View of Ventricular Muscle of the Heart

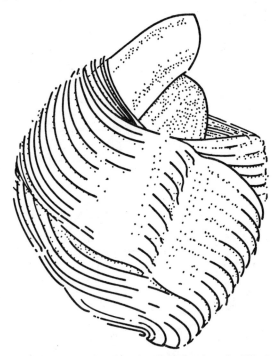

Ventricular muscle fibers are in circular bands that facilitate the pumping mechanism of the heart.

A thin wall of tissue, the *interatrial septum*, separates the atria and the *interventricular septum*, a thicker wall, divides the ventricles. The atria are separated from the ventricles by the atrioventricular (AV) valves, which are anchored in circular bands of fibrous tissue (the AV "rings" or septa) located at the junction of the atria and ventricles on each side of the heart.

The Valves. Four valves control the one-way flow of blood through the atria and the ventricles. (See Figure 9.3.) These valves are called:

    tricuspid valve
    mitral or bicuspid valve
    aortic valve
    pulmonic valve

The tricuspid and mitral valves control the flow of blood from the atria to the ventricles. The mitral, or left AV valve, separates the left atrium and left ventricle, while the tricuspid, or right AV valve, separates the right atrium and right ventricle. The mitral valve is so named because it resembles a miter, the two-cusped hat worn by bishops. Since it possesses two cusps, it is also

Figure 9.3: The Heart Valves

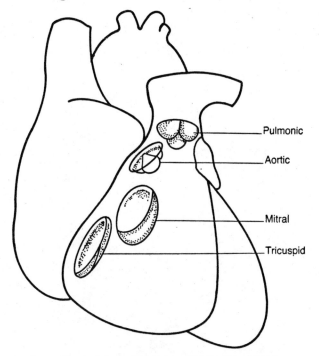

Location of heart valves within the heart.

called the bicuspid valve. The tricuspid valve, on the other hand, derives its name from its form: three cusps or leaflets. To sum up: the *left AV valve* is mitral and has two cusps; the *right AV valve* is tricuspid and possesses three cusps.

The aortic and pulmonic valves control the flow of blood from the ventricles to the so-called great vessels, the two large arteries that conduct blood away from the ventricles. Both the aortic and pulmonic valves are three-cusped, or tricuspid, valves. The cusps are shaped like half-moons; therefore, the aortic and pulmonic valves are known as *semilunar valves*. The aortic valve permits blood to flow from the left ventricle to the aorta, while the pulmonic valve allows the blood to flow from the right ventricle to the pulmonary artery.

What prevents the blood from flowing backward or into the wrong chamber? How is this continual process of unidirectional blood flow maintained by the heart? Fortunately, this group of heart chambers and valves is designed to function as a coordinated unit; when one set of valves (e.g., the AV valves) opens to permit the blood to flow from one chamber to the next, the other set of valves (the semi-lunar) automatically snaps shut to prevent backflow. In certain types of heart disease, the normal function of these valves may be disrupted, thereby impairing the pumping function of the heart, with consequent cardiac enlargement and heart failure. Before we discuss these abnormalities, however, let's examine the pathways of normal circulation.

Figure 9.4: How Blood Flows Through the Heart

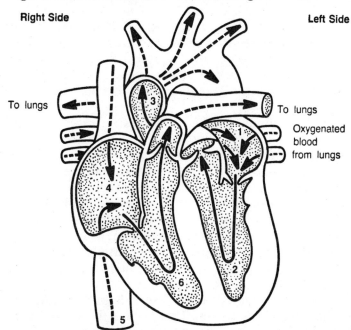

The left atrium (1) receives oxygenated blood from the lungs. Blood passes to left ventricle (2), which forces it via the aorta (3) through the arteries to supply the body's tissues and organs. Right atrium (4) receives blood from the vena cava (5) after it has passed through tissues and given up much of its oxygen. Blood passes to the right ventricle (6), then continues the cycle to the lungs, where it is oxygenated.

How Blood Circulates

Blood moves, or circulates, continuously throughout the body, supplying millions of cells with the important nutrients necessary to their viability and the performance of their functions. Ultimately, all blood must pass through the heart and lungs. The atria receive the blood, and then contract and send it through the open valves into the ventricles. Next, the ventricles contract, and the blood moves out of the heart's chambers and through the circulatory system. (See Figure 9.4.)

Blood that reaches the left atrium has passed through the lungs and picked up oxygen, the vital nutrient for all of the body's cells. This bright red, oxygenated blood then passes from the left atrium across the mitral valve and enters the left ventricle. The increased pressure in the left ventricle closes the mitral valves, when the left ventricle is filled, it contracts. Mitral valve closure prevents backflow of blood into the left atrium. Contraction of the left ventricle increases pressure in this chamber; as a result, the aortic valve opens and blood is ejected into the body's major arterial pipeline, the aorta. This phase of the cardiac cycle (when the ventricle contracts), is called *ventricular systole*, and the passive period (when the ventricle receives blood from the atrium is *ventricular diastole*. In normal circumstances, the entire cardiac cycle or heartbeat takes about one second; and diastole normally takes twice as long as systole.

After the blood circulates, the two largest veins in the body, the superior vena cava and the inferior vena cava, carry blood back to the right atrium. When the right atrium is filled with dark red venous blood—low in oxygen and high in carbon dioxide—that it has received from the systemic venous circulation, it contracts, and the blood is forced through the tricuspid valve into the right ventricle. As soon as the ventricle is filled, *it* contracts. In order to prevent blood from flowing from the right ventricle backward into the right atrium, the tricuspid valve, located between the right atrium and the right ventricle, is automatically forced shut by the increased pressure in the right ventricle. From the right ventricle, the blood is then pumped through the pulmonary valve to the pulmonary artery and into the lungs.

Oxygen-rich blood returns to the left side of the heart (the left atrium), through the pulmonary venins. This part of the circulatory pathway—the route from the right atrium through the right ventricle to the lungs and then to the left atrium—is called the *pulmonary circulation*.

To recap:

1. The ventricles contract, a process called ventricular systole, and the mitral and tricuspid valves close.

2. As the contraction continues, the blood in the ventricles is ejected through the pulmonic and aortic valves into the pulmonary and systemic circulations, respectively. Thus, the tricuspid and mitral valves control ejection of blood flow between the atria and the ventricles, while the aortic and pulmonic valves control ejection of flow between the ventricles and two major arteries.

3. The internal beginning with ventricular contraction—which builds up pressure to open the aortic and pulmonic valves and propels blood into the pulmonary and systemic circulations—continues through closure of the aor-

tic and pulmonic valves and ends with the opening of the AV valves. This is know as *systole*.

4. Diastole is the interval from the opening of the tricuspic and mitral valves to the moment when the ventricles contract; this time, the ventricles relax and blood moves from the atria to fill them. (The diastolic period of the cardiac cycle encompasses about two-thirds of each cycle, the systolic period about one-third.)

5. Therefore, there are two phases in each cardiac beat or cycle: a *diastolic phase*, in which the mitral and tricuspid valves are open so the ventricles can receive blood from the atria and fill, closing the AV valves, and the *systolic phase*, in which the ventricles contract, opening the aortic and pulmonic valves. This allows blood to be ejected from the right ventricle through the pulmonic valve and into the pulmonary artery to the lungs, and from the left ventricle through the aortic valve into the aorta and through the systemic circulation.

The Coronary Arteries

The coronary arteries supply the heart muscle with blood. There are two main coronary arteries, the right and the left. The left coronary artery divides into two large branches, the left anterior descending and the left circumflex arteries. Thus, the coronary artery system is usually referred to as having three major vessels: the right, left anterior descending and left circumflex arteries. (See Figure 9.5.)

The right coronary artery. This artery descends between the right atrium and ventricle from its aortic origin just above the heart, to the lower or inferior border of the right ventricle. It supplies the right atrium and right ventricle with blood and, in most individuals, the right coronary artery also supplies the inferior or lower wall of the left ventricle. As in many aspects of human biology, there is also some variation in the coronary artery system among different individuals.

The left coronary artery. This artery arises from the aorta opposite the right coronary artery and within 2 cm forks into the left anterior descending artery and the left circumflex artery. The left anterior descending artery supplies the anterior, or front surface of the left ventricle as well as the superior two-thirds of the interventricular septum. It also may supply the left anterior portion of the right ventricle. The anterior descending artery courses almost straight downward toward the tip of the left ventricle, giving off lateral wall branches to the left and interventricular septal branches below. The left circumflex artery supplies the lateral (side) portion of the left ventricle and in some people, the inferior surfaces.

If one or more arteries become partially stenosed (narrowed), the blood sup-

Figure 9.5: Coronary Artery Anatomy

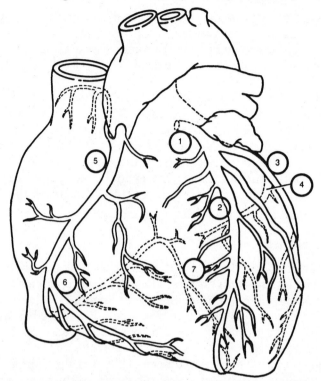

Coronary artery (CA) anatomy. 1–Left main CA; 2–Left anterior descending CA; 3–Left circumflex CA; 4–Posterior circumflex CA; 5–Right CA; 6–Marginal branch of #5; 7–Posterior descending artery.

ply to the heart may still be partially maintained, depending on the degree of stenosis, but don't be misled. Once an artery becomes stenotic, coronary artery disease is present. Stenosis of one artery constitutes "single-vessel disease"; when three coronary arteries are clogged or narrowed, "triple-vessel disease" exists, and so on. Stenosis of one or more of the coronary arteries makes you susceptible to angina pectoris, a heart attack or even sudden death, since these defects deprive the cardiac muscle of necessary oxygen and nutrients.

How the Heart Beats

Electricity! That's right, waves of bio-electrical currents literally keep your heart beating rhythmically, day in and day out. However, heart disease can disrupt this natural electrical activity, resulting in abnormal rhythms that can seriously disrupt cardiac function and even result in sudden death. In brief, here is how the electrical conduction system of your heart works;

The heart has a natural "pacemaker" called the *sinoatrial node* (or SA node). Actually, this is a tiny bundle of tissue—located in the wall of the right atrium. It is composed of specialized cells that have the inherent capacity to spontaneously and continuously discharge electrical activity at a regular rate. The SA node rhythmically generates waves of electrical impulses that spread through the myocardium (heart muscle) via a highly specialized tissue network: the *cardiac conduction system.* This electrical discharge and conduction is extraordinarily precise and causes the atria and the ventricles to contract in the proper sequence required to pump blood efficiently throughout the heart muscle and the body. (See Figure 9.6.)

Thousands of "pacemaker cells" make up the SA node. These cells automatically and rhythmically generate electrical impulses. The impulses, in turn, travel over the atria by radial spread through atrial muscle tissue and also via highly specialized conduction pathways located in the walls of the atria. (See Figure 9.7.) In only a very short time, about 0.08 seconds, this electrical impulse reaches the *atrioventricular node* (or AV node), located at the top of the interventricular septum in an area of the heart called the atrioventricular junction (the point at which the atria and ventricles are joined). The bundle of His is also located in this area. This band of cardiac fibers gives rise to the

Figure 9.6: The Cardiac Conduction System

Right Side

Left Side

1) SA node

2) Internodal pathways

4) Bundle of His

3) AV node

Right bundle branch

5)

Left bundle branch

6) Purkinje fibers

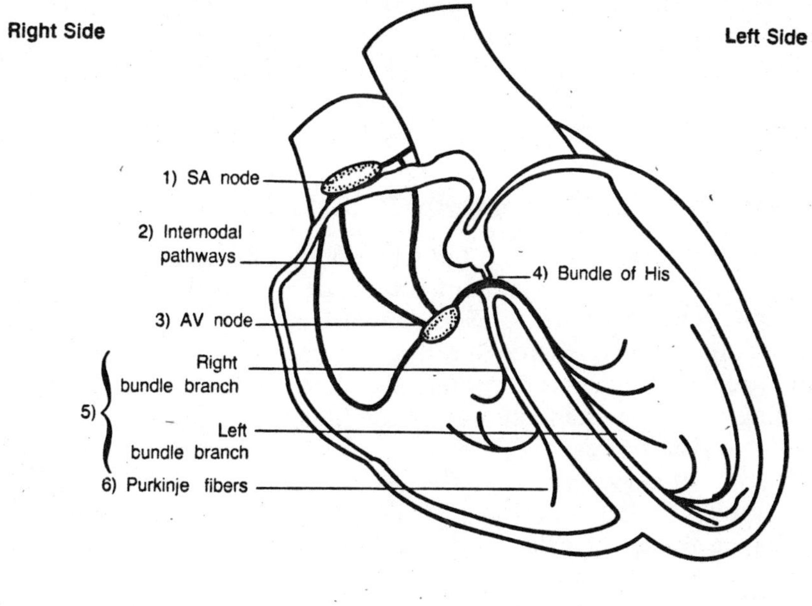

common bundle from which, in turn, originate the left and right bundle branches—important segments of the conducting system that convey cardiac impulses to the left and right ventricles, respectively. The bundle branches subdivide into smaller constituents which terminate in the Purkinje fibers— named after Johannes E. Purkinje, a nineteenth century Bohemian physiologist. These terminal fibers convey the electrical impulses to each cell in the ventricles.

If interruption occurs at any point in the entire conduction system—from the SA node to the bundle branches or their divisions (due to disease or other factors such as drug toxicity—electrical conduction can suffer and "heart block" can occur. In heart block, all or a portion of the impulses from the atrium do not reach the ventricles, resulting in slowing of ventricular contraction rate which, if severe, can seriously impair heart function. In addition to heart block, excessively slow heart rate can also occur if the pacemaker of the heart, the SA node, fails to generate an appropriate frequency of impulses due to disease or other factors.

What triggers the SA node to initiate this electrical impulse?

The mechanisms by which the SA node produces its rhythmic electrical activity are extremely complex and involve chemical reactions within the cells and the movements of certain elements such as sodium and potassium into and out of these cells. Certain cells such as the SA node and the cells of the entire specialized cardiac conduction system down to the Purkinje fibers contain the unique property of spontaneous electrical discharge. The spontaneous electrical discharge of the areas in the conduction system—other than the SA node—only function as "pacemakers" when the SA node fails to function. In these other areas of the conduction system, the spontaneous rate of discharge is less than that in the SA node.

How the Nervous System Helps Pace the Heart

Of course, your heart does not function autonomously; it has to work in unison with the other organs in your body. To do this, the heart muscle is linked with the brain, the master control center of all bodily functions, via a network literally consisting of billions of nerve cells. Two highly specialized components of the nervous systems control your body's voluntary (running, walking, talking) and involuntary (breathing, glandular secretions, digestion, circulation) activities.

The central nervous system (CNS) controls all voluntary muscle activities. The autonomic nervous system (ANS) controls involuntary functions. The ANS is subdivided into the sympathetic (adrenergic) system and the parasym-
(Text continues on page 134.)

Figure 9.7: How the Heart Beats

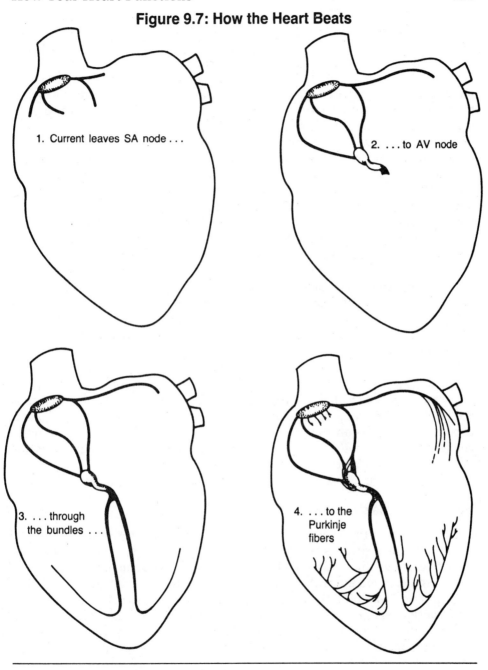

1. Current leaves SA node . . .

2. . . . to AV node

3. . . . through the bundles . . .

4. . . . to the Purkinje fibers

(Text continued from page 132.)
pathetic (vagal or cholinergic) system. These systems are generally antagonistic—they balance each other to regulate body functions such as breathing, heart rate, and blood pressure. (See Figure 9.8.)

Two distinct nerve centers, the cardioinhibitory center, which is part of the parasympathetic nervous system, and the cardioaccelerator center, which is part of the sympathetic nervous system, are situated in an area at the base of the brain called the *medulla*.

These centers are responsible for nervous control of the heart. Impulses are relayed to them from all parts of the body, communicating any changes in the body's need for blood. For example, more blood is needed in the gastrointestinal tract during digestion than during periods when that system is at rest. Impulses relaying the message for more or less blood are transmitted from the digestive system to centers in the brain, then through the sympathetic and parasympathetic nerves, which terminate in the electrical conduction system and muscle fibers of the heart.

Various chemical substances are released at nerve endings; the most important of these are acetylcholine and norepinephrine. Nerves are often classified according to the chemical substance they release. Those nerves that release acetylcholine when stimulated are classified as *cholinergic* nerves (parasympathetic and sympathetic nerves), while nerves that release norepinephrine are called *adrenergic* nerves (sympathetic system). Epinephrine, which is chemically related to norepinephrine, is produced by the adrenal gland.

When the sympathetic nervous system is stimulated, both the electrical activity and force of cardiac contraction are increased. Thus, the firing rate of the SA node is increased, the electrical conductivity through the AV node is enhanced, and the contractions of the atria and the ventricles are strengthened. Stimulation of this system results in a faster heart rate and an elevation in blood pressure. When the parasympathetic nervous system is stimulated, the opposite occurs. Heart rate drops and force of contraction may decrease.

Functional Characteristics

The parasympathetic nervous system is involved with restorative and vegetative functions, such as rest and digestion, while the sympathetic nervous system activates the body's protective mechanisms during periods of stress. For example, if you are resting on the beach and hear a child scream for help, you respond immediately by jumping up and running to his aid. To produce this reaction, your cardiovascular, perspiratory and musculoskeletal systems are activated by the sympathetic nervous system. More oxygenated blood is pumped to the muscles to facilitate reaction to the emergency.

(Text continues on page 136.)

Figure 9.8: Divisions of Nervous System

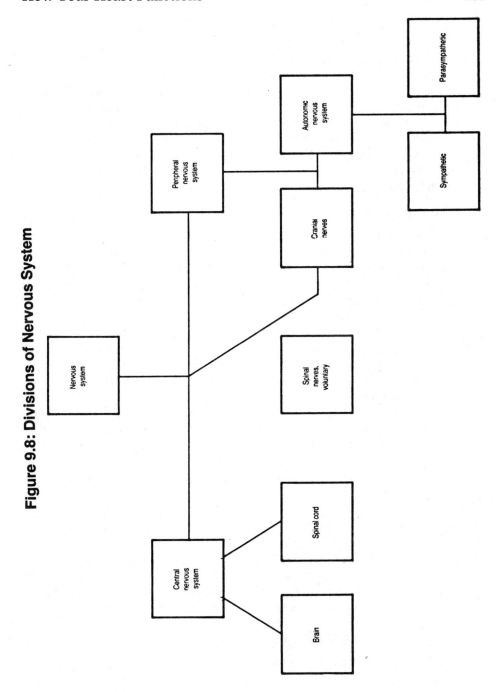

(Text continued from page 134.)
The Respiratory System

Blood circulates throughout the body in order to carry nutrients, such as oxygen, to the cells, and to remove waste products, such as carbon dioxide and water. Carbon dioxide is ultimately eliminated via the lungs when we exhale, whereas other waste products are removed via the kidneys, liver and skin. Oxygen enters the circulation through the lungs when we inhale. Inhaling and exhaling are separate parts of an involuntary process controlled by the autonomic nervous system. Since it's likely that you inhale and exhale over 100,000 times a day, it's a good thing you don't have to think about it in order for it to happen!

How You Breathe

Respiration begins with the nose and mouth—passageways to the lungs. Air passes from the nose and mouth to the pharynx (throat), larynx ("voice box") and into the trachea, a flexible tube that divides into the two branches that each lead to one of the lungs. Once the bronchus meets the lung, it subdivides into many smaller branches, called *bronchioles*. The smallest bronchioles lead to the *alveoli*, or air sacs of the lung. Each lung contains approximately 750 million alveolar sacs, all of which are in direct contact with the capillary bed of the pulmonary circulation. Since the alveoli are surrounded by walls of lung tissue only one cell thick, it is easy to see how an exchange of gases can occur between the air in the alveoli and the blood in the capillaries.

The Lungs. The primary function of the lungs is to oxygenate the blood and eliminate waste products, most notably carbon dioxide and water vapor, from the body. This process cannot be accomplished without breathing. When you inhale, the diaphragm, a large concave muscle, descends, the pressure in the chest cavity decreases, and air then enters the lungs. When you exhale, the diaphragm relaxes, rises, and air is then expelled. Pulmonary ventilation occurs as a result of this continuous inhaling and exhaling. In breathing, air containing oxygen moves in and out of the alveoli due to the expansion and contraction of the lungs. Through the alveolar and capillary membranes, oxygen is diffused from the alveoli to the capillary blood, and carbon dioxide passed back from the capillary blood to the alveoli. The pulmonary circulation provides blood that is high in oxygen and low in carbon dioxide for delivery to the body's tissues, and returns venous blood—high in carbon dioxide and low in oxygen—to the alveolar capillaries for expulsion from the body.

The Body's Vital Fluid: Blood

Up to this point, we have spent most of our time talking about how the heart manages to pump blood continuously to all of the body's organs and tissues, and how the lungs supply the blood with oxygen, but one important question remains: What elements does blood contain that make it so vital? That answer is readily available.

Blood is really nature's best example of liquid tissue. It acts as a "messenger" tissue and needs to be liquid so it can flow through virtually every part of the body, delivering a wide variety of substances, such as hormones from the brain, to "target" or specific organs. In effect, the blood is the messenger service that carries these substances to the appropriate organs, such as thyroid-stimulating hormone from the pituitary gland to the thyroid gland. Similarly, blood carries waste products; it takes carbon dioxide from the body's cells to the lungs to exchange it for oxygen, and carries other metabolic waste products from the cells to the kidneys for excretion.

What Is Blood?

Blood is a complex substance composed of a liquid called *plasma*, blood cells, inorganic salts, and certain types of proteins (some regulate clotting, others act as carriers of chemicals such as fats and a variety of other substances, such as hormones and enzymes), and the waste products of tissue metabolism such as urea. Plasma is the major liquid component of blood, in which the blood cells are suspended. Blood cells consist of red corpuscles, white corpuscles and platelets.

Red blood cells, *erythrocytes*, are shaped like bioconcave disks and are filled with a very specialized iron-rich protein, *hemoglobin*, which gives the cell its oxygen-carrying ability. This chemical accounts for the typical red color of blood.

The red blood cells carry oxygen from the lungs to the organs and tissues of the body. Once the hemoglobin gives up its oxygen to the cells, the red blood cells return to the lungs, where reoxygenation occurs. White blood cells are part of the body's defense system against infection.

Blood platelets are very important in terms of coagulation, or blood clotting. When a blood vessel breaks, platelets collect at the site where the break occurs, then release chemicals that promote rapid clot formation, and cause the injured blood vessel to constrict so that blood loss from the injury is prevented.

In summary, red and white blood cells and the platelets are all suspended in the plasma, the liquid portion of the blood. Plasma contains many other components, including vitamins, inorganic salts, hormones, and proteins. The red blood cells are responsible for delivering oxygen to the tissues and transporting carbon dioxide away. Other waste products, such as urea, are also transported from the sites of origin.

PART III
Diseased Hearts

Understanding the "Language of the Heart"

A person who adheres to a moderate life-style, in the form of a prudent diet, not smoking, and exercising regularly will often be rewarded with a long and healthy life. In some cases, however, coronary heart disease may develop despite the best efforts. In others, an unrelated cardiovascular disorder, such as an arrhythmia (an abnormal heart rhythm), a cardiomyopathy (a disorder of the heart muscle) or valvular heart disease may occur.

The following section comprises a complete discussion of diseases of the heart. In it, the causes and mechanisms involved in the development of coronary artery atherosclerosis, (more commonly known as coronary artery disease), angina, and heart attack are reviewed. Other cardiac problems such as tachyarrhythmias (rhythm abnormalities in which the heart beats too fast), bradyarrhythmias (rhythm abnormalities in which the heart beats too slowly), common cardiomyopathies, and congestive heart failure are also covered. In addition, this section includes the most recent information pertaining to heart disease in women, especially as it relates to the Pill, pregnancy, and the menopause. Finally, parents of children with heart disease should find pages 196–205 both reassuring and informative.

Our primary objective has been to remove the mystery that shrouds many cardiovascular diseases. In fact, in researching this book, we were struck by an editorial in an issue of a medical journal appropriately entitled "The Language of the Heart."* The two cardiologists who wrote it observed that many of the terms that they and other physicians routinely use to describe various

---

*R.S. Blacher and H.J. Levine. "The Language of the Heart," JAMA, 236 (15) 1699, 1976.

cardiac disorders are frequently alarming to the patient. They pointed out that the term "heart failure" often implies cardiac doom to the patient, although it simply means the heart muscle lacks the ability to contract regularly at full force. Numerous medications may be prescribed to alleviate this condition.

Similarly, the term "heart block" suggests that blood flow to a major artery is obstructed, and death is imminent, whereas it actually means that there is some disturbance, often minor, in the electrical conduction system of the heart. The terms *flutter* and *murmur* imply that the heart is about to take off on its own any minute; again, these conditions may actually be quite benign. Other clinical descriptions such as "leaking valve," "split-heart sound," "mitral regurgitation," "floppy valve," and the "click-murmur syndrome" all bring to mind rather gruesome pictures, which the imagination might use to conjure up a condition far worse than is warranted.

In the following pages, we hope to clarify some of the more regularly used terms as we discuss a wide variety of cardiac disorders and diseases.

10
The Biggest Killer: Coronary Heart Disease

Coronary heart disease, which some physicians consider the epidemic of the twentieth century—makes its initial presentation in one of three distinct clinical forms, or "coronary events." These are: myocardial infarction (heart attack), angina pectoris, and sudden death. Myocardial infarction is the most common *initial* manifestation of coronary heart disease; it occurs as the *first* sign of the disease in over 50 percent of the men who have coronary heart disease. Angina is the first event in about one-third of the men (in women angina is a more frequent initial finding than is myocadial infarction); and sudden death (death within seconds, minutes or hours of onset of symptoms) heralds the disease in about 15 to 20 percent of all victims. Sudden death is the result of a lethal cardiac arrhythmia (ventricular tachycardia or ventricular fibrillation) and accounts for the majority of deaths in all patients with coronary heart disease, including those who have chronic angina pectoris or a prior myocardial infarction.

Clearly, the course of coronary heart disease is variable. For example, myocardial infarction may be followed by angina, or an infarction may occur only after months or years of angina, or not at all. The risk of sudden death is highest in those patients with the most extensive coronary artery disease, complications from a prior myocardial infarction and a chronically unstable clinical course.

Myocardial infarction, angina pectoris, and sudden death all stem from a single basic abnormality—obstruction of the coronary arteries that supply the myocardium (heart muscle) with blood. The obstructive process, known as coronary artery atherosclerosis, deprives the myocardium of oxygen-rich blood. If this deprivation is temporary, angina pectoris may occur and usually lasts for a few minutes; if, on the other hand, coronary artery obstruction is total and longstanding, such as frequently results when a blood clot is suddenly

141

superimposed on a site of atherosclerosis, a myocardial infarction typically results. Finally, at any time during the course of significant coronary atherosclerosis, a lethal arrhythmia can occur, causing cardiac arrest and sudden death.

It is alarming that in more than 60 percent of victims, coronary heart disease makes itself initially known in the form of a lethal or very serious event, such as sudden death or myocardial infarction. This phenomenon explains part of the shock and incomprehension of family members on learning that a loved one has suffered a myocardial infarction or a sudden fatality. The initial reaction is one of incredulity because the victim has frequently "never before had any evidence of heart trouble." However, our knowledge of the natural history of coronary heart disease has demonstrated to us that in a majority of its victims, there is no obvious history of the condition prior to myocardial infarction or sudden death. Why the disease surfaces as myocardial infarction in some patients, angina in others, and sudden death in still others is not understood. Associated factors may play a role. For example, cigarette smoking increases the likelihood of severe complications of coronary heart disease such as sudden death and may account for at least some cases in which the first manifestation is a fatal arrhythmia. The fact that a major complication is usually the first sign of coronary heart disease makes early detection of this condition, *before* the occurrence of serious consequences, a crucial objective of modern medicine. Indeed, conquest of the problem of sudden death is the focus of major efforts by leading cardiologists today who are striving to develop new methods of early detection of those at risk and improvements in methods of prevention.

ATHEROSCLEROSIS: THE DOCTOR'S NAME FOR CORONARY HEART DISEASE

What is it? When does it begin? Essentially, atherosclerosis involves a buildup of fatty deposits in the arteries. The term *atherosclerosis* was derived from the Greek *athera* (gruel) and *sclerosis* (hardening).

Initially, the buildup starts out as a thin streak or plaque inside the normally smooth lining of the artery. As it develops, a "patch" forms, called an *atherosclerotic plaque*. (See Figure 10.1.) These lumpy plaques obstruct blood flow through the arteries; ultimately the vessel may become severely or totally occluded, and a heart attack can result. (See Figure 10.2.) Many medical scientists believe that some "streaks" in the coronary arteries may be a result of normal growth and development, but the excessive amount of atherosclerosis known to be present in the U.S. adult population has caused great concern because it is the culprit in the overwhelming majority of heart attacks.

As we pointed out earlier, since fats play a key role in the development of

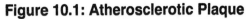

Figure 10.1: Atherosclerotic Plaque

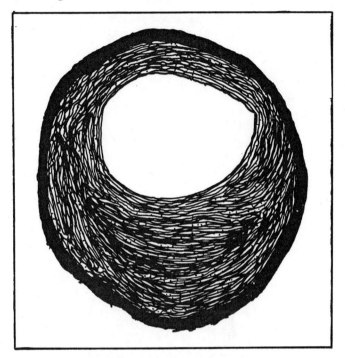

Plaque narrows the lumen, or passageway, of a human coronary artery. The plaque is a thickening of the artery wall composed of connective tissue and fatty debris.

this disease, many clinicians today urge their patients to reduce their dietary intake of saturated fats. Their hope is that this will help to cut down the incidence of coronary heart disease in later life. Needless to say, their advice is based on clinical evidence that atherosclerosis is a progressive disease that can begin early. For example, autopsy studies of men in their twenties who died in Korea and Vietnam showed a considerable degree of atherosclerosis. This buildup may be related to the typical American diet, which is often high in cholesterol.

The Anatomy of a Coronary Artery

In order to understand the pathogenesis, or development, of coronary heart disease, a close look at the anatomy of a coronary artery is required.

A coronary artery is composed of three distinct layers: the *intima*, the *media*,

Figure 10.2: Normal and Atherosclerotic Blood Vessels

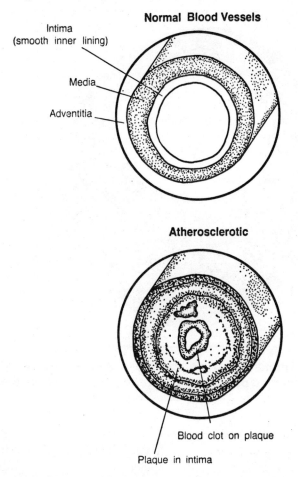

Normal Blood Vessels

Intima
(smooth inner lining)

Media

Adventitia

Atherosclerotic

Blood clot on plaque

Plaque in intima

and the *adventitia*. The innermost lining is the *tunica intima*, made up of *endothelial cells*, a few smooth muscle cells, and collagen, a fibrous substance. The next layer, surrounding the intima, is the *tunica media*, which is composed of elastic tissue. The outer layer is the *tunica adventitia*.

Two theories in particular have paved the way for intensive research on the cause of atherosclerosis; each theory may be traced to the nineteenth century. The theory that has received the most attention stems from work done by Rudolf Virchow, a German pathologist. According to his theory, atherosclerosis is caused by the infiltration of fatty substances from the bloodstream into the smooth wall of the artery. The result of this silent but potentially lethal process is the transformation of a once-smooth arterial wall

into a thickened, lumpy conduit through which it becomes increasingly difficult for blood to flow. Many investigations since then have supported Dr.
Virchow's reasoning. For example, subsequent studies already mentioned
(The Framingham Heart Study, The Seven-Nation study, and so on) support
the concept that an increased rate of coronary heart disease is associated with
an increased dietary intake of saturated fats.

The other theory of the development of atherosclerosis holds that a plaque
(an atheroma) starts as a *thrombus*, a small deposit of tissue that forms from
the aggregation or clumping of platelets, the components of blood vital to clot
formation. Over a period of time, the thrombus is replaced by fibrous tissue,
and a plaque is formed. In some instances, a thrombus can form at the site of a
plaque; then, the arterial channel can become totally occluded.

Today, medical scientists know that atherosclerotic plaques are composed
of lipid-rich debris, especially cholesterol. However, it is now also known that
lipoproteins, which carry cholesterol in the blood, play a role in regulating
cholesterol buildup. You may recall that high-density lipoproteins (HDLs)
help transport cholesterol away for elimination, whereas low-density
lipoproteins (LDLs) are not transported as readily. Thus, the high percentage
of cholesterol carried by LDLs can be caught for some time within the artery,
where it interacts with the smooth muscle cells, and plaque begins to form.

Regardless of the precise mechanisms involved in the origins of
atherosclerosis, it is known that once plaques are present, it is difficult, if not
impossible, to eliminate them—that is why it is important to eat prudently,
since a diet high in saturated fats has been implicated in the development of
atherosclerosis. Partially occluded coronary arteries may result in angina or
a heart attack. Unfortunately, the first sign of the presence of atherosclerosis
may be a heart attack; sometimes, a fatal heart attack. For this reason, it is important to be aware of the warning signs of an impending case of angina, or
heart attack, or both; these conditions are delineated in the following pages.

ANGINA: NATURE'S PAINFUL WARNING OF CORONARY HEART DISEASE

But there is a disorder of the breast marked with strong and peculiar symptoms, considerable for the kind of danger belonging to it, and not extremely
rare, which deserves to be mentioned more at length. The seat of it, and
sense of strangling, and anxiety with which it is attended, may make it not
improperly be called angina pectoris.

They who are afflicted with it are seized while they are walking (more especially if it be uphill, and soon after eating) with a painful and most disa-
greeable sensation in the breast, which seems as if it would extinguish life
if it were to increase or to continue; but the moment they stand still, all this
uneasiness vanishes.

So said William Heberden in 1768 in a lecture before the Royal College of Physicians of London; four years later, in 1772, his work, entitled "Some Account of a Disorder of the Breast," was published in *Medical Transactions of the Royal College of Physicians of London.*

However, well before Heberden's accurate clinical description of angina pectoris (Latin for "chest pain"), historians had described the same syndrome, but it was he who assigned the name "angina pectoris" to it. The next breakthrough came in 1912, when Dr. James Herrick, an American physician,

Figure 10.3: What's the Difference Between a Heart Attack and Angina Pectoris?

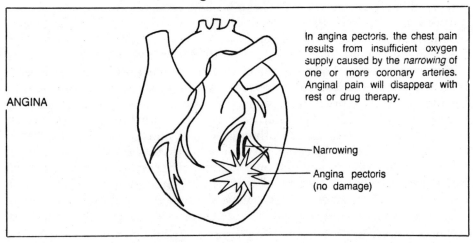

ANGINA

In angina pectoris. the chest pain results from insufficient oxygen supply caused by the *narrowing* of one or more coronary arteries. Anginal pain will disappear with rest or drug therapy.

Narrowing

Angina pectoris (no damage)

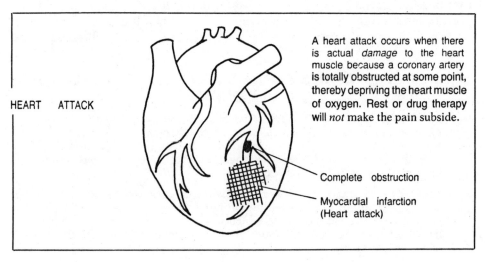

HEART ATTACK

A heart attack occurs when there is actual *damage* to the heart muscle because a coronary artery is totally obstructed at some point, thereby depriving the heart muscle of oxygen. Rest or drug therapy will *not* make the pain subside.

Complete obstruction

Myocardial infarction (Heart attack)

published his paper entitled "Clinical Features of Sudden Obstruction of the Coronary Arteries" in the prestigious *Journal of the American Medical Association*. In it, Dr. Herrick covered the total syndrome of coronary artery disease. Later, he wrote that arteries could be occluded, but sudden death did not always occur; anginal pain, however, was quite common.

What Is Angina?

Simply stated, *angina pectoris* is nature's warning sign of coronary artery disease. It is a disorder that is easy to understand if we utilize the following analogy: If you write more checks against your account than you have funds available, you create an imbalance; the supply of cash in your banking account cannot meet the demands—the checks come in for collection and your account is overdrawn. On the other hand, if you have enough funds available, there isn't any problem.

So it is for the heart, or myocardium, too. As long as myocardial oxygen supply can meet myocardial oxygen demand, angina pectoris will not occur. This does not necessarily mean atherosclerosis is not present, since most individuals have some trace of fatty deposits in the coronary arteries by the time they reach adulthood. Still, the heart may be able to pump sufficient amounts of blood through the coronary arteries so the myocardial tissue is nourished. When an adequate amount of oxygenated blood reaches the myocardial tissues, chest pain due to angina will not occur. However, when there is an imbalance in this black-and-white formula—in other words, when myocardial oxygen demand exceeds myocardial oxygen supply—anginal pain, heart attack, or potentially lethal cardiac rhythm disturbance can occur.

Thus, the pain of angina pectoris stems from the disease process described earlier: atherosclerosis. Once the coronary arteries are occluded, even partially so, it becomes increasingly difficult for the heart to pump the blood through them. When more oxygen-rich blood is required—perhaps because of exercising, excitement, and so on—than the coronary arteries can deliver, an imbalance in the oxygen supply/demand ratio occurs and chest pain develops. Generally, this type of anginal pain is transient and is relieved by rest. A reduction of 50 percent in the diameter of the coronary artery channel will prevent substantial increase in coronary blood flow, which may be required to meet increased myocardial oxygen demand; resting blood flow through the coronary arteries does not fall until the diameter is decreased by more than 80 percent of normal. Thus, angina is usually associated with greater than 50 percent narrowing of a coronary artery, and this degree of narrowing is usually considerd clinically significant.

This classic type of angina is often referred to as *stable angina*. Another kind of angina, called *Printzmetal angina* (named after the physician who first described the atypical form of the syndrome) caused by "coronary spasm," can also occur. Unstable angina is characterized by prolonged pain, even without exertion. Often, hospitalization is required to differentiate this type of anginal pain from myocardial infarction. We include these variant forms of angina in the following discussion even though their clinical significance is still somewhat unclear.

Stable Angina: The Classic Description

Anyone can develop angina pectoris, but it most often occurs in men in their prime (ages 45 to 65). Many of these patients live a normal life despite this syndrome; for others, some restrictions are necessary. In every case, the physician will work closely with the patient to determine his social and psychological needs, and to help the patient plan a life-style that is rewarding to him both personally and professionally and which adheres to the necessary restrictions.

Most physicians would agree that, more important than any physical examination or laboratory test in the diagnosis of angina pectoris, is the patient's own description of the pain. The formula which describes the pathophysiology of anginal pain is straightforward: myocardial oxygen demand exceeds myocardial oxygen supply. The patient's description of the syndrome is usually classic: chest discomfort after exertion (physical or emotional), which is relieved by rest. Here are some typical symptoms:

Table 10.1. Complaints Usually Associated with Angina

Ache	Indigestion
Burning in the chest	*Pressure in the chest
*Constriction in the chest	Soreness in the chest
*Dull chest pain	*Sensation of squeezing of the chest
Feeling of fullness in the chest	Sweating
*Heaviness in the chest	*Tightness in the chest
Heartburn	*Weight on the chest

*Most typical.

Table 10.2. Complaints Not Usually Associated with Angina	
Jabbing pain	Stinging pain
Knifelike pain	Throbbing
Stabbing pain	Tenderness
Shooting pain	Tingling pain

Site of discomfort. Generally, patients with angina have pain or a feeling of discomfort in the midchest. Few patients simply point to one isolated area; instead, most sweep their arms across their chest to indicate where the pain is felt. Some even describe pain in the neck, wrists, arms, and jaw. Most often, the pain radiates to the left arm.

Radiation of discomfort. The entire upper torso may be involved. Usually, the patient says he or she has discomfort, sometimes throughout the chest, arms, and neck.

Duration of discomfort. Typically, the pain is over in five minutes or so—pain that lasts more than thirty minutes is often indicative of injury to the myocardium.

Provocation of discomfort. For some, the list seems endless—even mild excitement, such as a wedding, may exacerbate angina. For others, the pain may be precipitated only by fairly strenuous exercise, such as an intense tennis or racquetball game. Most frequently, walking fast, climbing a flight of stairs or sexual intercourse can produce angina.

Diagnosis. In addition to ascertaining the description of symptoms, the physician will evaluate the patient for the presence of coronary risk factors, and usually obtain a resting and often, a stress electrocardiogram (ECG). In some cases, the physician will also order arteriography, a more sophisticated test, in order to document the extent of disease.

Today, physicians still argue about the exact association between angina and the extent of coronary artery disease that may be present, but most agree that typical anginal pain is usually indicative of a significant degree of coronary artery disease. For example, two fairly recent comprehensive studies show that three-fourths of patients with typical angina pectoris (chest pain characterized by discomfort, brought on by exertion, and alleviated by rest) have a significant stenosis (narrowing) of the coronary arteries. Patients who are symptomatic generally have disease involving several of the coronary arteries—prognosis is related to the extent and severity of the disease in the coronary arteries.

Fortunately, effective drug therapy is available to relieve the symptoms of angina pectoris, but no drug can wipe out the disease. Sometimes, the physicians recommend coronary artery bypass surgery, a surgical technique in which the severely occluded vessels are "bypassed" by inserting a portion of a clear vessel (a vein) from the leg, thus "reestablishing" coronary blood flow. (A discussion of drug therapy for angina pectoris appears on page 229; a discussion of coronary artery bypass surgery begins on page 250).

A Checklist of Anginal Pain

Site	Generally begins in front of chest.
Radiation	Arms, shoulders, jaw, head.
Quality	Sense of pressure, constriction, weight, tightness, discomfort, squeezing, burning.
Duration	A few minutes—usually not more than five; very rarely either prolonged or just a few seconds.
Provocation	Climbing stairs, tennis, heavy gardening, shoveling snow, a brisk walk, running, moving furniture, picking children up, cold, meals, smoking, stress, hypoglycemia, alcohol, excitement (even at a sports event).

A Chip off the Anginal Block: Prinzmetal Angina

> There is [a] type of angina pectoris which appears to be a separate entity.... It does not show the two major characteristics of the classic form, and [there are] other important clinical and experimental differences. In this variant form of angina the pain comes on with the subject at rest or during ordinary activity during the day or night. It is not brought on by effort.... The attacks almost always terminate spontaneously, but if long continued, they may lead to death.

Heberden's classic description of angina pectoris in 1768 stood unchallenged until 1959, when an American clinician named Prinzmetal published the above finding in a medical journal; thus, the solid block of knowledge about angina pectoris was splintered in two. Dr. Prinzmetal hypothesized that this new syndrome might be due to "spasm" in a diseased major coronary artery. Later, when angiography was introduced, Prinzmetal's hypothesis was proven to be correct. To complicate matters further, other clinicians began to note that sometimes patients who complained of chest pain typical of angina pectoris and who had spasm also had normal coronary arteries as shown by angiography. It is now known that variant angina may occur when all of the coronary arteries are normal *or* in the presence of minor or severe atherosclerotic disease. Further, spasm of coronary arteries may contribute not only to Prinzmetal-type rest angina, but recent studies have shown that it may be involved in myocardial infarction, exertional angina, and even sudden death.

WHAT HAPPENS TO YOUR HEART WHEN YOU HAVE A HEART ATTACK?

A heart attack goes by many names: "a coronary," an "MI" (myocardial infarction), an "AMI" (acute myocardial infarction), a "coronary occlusion," or even a "heart seizure." Despite the various terms in use, a heart attack means only one thing: The myocardium, or heart muscle, does not receive enough oxygen-rich blood to sustain the heart's tissues. This usually occurs because one or more of the coronary vessels is occluded, the result of an insidious disease process known as atherosclerosis. Once the myocardial tissues are deprived of nutrients, the cells die.

In some cases, a physician will notice—based on a routine ECG—that the patient has had a heart attack at some time in the past even though he may not have realized it. In these cases, even if the patient was free of chest pain, he had some minor symptoms that he ignored, such as fatigue, "indigestion," or a general feeling of slight malaise.

Remember, numerous risk factors have been identified as potentially significant in the development of atherosclerosis, and the presence of this condition can result in a heart attack. In fact, when a patient has a heart attack as his first "sign" of coronary heart disease, he almost always has double- or triple-vessel coronary artery disease—significant atherosclerosis involving two or three coronary arteries.

Physical activity, of itself, does not usually cause a heart attack; in fact, approximately half of all heart attacks occur while the individual is resting or asleep. On the other hand, it has been established that physical exercise, emotional strain, and heavy meals may aggravate coronary heart disease. Emotional stresses in particular have been linked with heart attack. Many patients frequently report considerable emotional duress in the few days or weeks prior to their heart attack.

When a heart attack occurs, it can affect any part of the heart muscle. (See Figure 10.3.) In approximately half of all heart attacks, for example, the anterior descending branch of the left coronary artery is the involved vessel; thus, the blood supply to the front part of the heart may be diminished and a heart attack—death of the myocardial cells—occurs. This is referred to as an *anterior infarction*. Similarly, an *inferior infarction* may result from occlusion of the right or occasionally the left coronary artery, in which case the *inferior* or the diaphragmatic wall of the heart muscle is affected. A physician can determine the location and estimate the extent of the damage to the heart muscle through a variety of diagnostic tests. These tests are discussed in Part IV.

The important point we wish to make is that both angina and heart attack can be treated—provided that you seek medical treatment early. As such, you should thoroughly familiarize yourself with the warning signs of heart attack and angina; if you or anyone you know has any of these symptoms, medical attention is advised. (See Tables 10.1 to 10.4).

Table 10.3. Descriptions of Pain Associated with a Heart Attack

Heavy pain in the center of the chest, under the breastbone
Heavy chest pain that lasts for five to ten minutes or more
A severe crushing feeling of chest pain
Sweating
Weakness
Nausea and vomiting (or feelings thereof)
Ashen, clammy appearance
Rapid, shallow breathing
A rapid or slow pulse rate
Pain that starts in the chest and may radiate to shoulders,
    neck, jaw, and one or both arms

Table 10.4. Descriptions of Pain Not Usually Associated with a Heart Attack

Numbness
Heart seems to skip beats
Tenderness
Tingling sensations
Chest pain of short duration—less than five minutes
Very sharp or shooting pains that last only a few seconds

What It Feels Like to Have a Heart Attack

To understand better what if feels like to have a heart attack, listen to what some of the victims have to say:

I remember it very clearly. It was in 1967, at a warm-up game in Fresno, California. We were all pretty excited because it was the first time the Knicks had made the play-offs in several years. During the game, I started to notice a shortness of breath, and slight chest pain, but after a few minutes of play, it felt like someone was sitting on my chest. I just thought it was indigestion. The team physician ordered an ECG in San Francisco, but it turned up negative, so I played in another game. I still felt some pressure in my chest, but it wasn't as tight. I was injured early in that game, and taken out of play for the rest of the evening. When we got back to New York, the team physician sent me to St. Clare's Hospital for more tests. I ended up in the hospital for thirty-four days—I had had a heart attack. After five days of drug treatment, the pressure in my chest was relieved, but, they told me, basketball was out for good.*

> David Stallworth, age 25,
> former forward for the New
> York Knickerbockers,
> professional basketball team.

I knew my father had died of "heart trouble" at 58. I didn't smoke, and I've taken pills to control my blood pressure ever since I learned it was high. I keep my weight down by eating nutritious low-fat foods and I exercise vigorously—tennis or racquetball four or five times a week. Even so, I was troubled by the breathlessness I began to experience while exercising. I had nine separate attacks before I went in for tests, and the verdict was what I had suspected: coronary artery obstruction—heart disease. I was eligible for coronary bypass surgery, which I had in the summer of 1975, and I've been here at the Clinic practicing medicine, and traveling and writing ever since.

> William A. Nolen, M.D.
> General Surgeon at the
> Litchfield, Minnesota Clinic
> and author of *The Making of a
> Surgeon* (New York: Random
> House, 1970) and *Surgeon Under
> the Knife* (Coward, McCann &
> Geoghegan, 1976).

A New York star athlete and a prominent Midwestern physician—each with very different careers and life-styles, but with one thing in common: coronary

---

*Stallworth returned to basketball and played with the Knickerbockers until he was traded to the Baltimore Bullets in 1971.

heart disease. Their stories are far from unique. Every day, similar dramas unfold in hospital emergency rooms. A patient comes in, complaining of "indigestion," tightness in the chest, or shortness of breath. Often, the evaluation confirms what the doctor on call suspects—angina or heart attack. Although we have made considerable progress in the diagnosis and management of coronary heart disease, more than 2,000 heart attacks still occur *each day* in the United States alone.

Chances are, if you think about it, you probably know someone who has had a heart attack. You need only think back over the last few years to realize that anyone—in any country, at any age—can have a heart attack. Some victims continue to lead productive lives; others must curtail their activities somewhat; still others die.

Bing Crosby "dropped dead" on a golf course in Madrid; James Daly, a 59-year-old actor who played Dr. Paul Lochner on the television series *Medical Center*, died of a sudden heart attack while he was preparing to perform in a New York suburban summer theater with his son. Robert Shaw, who starred in the movies *The Sting* and *Jaws*, died shortly after getting out of his car on a road in Ireland at the age of 51. Frank Fontaine, a veteran vaudevillian best known as "Crazy Guggenheim" on the Jackie Gleason show, dropped dead of a heart attack in Spokane, Washington. And Totie Fields, a popular comedienne, died of a heart attack at 48 years of age in the same week. Peter Finch, who starred with Faye Dunaway in *Network*, also died of a sudden heart attack shortly after that film was completed. And actors David Janssen (*The Fugitive*) and Peter Sellers were also victims of sudden death due to coronary heart disease. Nelson Rockefeller "dropped dead" in January, 1979. Van McCoy, a 38-year-old disco composer known for his 1975 hit "The Hustle" died of cardiac arrest after suffering a heart attack a week earlier. Charles (Chic) Anderson, a nationally known caller of Thoroughbred races, died suddenly of a heart attack at age 47. And Mendy Rudolph, who officiated a record 2,112 games in twenty-two years of pro-basketball died suddenly of a heart attack in his home at 53 years of age. Finally, I. Rodale, a noted nutritionist, dropped dead on the Dick Cavett Show, shortly after being interviewed. (The show was never telecast as a result.)

Other television and movie personalities also have coronary heart disease, but they have fared better. Jackie Gleason and Walter Matthau have had coronary bypass surgery. Pearl Bailey also has coronary heart disease and still manages a flourishing career; George Carlin, a well-known comedian and frequent guest on the *Tonight Show*, had a heart attack and later discussed his experience candidly on national television.

Several politicians are also victims of coronary heart disease. Most notable today, perhaps, is Menachem Begin, Prime Minister of Israel. Presidents

Eisenhower and Johnson had heart attacks but continued to pursue extremely active political careers. Adlai Stevenson, on the other hand, dropped dead of cardiovascular disease on the street in London, where he was serving in a diplomatic capacity.

Despite the high incidence of "sudden death," most heart attacks are preceded by warning signs. Most victims describe very similar symptoms—regardless of their sex or age. Table 10.1 lists the most frequently encountered complaints; Table 10.2 lists symptoms not generally associated with heart attack.

Although atherosclerosis is an insidious process that silently ravages the coronary arteries, nature does have a way of providing potential victims of heart attack with clues. Sometimes these "tips" precede heart attack by only a few minutes. More often, however, the typical victim of heart attack has experienced one or more symptoms for at least a few days, and sometimes even for weeks or months.

One of the most important things you can do for yourself is learn to recognize the symptoms of angina and the early warning signs of a heart attack. If you or any member of your family, or an associate at work, has any of these symptoms, call your physician immediately. If your physician is not available, the patient should go to the nearest emergency room. Remember, not every pain in the chest is indicative of angina or an impending heart attack—some symptoms are far more common than others and they may be meaningless. On the other hand, it is vitally important to keep in mind that, of the approximately 350,000 people each year who die from heart attack before they reach the hospital, the average victim experiences one or more symptoms, often three hours or so before the "sudden" fatal event occurs.

Our best advice is: Keep your physician's phone number and a number to call for an ambulance near your phone, and don't waste precious time if you have troublesome symptoms. It is far better to learn that your chest pain is truly a case of indigestion than to postpone diagnosis and, possibly, regret it.

To summarize:

1. Your heart is located close to the center of your chest, not on the left side. Pain usually starts here—sometimes it feels like a weight—as though someone or some object was pressing on your chest. The feeling of pressure or tightness in the chest is very common.

2. If you are having either a heart attack or an attack of angina, the pain can radiate or spread down the left arm.

3. Pain due to heart attack or angina can also radiate to the shoulders, neck, jaw, and both arms. Sometimes, a feeling of fullness in the abdo-

men and a burning sensation accompany this pain. Unfortunately, these feelings may be mistaken for indigestion.

4. Pain can occur in all of these areas at once, or it may vary. Shortness of breath, a feeling of nausea, and sweating may also occur.

SUDDEN DEATH

As noted previously, the majority of deaths from coronary heart disease are sudden, and by far the most common cause of this catastrophe is a lethal cardiac arrhythmia, i.e., ventricular tachycardia or ventricular fibrillation. During these arrhythmias, which result in disorganized, chaotic electrical activity consisting of uninterrupted trains of abnormal ventricular beats, effective pumping action by the heart ceases and its mechanical action consists of little more than a quivering of its muscle. This situation is termed "cardiac arrest." When ventricular tachycardia or ventricular fibrillation occur, they must be abolished and normal rhythm reestablished within three to five minutes or the consequence is usually permanent brain damage and irreversible coma, even when heart rhythm is restored later than the crucial three to five minutes

These lethal arrhythmias can be caused by a myocardial infarction or may emanate from an area of localized myocardial ischemia (inadequate oxygenation), which results in electrically unstable cardiac tissue, even in the absence of an infarction. Frequently, in fact, the condition of the heart muscle is actually quite good because no myocardial infarction has occurred, and thus, no permanent damage or scarring is present. However, there may be considerable ischemia from extensive coronary artery disease with marginal blood flow to one or more areas of heart muscle. Such a condition has been described as one of the "hearts too good to die," in other words, the heart muscle itself possesses normal or near-normal pumping ability but a lethal interruption can occur, caused by ventricular tachycardia or ventricular fibrillation. Impairment of cardiac pump function during a lethal arrhythmia is secondary to the arrhythmia itself and not to damage or destruction of cardiac muscle. Therefore, the pumping ability of the heart can be restored *providing* the abnormal rhythm is terminated quickly. Very often, it is possible to stop the abnormal rhythm by cardiopulmonary resuscitation (CPR), which is discussed in the following chapter. This condition is very different from the clinical situation that results when a large myocardial infarction occurs. An extensive infarction can cause considerable damage to heart muscle and thereby reduce permanently the heart's pumping ability; it can also cause shock or chronic congestive heart failure. If a lethal arrhythmia occurs in this setting, CPR is less likely to be effective because of the extensive pre-existent damage to cardiac muscle.

Premature Ventricular Contractions (PVCs): In most patients with coronary heart disease who are at a risk of lethal arrhythmia, cardiac arrest, and sudden death, evidence of electrical instability of the heart in the form of premature ventricular contractions or beats (PVCs or PVBs) is frequently present for a considerable period (weeks or months) preceding the event. These abnormal beats, which are rhythmically out of step with the normal sequence of cardiac beats, originate in ischemic ventricular muscle, in contrast to the normal source of cardiac electrical activity, the sinoatrial node, in the right atrium. PVCs, which usually occur one at a time, may arise in scores, hundreds or even thousands of times each day, and they may be unknown to the patient, who may or may not sense "skipped" beats or palpitations. While PVCs are usually of no consequence in themselves, they may signal electrical instability and the possibility of degeneration into ventricular tachycardia or fibrillation. (It is important to distinguish ventricular tachycardia and ventricular fibrillation from tachycardia and fibrillation originating in the atrium (atrial tachycardia and atrial fibrillation). Although the latter arrhythmias also require treatment, they are not, in themselves, life-threatening and do not carry the dire implications of ventricular tachycardia and fibrillation. Indeed, in some cases, atrial tachycardia and fibrillation may not require hospitalization for treatment and they may respond to oral medications which can sometimes be administered over a period of hours or days.

It is important to recognize that PVCs are a very common arrhythmia and *do not always* imply risk of sudden death. Remember this if your physician remarks that your electrocardiogram or exercise stress test reveals PVCs. These abnormal beats can occur in normal individuals and in patients with any type of heart disease. Precise evaluation of PVCs is best carried out by ambulatory electrocardiography (Holter monitoring), in which the patient wears a small portable electrocardiograph-tape recorder apparatus to which are connected electrocardiographic leads from the patient's chest. The entire system, which can be worn unobtrusively during all the patient's daily activities, provides complete, continuous 24- to 48-hour electrocardiographic data recorded on electromagnetic tape. The data can be analyzed on an electronic scanner in 1/60 or less of the time over which the tape was made. This record affords analysis of the presence of PVCs and their frequency, types and patterns, as well as the potential provoking factors or situations with which they are associated, as determined from the diary kept by the patient while wearing the apparatus.

The significance of PVCs is, to a large extent, determined by "the company they keep" and the forms in which they appear. Thus, if PVCs are associated with evidence of coronary heart disease (angina pectoris or a history of myocardial infarction), and they are what is termed "complex" (high frequency; e.g., occur at a rate of more than ten per hour; originate in more than one area of the ventricle; occur in bursts of two or more in a row; or occur at a crucial point in the cardiac cycle, as determined from the electrocardiogram), their significance increases and serious consideration will usually be given to abolishing them with drugs or other therapy. Occasionally, all that is needed to abolish or reduce the frequency of PVCs is elimination of certain provoking factors—such as cigarette smoking, alcohol, emotional stress—or, in some cases, correction of metabolic abnormalities—such as reduced blood potassium concentration, which may be caused by diuretic therapy. In other cases, specific antiarrhythmic drug therapy is necessary. The rationale for this approach is the hope that abolition or reduction of PVCs will prevent the occurrence of life-threatening arrhythmias, ventricular tachycardia and fibrillation.

When PVCs are infrequent and unassociated with evidence of cardiac disease, treatment is usually unnecessary. The detection of PVCs in otherwise completely normal individuals over age 40 is an indication to pursue diagnostic measures to determine whether or not the PVCs are due to coronary heart disease. In such cases, a basic non-invasive evaluation, consisting of ambulatory electrocardiography, echocardiography, and exercise stress testing, may be undertaken. PVCs which are unassociated with heart disease may warrant treatment if the individual is aware of and disturbed by the sensation of palpitations or skipped beats they produce. It is interesting to note, however, that no associated PVCs or other arrhythmias account for the symptoms. Such complaints usually merely reflect a heightened awareness of the normal heartbeat. Furthermore, most patients with PVCs are unaware of their presence, which is usually detected during a physical examination or electrocardiogram.

It is not known why individuals without evidence of heart disease, some of whom may be young, healthy adults, have PVCs, but it is not uncommon for PVCs to occur or increase in frequency during times of emotional stress, noncardiac illness, and in association with provoking factors such as cigarette smoking or psychoactive drugs. While the presence of these abnormal beats should induce screening measures to detect underlying cardiac diseases such as rheumatic heart involvement, mitral valve prolapse syndrome, or other conditions that may be present in the population below the age of coronary risk, including children, it is important to remember that these rhythm abnormalities are not rare in individuals shown to be completely healthy, and they appear to be associated with no risk in this group.

11
How to Help When Someone Has a Heart Attack

You are shopping in a busy store when, suddenly, without warning, a man nearby crumples to the floor, apparently a victim of a heart attack. Or you are simply sitting in bed with your spouse, reading, when he clutches his chest and slumps over, ashen and unconscious. You call to him, shake him—even slap his face—but you can't get a response. Then you fear he has had a fatal heart attack. Would you know what to do? In these cases, and thousands more like them, victims may be brought back to life, but they require help from a rescuer who knows exactly what to do immediately.

Each year in the United States, more than 650,000 Americans die of coronary heart disease—a heart attack or a lethal arrhythmia that occurs in the absence of an actual heart attack, and over half of these deaths—350,000—are "sudden." In other words, the victim dies within seconds, minutes, or hours after he is stricken and usually before he reaches a hospital.

Would you know how to help these victims, one of whom might be your spouse, father, mother, brother, sister, friend, work associate, or an acquaintance? Don't make the sad mistake of thinking something like this is *never* going to happen to anyone you know. Perhaps your spouse has told you about a co-worker or boss who literally keeled over on the job, or your son or daughter may have told you that their principal or teacher was rushed to the hospital by ambulance—the victim of a heart attack. Read this chapter carefully to learn more about what to do when someone has a heart attack.

Cardiopulmonary Resuscitation (CPR)

Today, thanks to intensive interest in a lifesaving technique called *cardiopulmonary resuscitation* (CPR), many people who have literally "dropped dead" from a heart attack are now walking around, alive and well. Fortunate-

159

ly, even children of junior high-school age can learn this technique. In fact, the three main steps of CPR are so uncomplicated that the American Heart Association has very appropriately named them the "ABC's;" "A" stands for Airway, "B" for Breathing and "C" for Circulation. In this chapter, you can learn in detail how to perform CPR properly—some day, this knowledge may help you save a life.

You can begin to learn CPR by carefully studying the illustrations that follow. These are the steps in the basic techniques that help restore life after cardiac arrest, the cessation of an effective heartbeat, has occurred. You may be familiar with mouth-to-mouth resuscitation, which is also used to revive victims of drowning, asphyxiation, and so on. In CPR, however, another major step, chest compression, is added. Chest compressions are applied to artificially stimulate the pumping action of the heart to maintain blood circulation to the brain and vital organs until the patient is revived or professional medical assistance arrives.

Before you administer CPR to anyone, ascertain whether or not the patient has actually suffered "cardiac arrest," or "complete heart stop." As noted by the American Heart Association's Subcommittee on Emergency Cardiac Care, "Cardiac arrest is recognized by pulselessness in large arteries in an unconscious victim having a death-like appearance and absent breathing." First, determine whether or not the person is conscious. Start by calling the victim loudly or jarring him to see if he will come around on his own. If he doesn't, call for help. Then kneel down next to the person's chest. Put your ear close to the person's mouth, and look toward the chest. If you're sure you can't hear or feel a breath, and the chest is not rising or falling, then take the next step:

> **A.** Begin *rescue breathing*. Start with the head-tilt maneuver, which consists of placing one hand on the victim's forehead and applying pressure to tilt the head backward. This will remove the tongue from the airway passage, ensuring that the windpipe is open. In some cases, the chin lift may have to be added to the head tilt to open the airway. To do this, bring the victim's chin forward with the tips of your fingers under the victim's jaw near the chin. This will help tilt the victim's head back.

> **B.** Now, begin *mouth-to-mouth breathing* (resuscitation). Pinch the victim's nose shut, take a deep breath, and put your mouth *completely* over the victim's to make an airtight seal. Blow into his mouth (this should feel somewhat like blowing into a balloon). Then, remove your mouth and look toward the victim's chest to observe whether or not it rises. When you turn your head to watch the chest, you'll also have your ear over the victim's mouth, so you should hear the air escape as the patient exhales. If the chest falls, you're performing mouth-to-mouth breathing properly.

> **C.** If the chest falls after the first breath, give three more quick breaths, called lung inflations, just like the first one, turning to watch the chest fall

each time. After these first four short, quick breaths, *check the carotid pulse in the neck.* This is the large artery in the neck. (You will actually feel blood being pumped through the carotid artery.) If there isn't any pulse, then you must go on to the third major step of CPR: the application of external chest compressions of the heart in order to maintain circulation of the blood. (The oxygen you are pumping into the lungs will be of no use if the blood is not transporting it to the tissues and organs throughout the body.) To do *chest compressions*, press down on the chest and release the pressure in a precise rhythmic manner. This action forces the heart to pump blood so the entire body can receive its blood carrying the vital oxygen supply. Without this oxygen, vital organs such as the brain will be irreparably damaged.

Start circulation by placing the heel of one hand about 1 to 1½ inches away from (above) the tip of the breastbone. Place your other hand on top of this one, and parallel to it, keeping your fingers *off* the chest and pressing only with the heels of your hands. It helps to interlock your fingers; do not cross your hands.

Next, bring your shoulders right over the victim's chest, as you press downward. Keep your arms straight by locking your elbows. Begin chest compressions. See figure on page 167. Depress the chest by about 2 inches; this means pressing rather hard, but each compression should be smooth and steady. Then relax, but don't take the heel of your hand off the chest, since you must compress the chest fifteen consecutive times. It helps to do this in a rhythmical, rocking manner, counting with each compression, "one down-up," "two down-up," and so on. After fifteen chest compressions, lean toward the victim's head, and start mouth-to-mouth breathing again, this time, using only two quick, full breaths. Follow this with fifteen more chest compressions. Continue this cycle—two breaths, fifteen chest compressions—until an ambulance or other help arrives, or until the victim recovers.

Like any motor skill, such as swimming or bicycle riding, you can learn basic motions by studying diagrams, but, of course, only accurate practice makes for perfect technique. And although you can perfect the mouth-to-mouth breathing technique pictured here on a family member or a friend, you can only practice and perfect the chest compressions on a manikin. Luckily, this is fairly easy to arrange. For example, both the American Heart Association and the American Red Cross sponsor training sessions in CPR. If you call a local chapter of either organization, they can tell you where to go for practice, and they will have an expert on hand to help you attain mastery of each step. You can also contact local police and fire stations, hospitals, and high schools. Some businesses sponsor courses to train their employees and they might open their program up to you and your neighbors. If you organize a group yourself, perhaps you may be able to get an instructor to come to your home, PTA meeting, or the like. The more people who know CPR, the better the chances of saving lives.

Expert instructors can also show you how to do CPR in other circumstances.

For example, when two rescuers are present, one person takes over breathing, the other does the chest compressions, and the sequence changes from two breaths, fifteen chest compressions for a single rescuer to one breath, five chest compressions for two rescuers. In addition, you will learn what to do when the victim's airway is blocked by food, dentures, and so on, how to do mouth-to-mouth on an infant or small child, and other practices and details.

According to the AHA, as many people as possible should learn CPR. It is *especially* important for you to know this lifesaving technique if your spouse or co-worker or, indeed, anyone with whom you spend considerable time is known to have heart disease. In fact, a woman in Seattle has successfully resuscitated her husband *twice*, and he was brought back to life a third time by a bystander in a store. By perfecting this technique, you, too, may become a lifesaver!

Seattle: One City Benefits from CPR

If someone collapses of a cardiac arrest in Seattle, the chances are now one in five that a passerby will know how to keep the victim alive until medical help is obtained. In 1970, Medic I, a research project, became operational in Seattle. In this program, teams of paramedics were trained in CPR; the aim of the project was to enable the city to deliver personnel with the capabilities of a sophisticated coronary intensive care unit to the scene of any cardiac or other medical emergency. These paramedics were trained in the use of numerous drugs, and they learned how to use portable electrocardiographs and other equipment very similar to that seen on television shows such as *Emergency!* Another program, Medic II, was introduced soon thereafter to provide 100,000 citizens of Seattle with training in CPR and the ability to recognize the early signs of acute heart problems. From 1971 to 1975, 65,000 people in Seattle were trained, at a cost of $1.25 per person. The training in CPR was then integrated into the curriculum of the Seattle public schools.

Some time ago, at an annual meeting of the American Heart Association, the doctors in charge of the program reported that their goal had been reached: over 100,000 people in Seattle had been trained in CPR, and in follow-up checks, the doctors found that most of the citizens who completed the three-hour course retained their skills. Also, in studies in which the doctors compared the progress of heart attack victims initially resuscitated by passersby to that of victims who had not received instant medical assistance, bystander-initiated CPR (BYCPR) was found to have the following effects:

1. Consciousness was regained considerably faster in those patients who had received BYCPR.
2. There were considerably fewer neurologic complications, such as stroke, noted in those who had been given BYCPR.

3. Most important, the death rate was lower among those who received BYCPR. Without BYCPR, 39 patients out of 118 remained comatose until discharge or death, compared to 7 of those receiving BYCPR. Of the remaining 72 patients who regained consciousness, prolonged disorientation was present in nearly half of those who did not receive BYCPR, compared to only one in 29 of those who did.

A recent Gallup Poll indicates that 12 million people in the U.S. have taken courses in CPR, and as many as 51 million others would like to. Perhaps you could organize a drive for such a program in your community.

The CPR Decision Tree

In 1973 members from several respected medical and scientific associations met in Washington, D.C., to outline a broad national program of life support measures in order to make the benefits of cardiopulmonary resuscitation available to everyone. Doctors from the American Heart Association and the National Academy of Sciences–National Research Council agreed to establish standards for teaching CPR. These doctors, many of whom are prominent cardiologists, realized that sudden death from coronary heart disease is probably the most significant medical emergency today, since over half a million deaths due to ischemic heart disease occur each year outside of the hospital— usually within two hours after the onset of symptoms. Actually, more people literally "drop dead" from coronary heart disease each year than are killed in auto accidents.

It is fairly easy to learn and remember the simple steps in CPR, but when an emergency strikes even the best of us might blank out momentarily, and the slightest delay could have serious consequences. The CPR Decision Tree diagram was approved by the American Heart Association and the National Academy of Science–National Research Council, and prepared by the National Conference on Cardiopulmonary Resuscitation and Emergency Cardiac Care. The steps you need to follow to perform CPR effectively are carefully outlined. Everyone who is trained in CPR should keep a copy of this diagram handy. At home, you might tape it inside your medicine cabinet door, or post it on a bulletin board in your kitchen, *especially* if any family member or neighbor has heart disease. You could also jot down on it the phone numbers of your local emergency medical services—your local hospital, the fire and rescue squad, and so on—and post it near your phone. And it might even be a good idea for you to make another copy of the CPR Decision Tree and keep it in your office.

(Text continues on page 165.)

Figure 11.1: CPR Decision Tree

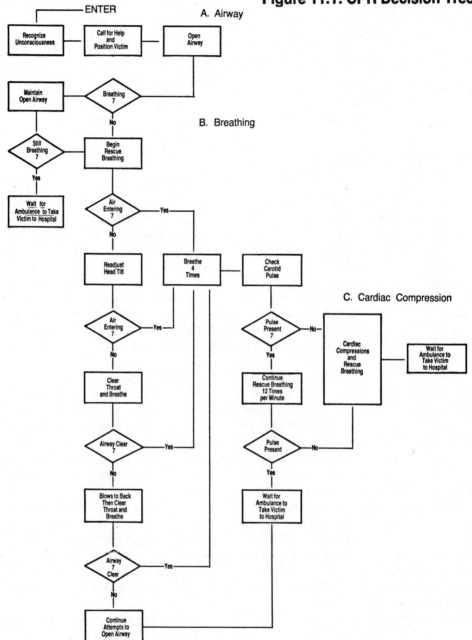

(Text continued from page 163.)

How to Perform Cardiopulmonary Resuscitation *(CPR)*

Read the captions and study the following illustrations very carefully. All of the instructions here presume that you will have to attempt to revive the victim on your own, without any assistance from anyone else. Instructions are given later for those instances in which two rescuers may be present, and instructions for resuscitating infants and small children also appear here.

Remember, you cannot practice the chest compressions on another person; you must use a manikin. It doesn't take more than a few hours to learn, and it is a lifelong, lifesaving investment.

Cardiopulmonary Resuscitation (CPR)

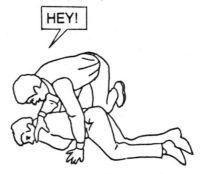

Recognize unconsciousness. Shake or shout at patient.

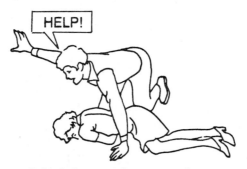

Call for help. Lay the victim face up.

All drawings and guidelines to perform CPR have been adapted from Supplement to JAMA, Standards for Cardiopulmonary Resuscitation (CPR) and Emergency Cardiac Care, Feb. 18, 1974, vol. 277, No. 7 and from the *Journal of the American Medical Association*, Aug. 1, 1980, vol. 244, No. 1, pp. 453–509; with permission.

A. AIRWAY

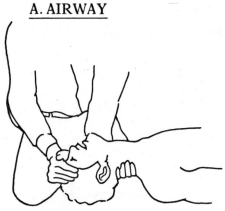

Open the airway. Do not place any object, such as a pillow or coat, under the victim's head. Instead, place one hand on the victim's forehead and apply firm, backward pressure with the palm of your hand, so the victim's head tilts backward. The chin lift may also be necessary.

B. BREATHING

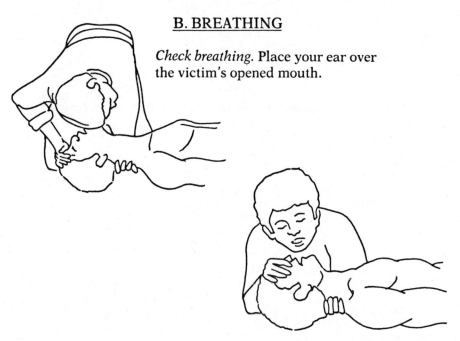

Check breathing. Place your ear over the victim's opened mouth.

Begin rescue breathing. If the victim is not breathing, pinch the nostrils shut. Blow four quick breaths into the victim's mouth. If performed properly, the victim's chest will rise.

C. CIRCULATION

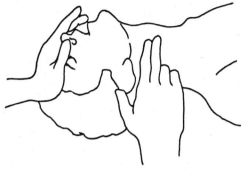

Check the carotid pulse. To find it, run your finger along the victim's throat, until you feel the Adam's apple. Slide your fingers into the groove beside the Adam's apple. (The *Adam's apple* is a projection formed by the largest cartilage of the larynx, which is the upper part of the windpipe.)

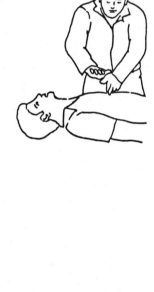

External Cardiac Compressions
1. Locate the point for chest compressions.
Move so your knees are opposite the chest.

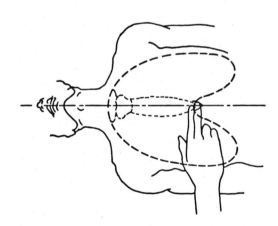

2. Positioning the hands for chest compressions.
Run your fingers up the rib cage until your middle finger fits right into the notch in the center of the chest, and your index finger is lying beside it across the lower end of the sternum.

HEEL IN CONTACT

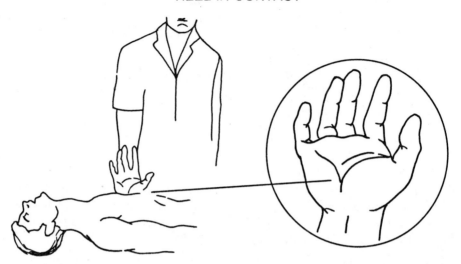

Then lay the heel of your left hand on the victim's chest. Center it over the midline of the sternum, right beside the index finger. Once the heel of your left hand is on the victim's sternum, you must position both your hands in a way that will prevent them from inadvertently pressing on the rib cage and at the same time ensure a quick, effective downward thrust and release when you wish to apply pressure. The heel of your left hand should be positioned on the victim's chest 1½ to 2 inches above the tip of the sternum. *Only the heel* of this hand should be in contact with the chest.

HEELS PARALLEL

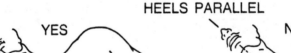

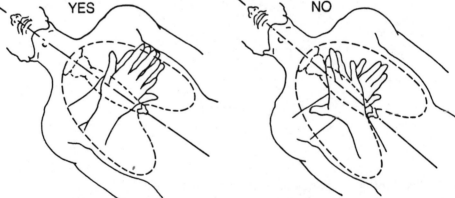

Place the heel of your right hand directly over the heel of the left and parallel to it. Interlock your fingers. This will give maximum control and enable you to perform firm, even compressions rapidly. Do not cross your hands over one another. If you do, the top hand will force the fingers of the bottom hand to press against the ribs and you risk cracking them. Crossing your hands will also reduce the effectiveness of your compressions, thereby decreasing artificial blood circulation.

3. Positioning Your Shoulders and Arms for Chest Compressions.

The positioning of the rest of your body is as important as the placement of hands in achieving maximum effectiveness with minimal strain. External cardiac compression requires a good deal of exertion, and you must do it as efficiently as possible to preserve your own energy and strength long enough to keep the cardiac arrest victim alive.

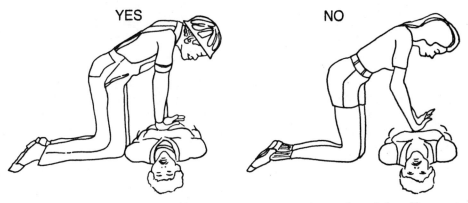

YES

NO

Keep your elbows straight; position your shoulders over the victim's sternum.

Do not bend the elbows.

While keeping your hands in place, position your shoulders directly over the victim's sternum (chest) and straighten out your arms. If you have short arms, you may have to kneel very close to the victim. Or, if you are relatively tall, you may need to kneel several inches away from the victim to achieve the proper position.

You must keep your arms straight throughout compressions. Bending the elbows tires you out much more quickly and requires a great deal more arm and shoulder strength than using your whole body to exert the downward pressure. Remember, keep your elbows locked, your arms straight, and your shoulders over the sternum.

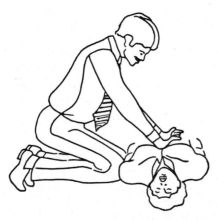

This position is wrong because the shoulders are not over the sternum.

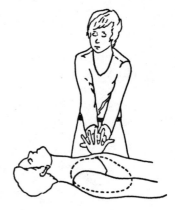

Perform 15 external chest compressions.

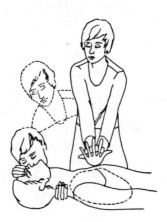

Lean over quickly and open the airway again. Take a deep breath, seal the nose, and perform mouth-to-mouth breathing 2 times, using quick, forceful breaths to fill the lungs.

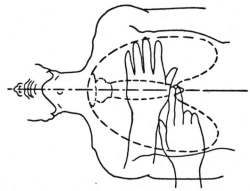

Lean back, locate the lower half of the sternum, and reposition your hands, arms, and body to do 15 more chest compressions.

Remember the ratio, 15:2. That's 15 chest compressions, 2 quick breaths, 15 chest compressions, 2 breaths, and so on. Because of the interruptions for lung inflation, the single rescuer must complete each series of 15 compressions at a rate of 80 compressions per minute. The 2 lung inflations must be delivered in rapid succession, within a period of 5 or 6 seconds, without allowing full exhalation between the breaths. If you exhale completely, the additional time required would reduce the number of compressions and ventilations that you could perform in a one-minute period.

Two Rescuers

The National Conference on Cardiopulmonary Resuscitation and Emergency Cardiac Care recommends that, when two rescuers are present, each should be on a different side of the victim. Thus, the rescuer who will take over breathing can kneel near the victim's head on the left side, while the rescuer who will perform chest compressions kneels on the victim's right side. In this way, it is easy for the rescuers to switch roles; that is, the rescuer performing the breathing takes over the chest compressions, and the other rescuer assumes responsibility for breathing. Because they do not have to physically change position, they can switch responsibilities when necessary without any significant interruption in the CPR rhythm. Two rescuers will often alternate roles in this way, for it is very tiring to perform chest compressions (once you have practiced on a manikin, you will fully appreciate this).

When two rescuers are present, the ratio is five to one. In other words, five chest compressions are performed, followed by one inward breath (lung inflation). There is no pause for the lung inflation, and the compressions must be performed at the rate of sixty per minute.

Table 11.1 Rescuers and Rates of Compressions

Rescuers	Ratio of Compressions to Breaths	Rates of Compressions
One	15:2	80 times/minute
Two	5:1	60 times/minute

How to Help a Victim of Choking

Thanks to a simple technique devised by Henry Heimlich, a surgeon in Cincinnati, Ohio, many choking victims are now being saved out-of-hospital without the aid of paramedics or physicians.

Here's how it's done. First, it is always important to ascertain whether the victim is choking or experiencing a heart attack. Often, when an adult begins to choke, particularly if it is a middle-aged male dining in a restaurant—many automatically think that the victim is having a heart attack, since the breathing becomes blocked, and he or she may turn blue rather quickly. There is, however, a simple signal one should look for that usually indicates that someone is, in fact, choking, and not having a heart attack: choking victims often point to their throats to show those nearby what the problem is. A rescuer then positions himself behind the victim, puts his arms around the victim in bear-hug fashion, makes a fist, and places the side of that fist up against the victim's chest, in the middle, just beneath the breastbone. Then the rescuer places his other hand over the fist that is pressed against the chest, and presses hard and fast—one quick thrust to expel the food or any other item that may have been swallowed.

Blows to the back also may be delivered. Use the side of one hand and strike the victim between the shoulder blades on the back. You can alternate the abdominal thrust with the back blow until one is effective, or the person becomes unconscious. If the latter occurs, place the victim on his back, face up. Open his airway and attempt to ventilate. If this is unsuccessful, the AHA recommends that you deliver four back blows, then four abdominal thrusts. If this is not effective, finger probe, and attempt to ventilate again. Be persistent!

Your local Heart Association and/or your local chapter of the Red Cross can provide you with more detailed information.

12
Other Cardiac Conditions

Although many people are inclined to think only of a heart attack (myocardial infarction) when they hear about heart disease, there are numerous other cardiovascular diseases that warrant consideration. For example, impairment of the electrical activity of the heart can result in *arrhythmias*, or abnormal heart rhythms. One of the most common and serious cardiac disorders is congestive *heart failure*. It may occur as a consequence of any of the diseases that affect the heart such as myocardial infarction, chronic inadequately treated hypertension, cardiac valvular disease, serious cardiac arrhythmias and cardiomyopathies.

The heart valves may also be damaged, either at birth (a congenital heart defect) or later in life, by divergent causes such as rheumatic fever, endocarditis or myocardial infarction. Infections can also involve the heart: the pericardium can become inflamed *(pericarditis)*, as can the endocardium or myocardium (inflammation of these tissues is referred to as *endocarditis* and *myocarditis*, respectively). Finally, the heart muscle, or myocardium, can be damaged, not only by a myocardial infarction but by various other disease processes, some of which are grouped together under the term cardiomyopathies.

Treatment of infections of the heart and cardiomyopathies is discussed briefly here; since arrhythmias, congestive heart failure and valve disorders are more common cardiovascular problems, their specific treatments are outlined in more detail in Chapters 16 and 18.

HEARTS OUT OF RHYTHM

Remember, the mechanical action of the heart, that is the contraction and relaxation of the heart muscle that produces its pumping action, normally proceeds in a regular rhythm. The heart rate—the frequency of the heartbeat—is determined by the physiological requirements of the body for oxygen and other nutrients delivered by the blood and the actions of the nervous system and certain hormones that act on the heart. During periods of very light activity, while we are sitting down reading or asleep, the heart rate is usually in the range of 60 to 100 beats per minute. However, in response to the augmented metabolic needs of the skeletal muscles during vigorous physical exertion, or during emotional stress, the heart rate may climb to over 150 beats per minute.

The cardiac control center for heart rate and rhythm is the *sinoatrial node* (SA), a tiny bundle of tissue that is located in the right atrium and spontaneously and continuously produces regular electrical impulses. These impulses spread from the SA node in a radial manner (as the waves circling outward from the point at which a pebble is dropped into a pool of water), through both atria, and then by special electrical connections to the muscles of both ventricles. In this manner, the SA node, the master cardiac pacemaker, regulates the frequency of beating of the entire heart. In most individuals, the impulses initiated in the SA node are delivered to all areas of the heart in a smoothly integrated sequence from the atria throughout the ventricles to produce a coordinated pumping action that delivers blood to the body's tissues at a rate commensurate with their needs.

Failure or dysfunction of the SA node or any interruption or damage to the specialized conducting system that transmits the impulses throughout the heart can result in an abnormal heart rate and/or rhythm—an arrhythmia. A heart rate that is slower than normal (less than 60 beats per minute) is termed a bradyarrhythmia (*brady* is Greek for "slow"), and an abnormally rapid heart rate (greater than 100 beats per minute) is known as a tachyarrhythmia (*tachy* is Greek for "fast"). Finally, "heart block" occurs when the spread of electrical activity is blocked at a point along the conduction pathway between the atria and ventricles, that is, when the electrical activity from the atria cannot reach ventricular muscle to stimulate contraction.

Bradyarrhythmias. These can be caused by numerous factors, all of which result in suppression of or decrease in the rate of electrical impulse formation in the SA node, or decrease in transmission of the impulse through the heart's electrical conduction system. Such factors include:

- damage to the heart's electrical conduction system (due to myocardial infarction, scarring or inflammation, or other forms of heart disease);
- abnormalities in the chemical environment of the blood, and thus, of the heart cells;
- cardiac drug toxicity, such as may occur with digitalis, propranolol or quinidine.

Heart block is defined as first-, second- or third-degree on the basis of the severity of impairment of conduction from atria to ventricles. In first-degree heart block, all impulses are conducted from the SA node to the atria and thence to the ventricles, but there is a slight delay in transmission from atria to ventricles. The heart rate is not altered in first-degree heart block. In second-degree heart block a variable number of impulses from the SA node and atria do not reach the ventricles, but at least some do. The ratio of atrial to ventricular beats may be of any order (2:1, 3:2, 3:1, 5:2, etc.). The ventricular rate thus falls, and flow of blood from the heart to the body may be seriously reduced. In third-degree or complete heart block, no SA node impulses reach the ventricles from the atria and the ventricles are driven by an "auxiliary" pacemaker that is located in the junctional area between the atria and ventricles or in the ventricular electrical conducting system, which have inherently slower rates of discharge than that of the SA node, varying from 15 to 20 beats per minute to as high as 60 beats per minute, depending on the site of the pacemaker in the ventricular conducting system. When the ventricular rate falls into the lower levels of this range, serious clinical problems usually result, such as fainting, heart failure or even death. (See Table 12.1.)

Tachyarrhythmias. These arrhythmias are either due to increased rate of electrical impulse formation in the SA node or to ectopic, abnormal pacemakers that take over the pacing function of the heart. These abnormal pacemakers can be located in atrial muscle outside the SA node, in the junctional tissues or in the bundle branches or Purkinje system in the ventricles. They can produce isolated, irregular beats or sustained rhythms of very high heart rates. These sustained tachycardias can cause serious impairment of the pumping function of the heart, and when they originate in the ventricles, they are life-threatening medical emergencies that must be immediately corrected. Tachycardias originating in the atria can be managed either by converting the heart's rhythm to normal through several different modes of therapy or, as is done in many patients when this cannot be accomplished, controlling the ventricular rate at a reasonable level by drugs that allow only a desired proportion of the impulses from the atria to reach the ventricles. Such patients may be satisfactorily managed by the latter approach for many years with a tachyarrhythmia originating in the atria.

Factors that may cause tachyarrhythmias are frequently similar to those implicated in the bradyarrhythmias. Thus, the reaction of the heart's rhythm to a given noxious condition or agent is not always predictable. Table 12.2 lists the most common types of tachyarrhythmias with their causes, signs and symptoms and some general remarks.

As can be seen, there is a wide array of cardiac arrhythmias. Many have similar causes, signs and symptoms. Still, physicians can identify these abnormalities of heart rhythm by simple clinical examination or, if necessary, sophisticated diagnostic tests. Treatment can then be tailored accordingly. In each table presented here only some of the causes, signs and symptoms, and general remarks pertaining to arrhythmias are included, since all the cardiac rhythm disturbances and their causes and symptoms are too extensive to list.

Table 12.1

Bradyarrythmias	Site of Dysfunction Within the Heart
Sinus bradycardia Sinoatrial arrest or block	SA node
Slow junctional rhythm Second-degree heart block Third-degree (complete) heart block	AV junction

Second-degree heart block
Third-degree heart block
	Ventricle
	  (bundle of His and
	  His-Purkinje System)

Table 12.2

Tachyarrhythmias	Site of Arrhythmia within the Heart
Sinus tachycardia	SA node
Paroxysmal atrial tachycardia (called "PAT") Atrial flutter Atrial fibrillation	Atria
AV junctional tachycardia	AV junction

Premature ventricular
  contractions (PVCs)
Ventricular tachycardia
  (called "V tach")
Ventricular fibrillation
  (called "V fib")
	Ventricle
	(His-Purkinje System)

THE FAILING HEART

Physicians frequently use the term "heart failure," which can be frightening to patients. However, contrary to its implications, it does not mean that the heart has totally "failed" or stopped working. Rather, it describes a chronic condition in which the heart can no longer pump an adequate amount of blood to supply the body's needs. Heart failure is not a disease in itself but is a syndrome that is a common end result of virtually any of the specific structural and functional defects that can affect the heart. It can therefore be caused by damage to cardiac muscle from myocardial infarction, cardiomyopathy (heart muscle disease) or from the chronic cardiac overwork, enlargement and subsequent damage resulting from hypertension, diseased heart valves or congenital abnormalities. Other conditions can also cause heart failure, including infection and inflammation of the heart.

Before clinically apparent heart failure ensues, compensatory mechanisms are called into play by the body and cardiovascular system to maintain the cardiac output (quantity of blood pumped by the heart per unit time, or rate of blood flow produced by the heart). These mechanisms include: 1) augmented stimulation of the heart by the sympathetic nervous system, increasing the force of contraction and elevating the heart rate; 2) cardiac muscle hypertrophy (increased cardiac muscle mass), which enhances cardiac pumping capacity; and 3) increased volume of the cardiac chambers (because of fluid retention in cardiac failure), which also contributes, to a degree, to a more forceful contraction.

These factors increase the pumping function of the diseased heart but they cannot normalize it. In addition, prolonged and intense activation of these compensatory mechanisms ultimately results in further deterioration of cardiac function. Thus, increase in heart muscle mass commonly leads to dilatation (excessive stretching) of the muscle, which, in itself, results in damage and scarring with further reduction in pumping capacity. Excessive sympathetic nervous system stimulation constricts the body's small arteries, raising blood pressure and increasing the resistance against which the diseased left ventricle must operate. In this manner, a chronic condition that reduces the heart's functional ability sets up a vicious cycle involving compensatory mechanisms that, while initially supporting cardiac performance, ultimately contribute to further cardiac impairment, additional activation of compensatory mechanisms and a deleterious situation that feeds upon itself.

The consequences of heart failure are several and serious. Interestingly, the problems posed for the patient are frequently not directly related, in terms of their subjective experience, to the heart or even exclusively to the chest, but occur in a widespread manner throughout the body, since the consequences of inefficient blood circulation ultimately involve all the body's organs. Inadequate ejection of blood from the heart results in excess residual blood in the ventricles after each beat, causing a "backup" of pressure and volume in the left ventricle that is transmitted to the left atrium, and in turn, into the veins and capillaries of the lungs. The increased blood volume in the lungs produces fluid congestion that impairs respiration and oxygen transport in the pulmonary system, which the patient experiences as shortness of breath and air hunger. The impairment of right ventricular function similarly produces increased blood volume and pressure "upstream" from it, i.e., in the right atrium and the veins and capillaries of the lower extremities and the organs of the abdomen, resulting in edema (swelling from fluid retention in the tissues) of the legs and abdominal organs such as the liver. Edema is aggravated by abnormal kidney function in heart failure, caused by the kidney's inability to eliminate adequately from the body excess sodium and, with it, water because of the reduced blood flow it receives in heart failure. Retention of sodium and water by the kidney further contributes to tissue fluid congestion and edema. Edema is not usually seen in the upper body because of the effect of gravity that promotes drainage of blood down to the heart. Because heart failure causes this congestion of the body's tissues with excess fluid due to inefficient circulation of the blood, physicians commonly refer to the condition as "congestive" heart failure.

In addition to fluid retention, lung congestion and edema, heart failure results in reduced blood supply to all the body's organ systems, which can seriously impair their function. Both components of heart failure—the congestive, fluid-retaining element, and the low cardiac output aspect—can produce major disability and severe illness.

The major *symptoms* of congestive heart failure are:

● *Shortness of breath* due to pulmonary congestion: the patient may have severe shortness of breath in the supine position because more of the excess fluid in the body is diverted to the lungs in this position, increasing congestion of these organs and causing some patients to sleep in an elevated posture.

● *Edema* of the lower extremities and abdominal organs. In severe cases, there is fluid retention in the abdominal cavity with swelling of the abdomen.

● Excessive and early *fatigue* with mild effort because of the inability of the heart to meet the increased blood flow required by the muscles of the body during exertion.

Depending on the severity of the foregoing factors, a range of disability can result. In mild cases the foregoing symptoms may occur only with strenuous effort, but in severe cases mild exertion may result in shortness of breath and extreme fatigue. In the most advanced cases of heart failure there are edema and shortness of breath even at rest.

Fatigue and a sense of breathlessness with severe physical exertion are normal and do not indicate heart failure. The latter is suggested by considerable shortness of breath and fatigue with mild degrees of exertion. But even in this instance the symptoms may be caused by a lack of physical conditioning (commonly referred to as being "out of shape") or by anxiety. Any concerns you may have in relation to exertional symptoms can be readily clarified by consultation with your physician.

DISEASES OF THE VALVES

These diseases can affect any of the four heart valves:

- Mitral valve—left atrioventricular valve; separates left atrium and left ventricle; its action imparts proper directional flow of blood between these chambers, i.e., from atrium to ventricle.

- Tricuspid valve—right atrioventricular valve; separates the right atrium from the right ventricle; directs flow of blood from the atrium to the ventricle.

- Aortic valve—situated at junction of left ventricle with aorta; directs blood flow from the ventricle into the aorta.

- Pulmonic valve—situated at junction of right ventricle with pulmonary artery; directs flow of blood from ventricle to pulmonary artery.

Valvular heart disease falls into two general categories: stenosis and insufficiency. Any heart valve can be affected by either of these conditions, which are caused by structural defects of the valves that prevent the normally precise mechanical activity that produces unimpeded opening and secure closure at the appropriate times in the cardiac cycle. *Stenosis* refers to inability of the valve to open completely, resulting in a narrowed valve orifice, which reduces the forward flow of blood through the valve. Consequently, the cardiac chamber which pumps blood through a severely stenotic valve must exert considerably increased contractile effort to maintain adequate flow. This may result in hypertrophy of its muscle with ultimate dilatation and failure, as previously described in this chapter. *Insufficiency* means that the valve does not close properly, which can cause blood to leak backward through the valve orifice during each cardiac beat, resulting in reduced forward flow and congestion of the area receiving the abnormal backward flow of blood. Again, the heart utilizes compensatory mechanisms to support forward blood flow, but the outcome in severe valvular insufficiency is ultimately heart failure. Stenosis and insufficiency frequently coexist in the same valve, and more than one valve may be diseased in the same patient. For example, a patient may have stenosis of one valve, insufficiency of another, both defects on several valves or one type of defect on several valves. Involvement of two valves is frequent, and disease of more than two, while it occurs, is uncommon.

An individual may be born with a valvular defect, or the abnormality may be acquired later in life. Many congenital valvular abnormalities are immediately evident at birth and produce the characteristic complications early in life. In other cases, a valve may be structurally abnormal at birth but not to an extent that its function is significantly impaired. However, its aberrant structure may ill suit it to withstand the wear and tear of years of circulatory stress under which the defect can become more marked, and significant stenosis or insufficiency can develop. In such cases, the congenital abnormality does not result in clinically significant valvular disease until adulthood. For example, in aortic stenosis related to a congenital bicuspid aortic valve (two valve leaflets instead of the normal three leaflets), serious overt complications related to the valvular abnormality may not occur until middle or old age. Indeed, the typical patient presenting the clinical manifestations of aortic stenosis is a male in his sixth decade or older, yet the abnormal valve has been present since birth. Mitral stenosis, on the other hand, generally produces resistant cardiac decompensation by the fifth decade, after acquisition of the disease from a childhood episode of rheumatic fever. Interestingly, patients with this specific valvular defect are usually female. An important factor determining the shorter interval between onset of the disease and decompensation in mitral stenosis than in aortic stenosis is the specific cardiac chamber directly affected by the valvular abnormality. The course in aortic stenosis is longer because the powerful left ventricle has a greater capacity to meet the increased work presented by the stenotic aortic valve than the left atrium has to meet the restriction to blood flow in mitral stenosis.

Valvular stenosis and insufficiency can vary considerably in severity. In mild cases, there may be no disturbance to the patient and the problem may be evident only by a heart murmur resulting from the turbulent flow of blood through the abnormal valve, detected by the physician listening with a stethoscope over the heart.

It is important to emphasize that all heart murmurs do not indicate a heart defect. There are a number of other factors, some quite benign, to which murmurs may be related. In children of elementary school age particularly, the prevalence of heart murmurs is very high—up to 50 percent in some studies!—and the great majority are "innocent," i.e., not associated with any cardiac abnormality. Most such murmurs disappear by adulthood.

Moderate and severe valvular disease increases the work of the heart, stimulating the compensatory mechanisms previously discussed. The latter finally become inadequate in many cases and heart failure supervenes. This sequence of events, even in severe valvular disease, may be very protracted and take years or, commonly, decades.

The complications of valvular disease, in addition to cardiac enlargement and heart failure, which can occur in all valvular lesions, depend on the particular valve and defect involved. However, they may include arrhythmias, angina pectoris, endocarditis and emboli.

Emboli (singular—*embolus*) are particles originating at one point in the body and carried through the blood to another area of the body where they produce complications. The emboli in valvular heart disease can originate either in a cardiac chamber through which the flow rate is markedly reduced because of interference to emptying by a stenotic valve, or on an infected cardiac valve, as in endocarditis. In the former instance the emboli are small blood clots that develop because of the stagnation, or stasis, of blood in the cardiac chamber blocked by the stenotic valve. In endocarditis, the emboli consist of inflammatory debris that collects at the site of involvement on an affected heart valve and can include bits of tissue, bacteria, clotted blood and blood cells. The particles that originate in the heart become emboli when they are carried away from their sites of formation by the blood. Emboli ultimately can lodge in and occlude small arteries in any organ in the body, obstructing blood supply and thereby causing infarction of the respective organ. An embolus to an artery of the brain can cause a stroke; likewise, bowel, kidney or myocardial infarction can result from emboli to the arteries of these organs, and an embolus to the artery of a limb can cause gangrene.

Aortic stenosis. Specifically, this term means that the leaflets of the aortic valve open inadequately, due to structural abnormalities resulting from any of several disease processes. The stenotic aortic valve is usually deformed, thickened, scarred and stiffened, and may frequently contain calcium deposits, a common occurrence in chronically damaged tissues, which add to the inflexibility of the valve.

The complications of aortic stenosis result from the hemodynamic burden this lesion places on the left ventricle, which must eject its blood through an orifice of inadequate size. The left ventricle is the most powerful pumping chamber of the heart with the greatest capacity for compensatory muscular hypertrophy. This reserve capacity can delay overt cardiac decompensation for a considerable duration, after which specific forms of therapy are mandatory. The appearance of certain major symptoms related to aortic stenosis heralds a serious inability of the left ventricle to function against the diseased valve.

The major symptoms of aortic stenosis, indicating severe valvular disease are:

- *Shortness of breath* (from pulmonary congestion caused by left ventricular failure) with exertion or when lying down and even sometimes at rest.

- *Lightheadedness* and/or *fainting* (due to inadequate blood flow to the brain).

- *Angina pectoris* (due to the excessive oxygen demand of the thickened left ventricle functioning at a markedly increased pressure).

Frequently, coronary artery disease is associated with aortic stenosis, since patients with aortic stenosis predominantly comprise a group of men over the age of 50. The occurrence of any of the three major complications—left ventricular failure, fainting or angina—signifies an ominous phase of the disease associated with rapid deterioration, frequently leading to death after a relatively short period. While the initial decades after the onset of the disease may be unassociated with significant symptoms because of the considerable capacity of the left ventricle to hypertrophy and function adequately even in the presence of severe aortic stenosis, when symptoms finally do occur, they indicate that the left ventricle has reached the limits of its compensatory capacity and that a rapid downhill course is imminent. The onset of the aforementioned symptoms is usually associated with a mortality of 30 to 50 percent within a two-year period.

Aortic stenosis also occurs as a congenital abnormality that may be severe in childhood, producing problems similar to those found in the older patient. In many patients, however, the presence at birth of an abnormal aortic valve (bicuspid—that is, a valve with only two instead of three leaflets) is not associated with severe stenosis for a number of decades, during which the structurally abnormal but initially adequately functioning valve becomes progressively more deformed, scarred, calcified and stiffened—finally resulting in severe aortic stenosis during middle or late adulthood.

Treatment. Heart failure, angina and arrhythmias should be treated by medical means, as discussed in Chapter 16. However, valve replacement should not be delayed after the appearance of these complications, for the reasons previously discussed. The timing of valve replacement is a critical issue that always receives careful consideration by the cardiologist and cardiac surgeon. Patients with valve disease in the early stages and no complications frequently ask, "Why wait until major symptoms appear before replacing a diseased heart valve when these complications might be averted by earlier surgery?" The answer lies in the current status of prosthetic heart valves, which, despite the tremendous advances in this field, still have significant limitations (see Chapter 18). The risks of surgery and the artificial valve are greater than their potential benefits to the patient early in the natural history of his disease when heart function is well maintained. However, when impairment of cardiac function and symptoms appear, the risks associated with valve replacement are less than those of delaying surgery. Thus, it is essential that valve replacement be performed at, or just before, the initial occurrence of overt cardiac decompensation, when the latter can be reversed by correction of the valve defect. Delay beyond this point is frequently associated with progressive, irreversible cardiac deterioration.

Aortic insufficiency. In this condition, the aortic valve does not close properly because of shortened, scarred, stiff leaflets with limited mobility. The resultant leakage of blood backward from the aorta into the left ventricle during diastole (the ventricle's rest period between beats) requires the ventricle to pump a greater volume of blood with each contraction in order to maintain an adequate systemic circulation. For example, if the left ventricle ejects 150 cc of blood with each contraction, and 50 percent (or 75 cc) leaks back from aorta to ventricle between ventricular contractions, the ventricle must pump 225 cc of blood with each beat to maintain normal flow. This is possible but only at the expense of left ventricular enlargement and the other compensatory mechanisms that ultimately result in heart failure and related complications.

Aortic insufficiency may be caused by a congenital abnormality of the valve, rheumatic fever, endocarditis, and untreated syphilis, and may be associated with certain systemic and genetic disorders. Management consists of medical treatment initially for the complications of cardiac failure, arrhythmia and angina (Chapter 18), and valve replacement by open heart surgery (Chapter 18), if indicated. Surgery should be performed before full-blown cardiac failure and irreversible heart damage supervene.

Mitral stenosis and insufficiency. The primary cause is rheumatic fever, but these valvular lesions can be of congenital origin. Mitral insufficiency may also result from endocarditis, can accompany certain systemic diseases, and is a complication of coronary heart disease, especially following myocardial infarction. In the latter case the valvular insufficiency is caused by damage to one or both papillary muscles, the small muscles within the left ventricle, to which the mitral valve leaflets are attached and whose contraction and relaxation maintain valve closure and allow its opening at the appropriate times in the cardiac cycle. Damage to a papillary muscle impairs its ability to hold the mitral valve shut during ventricular contraction, with resultant valvular insufficiency.

In mitral stenosis, blood flow from the left atrium to the left ventricle is decreased because of the narrowed valve orifice, and excess blood volume and pressure build-up in the left atrium and ultimately "upstream" in the pulmonary circulation, causing pulmonary congestion and the syndrome of left-sided heart failure. The resultant high pressures in the pulmonary circulation can also lead to failure of the right ventricle because of the increased pressure it must pump against to eject blood into the pulmonary system. With mitral insufficiency, instead of all blood flowing from the left ventricle into the aorta during each ventricular contraction, a certain proportion of blood in the left ventricle flows backward into the left atrium, thus reducing the normal volume of blood pumped to the body. A similar sequence of events results as in mitral stenosis relative to pulmonary congestion and subsequent right heart failure. However, in mitral insufficiency the left ventricle is presented with increased amounts of blood that it must pump because it receives the normal flow from the left atrium plus the additional amount of blood that leaked backward into the atrium during ventricular contraction. The increased work associated with this augmented blood volume pumped by the left ventricle can produce enlargement and failure from the chronic overload. In contrast, in mitral stenosis, the valvular defect reduces the amount of blood received by the left ventricle from the left atrium, and the consequences of the stenotic mitral valve are imposed on the left atrium and the right side of the heart in the form of increased pressure against which they must pump because of the block to flow produced by the valvular defect. Thus, in pure mitral stenosis there is no enlargement, increased work, or failure of the left ventricle. In both mitral stenosis and mitral insufficiency, there are congestion of the lungs and increased pressure in the pulmonary circulation faced by the right ventricle, and the flow of blood from the heart to the body is reduced.

Both mitral stenosis and mitral insufficiency can produce cardiac enlargement, heart failure and arrhythmias. Emboli from the left atrium are an important potential complication of mitral stenosis, because of the relative stasis of blood in the left atrium secondary to the reduced valve orifice. Endocarditis of the diseased valve can occur in either mitral stenosis or mitral insufficiency.

Heart failure and arrhythmias are treated as discussed in Chapter 16 and mitral valve replacement is performed when complications are not easily managed medically and before irreversible cardiac damage occurs (Chapter 18). In certain cases of mitral stenosis unassociated with mitral insufficiency, it is possible to perform a valvuloplasty, that is, surgical correction of the native valve without replacing it with a prosthesis. This approach is advantageous because the operation is simpler and of lower risk than valve replacement. Although repair by valvuloplasty cannot restore the valve to normal, the corrected native valve is, in several important respects, superior to the artificial device. Unfortunately, valve replacement is commonly necessary within a decade or less in most patients who have valvuloplasty because restenosis and other complications, such as surgically induced insufficiency, usually occur.

Tricuspid stenosis and tricuspid insufficiency. These disorders may occur in 10 to 15 percent of patients with chronic rheumatic heart disease and can also result from congenital defects of the valve. The most common cause of tricuspid insufficiency is actually right ventricular failure and dilatation secondary to marked left heart failure, usually resulting from severe, combined aortic and mitral valve disease. The latter situation results in markedly increased pressure in the pulmonary circulation, increasing the work burden of the right ventricle, which may ultimately dilate and fail. When the right ventricle is severely dilated, even a normal tricuspid valve cannot close properly during right ventricular contraction because the abnormal degree of stretching of the walls of the right ventricle prevents its papillary muscles from pulling the tricuspid leaflets to a position of complete closure.

The chief consequences of tricuspid stenosis and tricuspid insufficiency are failure of the right side of the heart (right ventricle and right atrium), with resultant retention of fluid, and occurrence of edema. Fatigue, arrhythmias and endocarditis can also occur. Pulmonary congestion does not result from tricuspid valve disease, since the back-up of blood is in the veins of the systemic circulation (all parts of the body except the lungs), and the amount of blood pumped by the failing right ventricle to the lungs is less than normal. Again, medical management is applied initially and surgery is indicated for severe valvular disease before irreversible cardiac damage occurs. In patients in whom tricuspid insufficiency results from right ventricular dilatation secondary to left heart failure from severe aortic and/or mitral valve disease, the insufficiency may be minimized or abolished after correction of the left heart valvular defects, if there follows significant reduction of elevated pressures in the pulmonary circulation and right ventricle.

Pulmonic stenosis and insufficiency. Pulmonic valve stenosis is one of the most common congenital cardiac defects while pulmonic insufficiency is uncommon and is usually acquired. In the latter case, it frequently results from severe elevation of pressure in the pulmonary artery from a variety of causes, most commonly marked left heart failure. Great elevations of pressure in the pulmonary artery can cause valvular insufficiency because of the considerable stress on even a normal pulmonic valve, which is structurally adapted to withstand relatively low pressures. Pulmonic valve disease is rarely caused by rheumatic fever. Pulmonic stenosis and insufficiency can lead to right heart failure in the same manner that aortic stenosis and aortic insufficiency adversely affect the left side of the heart. Arrhythmias, fatigue and endocarditis can also occur. Medical management is applied as required, and in certain cases surgery is indicated. Surgery is commonly performed in childhood for severe congenital pulmonic stenosis. The procedure usually consists of direct surgical correction of the abnormal valve rather than replacement by a prosthetic device. This operation is usually highly effective and of very low risk.

"ITIS" SPELLS INFLAMMATION OF THE HEART

You may recall from the discussion of anatomy that the heart is enclosed in a fibrous sac, the pericardium. The myocardium is the muscular portion of the heart, and the endocardium is the thin fibrous portion of flat endothelial cells that provides a smooth lining to the inner surface of the chambers of the heart and a smooth covering for the heart valves. Each of these may become inflamed, leading to conditions called "pericarditis," "myocarditis" and "endocarditis" ("itis" means inflammation). Inflammation can be caused by a wide variety of inciting factors, but the most common cause of inflammation of the heart's tissues is infection by any of the microorganisms (for example, bacteria, viruses or fungi) that can affect humans. Here is a brief description of these entities.

Pericarditis. This is an inflammation of the pericardium and may be caused by–in addition to viral, bacterial or fungal infections–myocardial infarction, chest trauma or systemic diseases such as rheumatoid arthritis or related conditions. Thus, pericarditis may be primary (resulting from a disease process that directly and chiefly affects the pericardium) or secondary (a result of a condition that primarily affects other areas of the body). Pericarditis also may be acute or chronic. In acute pericarditis the major problems experienced by the patient are fever and chest pain, but if the inflammation causes collection of a large volume of fluid in the pericardial sac surrounding the heart, the pumping action of the heart can be disturbed and heart failure may result. In chronic constrictive pericarditis, which in the past was most commonly caused by tuberculosis, heart failure with edema may be a consequence because of disruption of normal cardiac function by the thickened, scarred and restricting pericardium enveloping the heart.

Treatment varies depending on the type and cause of pericarditis, but rest, pain relievers and anti-inflammatory agents may be administered. If acute pericarditis causes severe heart failure due to the rapid accumulation of excessive pericardial fluid, a life-threatening medical emergency may result. Treatment consists of prompt removal of the fluid through a needle directly inserted into the pericardial sac through the chest wall. This maneuver typically results in immediate, dramatic relief of the cardiac dysfunction and clinical symptoms of heart failure. In the case of severe, chronic constrictive pericarditis with resultant heart failure, surgical removal of the diseased pericardium may be required.

Myocarditis. Like pericarditis, myocarditis may also develop from a wide variety of underlying disorders, such as infectious processes, systemic diseases (including rheumatic fever), and toxic chemical substances. In mild forms, symptoms may be absent; even more severe cases may be unrecognized until complications such as congestive heart failure develop.

Complications of myocarditis include chest pain, arrhythmias and heart failure. There are no typical signs or symptoms that can absolutely identify myocarditis. Management consists of bed rest, treatment of pain, and, if present, control of arrhythmias and heart failure.

Endocarditis. This is usually caused by bacterial or fungal infection of one or more of the heart valves. It also occasionally results from a noninfective inflammatory process associated with a systemic disease. The inflammation can damage or destroy the involved heart valve, seriously compromising cardiac function and resulting in heart failure. Endocarditis is most likely to occur on an abnormal heart valve, so patients who have valve damage from congenital, rheumatic or other causes are highly susceptible to this condition.

Thus, endocarditis typically occurs in patients with previously diseased heart valves in whom infectious agents gain entrance to the bloodstream, as after a wound, or major and even minor surgical procedure, e.g., dental cleaning or extraction and genitourinary examinations. However, in many cases of endocarditis no such preceding factors are obvious. The risk of endocarditis following procedures with the potential to introduce infection into the body can be minimized by administration of prophylactic antibiotics in conjunction with the procedure. It is thus essential that a patient's dentist or physician be aware of the presence of any cardiac valvular abnormality so that proper steps, when indicated, can be taken to prevent endocarditis.

A group of patients whose personal habits have made them particularly vulnerable to endocarditis, even in the absence of valvular abnormalities, are the drug addicts who practice self-injection of agents such as heroin. By their use of unsterilized needles, they frequently inoculate themselves with very virulent bacteria and fungi that can infect and destroy even normal heart valves. Endocarditis generally occurs in its most malignant form in these individuals and has a considerable mortality in them.

Symptoms of endocarditis include chills, fever and serious complications such as heart failure and emboli. Emboli are discussed earlier in this chapter. Treatment includes bed rest, antibiotics to eradicate the infection, and management of heart failure, arrhythmias and other complications, if present. In severe, resistant cases in which the endocarditis produces life-threatening complications and fails to respond to antibiotic therapy and other measures, emergency open-heart surgery, to replace the diseased valve with an artificial one, may be required.

DISEASES OF THE HEART MUSCLE: CARDIOMYOPATHIES

From the Greek (*cardio*, heart; *myo*, muscle; and *pathos*, disease), *cardiomyopathy* is a catchall term describing those conditions that produce a direct, chronic disease process of the heart muscle that is not related to associated coronary artery, valvular or hypertensive disease. Thus, the abnormality is in the heart muscle itself and is not related to a defect of other cardiac structures as, for example, in myocardial infarction the damage to heart muscle is directly related to coronary artery obstruction. The precise causes of the cardiomyopathies are frequently undefined. In some cases, infectious agents (bacteria and viruses), systemic diseases (metabolic abnormalities, inflammatory conditions or genetic abnormalities) or toxic substances, such as alcohol, may cause cardiomyopathy. The cardiomyopathies are frequently but not always characterized by enlargement of the heart, cardiac failure and arrhythmias. In some patients, angina pectoris may be present.

Physicians classify cardiomyopathies into three general groups:

Congestive cardiomyopathy—characterized by cardiac enlargement, heart failure and arrhythmias.

Hypertrophic cardiomyopathy—characterized by thickening, primarily of the interventricular septum, the muscular wall that separates the left and right ventricles; it is commonly associated with one or more of the following problems: obstruction to outflow of blood from the left ventricle, mitral valve dysfunction (regurgitation, or leak), arrhythmias, dyspnea, angina, fatigue, lightheadedness and fainting.

Restrictive cardiomyopathy—characterized by a symmetrical thickening of the left ventricular muscle which is non-compliant (stiff) and results in restriction to left ventricular filling. Complications include heart failure and arrhythmias. Restrictive cardiomyopathy is not uncommonly associated with a general, systemic disease that involves many of the tissues of the body and that can result in abnormal deposits of certain substances in these tissues, including the heart. Hemochromatosis, an inability of the body to metabolize iron properly, resulting in deposition of excessive amounts of iron in many organs, is an example of a systemic disease that results in a restrictive cardiomyopathy through its effects on the heart.

Whether the cardiomyopathy is due to infection, a toxic substance, a metabolic abnormality or another type of disease process, the end result is generally the same: impaired contractile ability of the heart muscle and reduced pumping capacity that, if sufficiently severe, results in heart failure.

Today excessive alcohol consumption is considered to be a cause of one type of cardiomyopathy (congestive cardiomyopathy), since it has been found that there is a relatively high rate of this condition among chronic alcoholics and that abstinence from alcohol frequently results in improvement. Further, it has also been shown in laboratory studies that alcohol can severely depress the function of even normal heart muscle, just as it may depress the activity of all cells in the body. Even chronic consumption of what might be considered "moderate" amounts of alcohol can sometimes be implicated as a potential factor in cardiomyopathy (two or three shots of liquor daily for many years, for example, may be associated with evidence of cardiomyopathy in some individuals).

Overall, the treatment of cardiomyopathies consists primarily of supportive therapy such as reduced activity, proper diet, management of heart failure and arrhythmias, if present, and removal of any causative factors, such as alcohol, if identifiable.

13

The Pill,
Pregnancy, Menopause,
and the Heart

Do we need a section devoted especially to heart disease in women? After all, heart attacks are basically a problem for men to worry about, right? Although the very words "heart attack" bring to mind an image of a man in his prime who suddenly drops dead, this stereotype is not accurate. True, every year men suffer more heart attacks than women do; nevertheless, it is also true that heart disease is the major cause of death among women.

Although statistics show that premenopausal women are far less likely to have a heart attack than postmenopausal women (this is often attributed to the idea that *estrogens*, the female hormones that help regulate the menstrual cycle, provide some "protection" against the development of coronary heart disease), experts agree that the same factors that contribute to the development of coronary heart disease in men also may have an unfavorable effect on women. In addition, in the last few years researchers have spent more time analyzing the incidence of stroke and heart attack among women, primarily as a result of the number of women who take oral contraceptives, smoke, etc. In this chapter, we discuss some of their most recent findings, as well as the effects that physiological changes unique to women—pregnancy, childbirth and menopause—have upon the heart.

CORONARY HEART DISEASE IN WOMEN

Although it is true that there are marked differentials in mortality rates for coronary heart disease, it is also known that risk of a cardiovascular event such as a heart attack or stroke, increases for women—just as it does for men—in proportion to the number of risk factors present. For example, re-

189

searchers at the Montreal Heart Institute conducted a study involving 239 women. Coronary arteriography (a diagnostic technique that permits one to visualize the coronary arteries) was performed in each of these women because of suspected coronary artery disease. In women under forty-five years of age, the investigators found a correlation between the presence of certain risk factors and coronary artery disease.

Specifically, in the 104 women who were found to have obstruction of one, two, and three coronary arteries, the existence of risk factors such as hypertension, hyperlipidemia, diabetes, cigarette smoking, and a positive family history of heart disease was significantly more frequent than in the 112 women with normal coronary arteries and the 23 women with insignificant coronary artery disease. Thus, this survey emphasizes that it is as important for women to be mindful of risk factors as it is for men.

Your Heart and the Pill

To date, much has been written about the role of oral contraceptives in the development of heart and arterial disease; or, more specifically, about the relationship between the use of oral contraceptives and the incidence of stroke and heart attack in young women. Is there any truth in these newspaper reports? Or are they just "headlines"? Regrettably, there is evidence to back these stories up. For example, reports have indicated that use of oral contraceptives can cause numerous circulatory problems, such as an embolism (blood clot), high blood pressure, stroke, heart attack, and hemorrhage in a small but significant percentage of women. In one study of 46,000 women in Great Britain, begun in 1968 and published in 1977, the researchers concluded that women who used oral contraceptives faced a 40 percent higher risk of death than nonusers of the same age—and that the excess risk could be primarily ascribed to circulatory diseases. However, this survey also showed that the risk of developing these problems is usually confined to women over the age of thirty-five and to those who smoke cigarettes.

As a result of this report, the Royal College of General Practitioners and the Royal College of Obstetricians and Gynecologists issued the following guidelines:

no change in use of oral contraceptives in women under age 30

no change in use of oral contraceptives in women age 30 to 35 unless they have been taking the Pill for five years or longer or they smoke cigarettes (in which case, they can either discontinue smoking or select an alternate method of contraception)

women over age 35 should reconsider their use of the Pill.

Heart attack. At a meeting of the American Heart Association in November 1977, it was reported that a twenty-one-country review showed that, in women aged 15 to 44 who did not use oral contraceptives, the risk of death from heart disease was 7.8 per 100,000. However, the risk rose to 27.5 per 100,000 when oral contraceptives were used—a difference of almost 20 deaths per 100,000. This may seem slight, but when you consider the fact that as of 1977 about 50 million women were taking oral contraceptives, it means approximately 10,000 deaths per year. Other studies show that the risk of nonfatal myocardial infarction in women who take the Pill, particularly those over 35 who also smoke, is higher than in those who don't use oral contraceptives.

Smoking and the Pill. In terms of the risk of developing cardiovascular problems, this combination is particularly deleterious. In fact, the Food and Drug Administration has issued new warnings about the debilitating effects of smoking while using oral contraceptives. Since April 1978, the FDA has required that oral contraceptive labels and information leaflets for patients carry this warning: "Cigarette smoking increases the risk of serious cardiovascular side effects from oral contraceptive use. The risk increases with age and with heavy smoking (fifteen or more cigarettes a day) and is quite marked in women over 35 years of age. Women who use oral contraceptives should be strongly advised not to smoke."

Other studies have also confirmed the risk of developing a cardiovascular problem for women who smoke cigarettes and take oral contraceptives. For example, the results of a study published in 1978 showed that there was a dose-response relationship involving smoking in women who had a heart attack before the age of 50. In fact, from this study the investigators estimated that women who smoke 35 or more cigarettes per day have a rate of heart attack that is twenty times higher than among women who have never smoked.

Hypertension. Most studies show that practically all women experience some elevation in blood pressure as a result of taking oral contraceptives, but the long-term effects of this rise in blood pressure are unknown. Therefore, physicians often encourage women on birth control pills to have their blood pressure checked frequently. Generally, the rise in blood pressure does not reach a level that is considered "hypertensive," but it is an increase, nonetheless, and in some cases, the level of blood pressure can rise high enough to indicate the need for discontinuation of the Pill.

Stroke. The incidence of stroke among young women taking oral contraceptives has been researched by several groups. Reports show that the use of oral contraceptives—even when other cardiovascular factors such as cigarette smoking and high blood pressure are absent—significantly increases the relative risk of stroke.

Finally, one of the most recent studies, reported in late 1980, should be discussed in detail, because of its noteworthy findings. It was conducted by the Kaiser-Permarente Medical Center, Walnut Creek, Calif. From 1969 to 1977, 16,638 women were observed to determine the relationship between taking oral contraceptives and the incidence of coronary heart disease, cerebrovascular disease and diseases of arteries and veins. The role of smoking, taking oral contraceptives and the incidence of the diseases just cited were also investigated. The findings of this study were striking, and in marked contrast to the results of numerous other studies, some of which we have just reviewed here. In this study, no significant differences were found in the mortality rates, cause-specific or overall, between women who never used oral contraceptives and those who did. These investigators concluded that there was no definitive evidence of an increased risk of death from cardiovascular diseases in users of oral contraceptives, compared to non-users.

Although its findings contrast sharply with the results of other studies, this study should not be considered the "last word" either. For the safest, most effective use of oral contraceptives, you should see your physician regularly and report any complaints or symptoms to him.

Diabetes. Use of the Pill can precipitate the onset of this disease in women who are predisposed to it. In women with known diabetes, generally, the Pill should be avoided because the diabetes itself poses an increased risk for the development of coronary heart disease.

No one would argue that the Pill is a very effective, convenient contraception method involving little risk in absolute terms. But every woman on the Pill should be checked routinely for blood pressure changes; any other symptoms or signs, such as headache, dizziness, and palpitations, should be reported to a physician immediately. Women who already have one or more cardiovascular risk factors, such as high blood pressure, diabetes, or cigarette smoking, should opt for another contraceptive. Women over 35 should also find alternate contraceptive means.

Pregnancy in Women with Healthy Hearts

The female body undergoes a wide range of physical changes throughout the course of pregnancy. The most obvious is simple weight gain, but even this normal change affects the heart. As the fetus develops, its nutritional needs and oxygen requirements increase. Consequently, a pregnant woman's heart rate increases progressively throughout pregnancy, generally reaching a peak that is about fifteen beats per minute above nonpregnant level.

For most women, however, such changes do not cause any problems. In fact, with a proper diet and exercise program, the average woman has little, if any, difficulty in meeting the increased physiological demands of the growing fetus. Fortunately, this extra workload is easily managed by most women and there aren't any ill effects upon the mother's heart. Generally, the maternal heart and circulation return to normal patterns about two weeks after childbirth. There are other women, however, who may already have heart disease or a history of heart disease; for them, special instructions and care are required.

Preparing for pregnancy. Whether you have heart disease or not, your doctor will want to know all of your medical history and, in particular, whether or not you or any family member has had any type of cardiovascular disease. Be prepared to provide as much information as possible regarding your family medical history.

Your diet and any medications you take should be supervised by your physician. Furthermore, any medicinal products you buy in the supermarket or drug store, including aspirin, cold remedies, antacids, and mild sedatives, should be considered drugs, and you should let your physician know if and when you take any such medication.

Exercise is also important, and an appropriate regimen will be recommended for you. Today, many women continue to swim, play tennis—even jog—right through the ninth month! Cigarette smoking is definitely out, and recent evidence also suggests that even moderate alcohol intake may be harmful to the fetus. Consult your physician for specific instructions.

Pregnancy in Women with Heart Disease

The two most common classes of cardiac disorders in women of childbearing age today are congenital heart disease and valvular heart disease (the latter most commonly involves the mitral and aortic valves). In each case, you should discuss childbearing with your physician. For some women, the risk may be minimal; for others, surgery may be recommended prior to a pregnancy to correct defects.

Although pregnancy is a normal physiological condition in a female, her body does undergo many changes to adapt to this altered state. For example, circulatory needs increase in order to supply nutrients to the fetus; in a woman with a diseased heart, however, cardiac failure may develop, since her diseased heart cannot meet the increased demands placed upon it by the state of pregnancy. As such, hospitalization and special treatment may be required.

In general, the advances in cardiac surgery now make it possible for many women with congenital heart defects to have these lesions corrected if necessary; thus, a normal, uneventful pregnancy is possible. In other cases, however, careful evaluation must precede decisions regarding pregnancy.

Valvular and congenital heart disease. The wisdom and safety of pregnancy in the presence of these problems is determined by their severity. Pregnancy may not be an undue stress on the minimially impaired heart; however, in the presence of more severe disease, pregnancy may be contraindicated unless prior surgical correction, if possible, of the cardiac defect is carried out. It is important to understand that cardiac disease which may cause no major symptomatology in the non-pregnant woman can still pose a high risk of heart failure and its consequences to mother and fetus under the increased burdens of pregnancy, and particularly during the delivery process, when the stress on the heart is greatest. Each woman with cardiac disease must be evaluated individually in terms of the risks of pregnancy and its management. In many situations, joint consultation by an obstetrician and cardiologist provides the best guidance.

Hypertension. This common cardiovascular disorder rarely is a contraindication for pregnancy unless it has been unresponsive to drug therapy. However, most hypertensive pregnant women require special care throughout their pregnancy because the drugs needed to control blood pressure can have adverse effects on the fetus. A hypertensive woman should consult her physician about pregnancy before making a final decision.

Toxemia of pregnancy. This condition, which consists of rapid development of high blood pressure, edema, and impaired kidney function, may develop in women with normal hearts—with previously normal blood pressure—as well as in pregnant women with known histories of hypertension. Toxemia usually develops late in the pregnancy—often after the thirty-second week. It affects about 7 percent of all pregnant women, and is more common in women with diabetes, pre-existing renal disease, and twin pregnancies. Toxemia is also referred to as *eclampsia* (from the Greek *eclampsis*, meaning "a sudden flash"). The onset of this condition is insidious but progressive. Typically, the edema and high blood pressure develop rapidly—abdominal pains, headaches, visual disturbances, nausea, and vomiting are also common, and indicate progressive involvement. In severe cases, convulsions and coma may result.

The cause of eclampsia is unknown. In mild cases, simple treatments, such as rest, sedation, and a low-sodium diet, are usually effective. In more severe cases, hospitalization and intensive medical therapy are required.

Coronary artery disease. Although angina and heart attacks are rare in women of childbearing age, any woman who has a history of ischemic heart disease must be monitored very carefully while she is pregnant. Each patient must be evaluated individually. For some women with coronary artery disease, a pregnancy may not be an undue strain, but childbearing may be contraindicated for others.

Your Heart and the Menopause

It is interesting to note that women seem to be "protected" from the development of coronary heart disease throughout their premenopausal years. This

"immunity" has, in part, been attributed to the amount of estrogen circula-
ting in the blood. On the other hand, estrogens have also been implicated in
contributing to the occurrence of stroke and heart attack in young women who
take oral contraceptives containing them and in postmenopausal women
who take them as replacement therapy. Is it possible that the same hormones
can both protect you and predispose you to heart disease?

Again, one of the most comprehensive surveys of the incidence of coronary
heart disease to include women is the Framingham Heart Study. Among 2,873
women whose histories were followed for twenty-four years, researchers
found that no premenopausal woman developed a myocardial infarction or
died of coronary heart disease, but that such events were not uncommon in
postmenopausal women. In fact, the researchers noted, among the age groups
aged 45 to 49 and 50 to 54, incidence rates in menopausal and postmenopausal intervals were more than double those in premenopausal intervals,
whether menopause was natural or surgical. The researchers also observed
that postmenopausal women on estrogen replacement therapy had a doubled
risk of coronary heart disease.

14

Heart Disease in Children

As any parent of a child with heart disease can tell you, cardiovascular disorders are not confined to adults. Most of us realize that cardiovascular disease is a serious medical problem, no matter when it is detected, so we would agree that cardiovascular problems take on a special significance when they occur in childhood. Happily, however, the prognosis today for most children with heart disease is a good one.

For example, just twenty years ago the prognosis for a "blue baby" (clinically referred to as "cyanotic," due to inadequate oxygen in the blood), or a baby with a "hole in his heart," was ominous. Now, new developments in diagnostic procedures, refined surgical techniques, and the introduction and use of additional drugs have helped to reverse these prognoses in the majority of cases.

Fortunately, physicians are also better equipped today to prevent as well as treat rheumatic fever, formerly a major cause of heart damage in children. In this chapter, we will discuss these diagnoses, as well as "innocent" heart murmurs (murmurs that raise the possibility of disease but actually are not associated with any abnormality of the heart), and tell you what treatments are available for each.

CONGENITAL HEART DEFECTS

Incidence. Overall, the American Heart Association recognizes thirty-five types of congenital heart defects affecting approximately 25,000 babies born each year. The American Heart Association's 1981 "Heart Facts" booklet listed an estimated post-natal mortality from congenital heart defects in 1978 at 6,500. It is hoped that this number will continue to be reduced, as more medical gains are made.

Approximately 100,000 children are afflicted with rheumatic heart disease,

196

but due to effective antibiotics, the mortality rate of this disease has dropped off sharply in young persons aged 5 to 24. The prevalence of heart murmurs and high blood pressure in children is unknown, although hypertension has been detected even in infants.

An infant may be born with any one of the thirty-five types of congenital heart defects recognized by the AHA, but those discussed in the following pages are the most common. In almost every case, the cause is not known, although the mother's having German measles during the first three months of pregnancy (when the fetal heart is being formed) can adversely affect the development of an infant's heart. Each of the seven disorders listed here may be treated surgically. In some cases, such as patent ductus arteriosus, drugs may be used instead or, as in ventricular septal defect, the "hole" in the heart may close spontaneously.

In most cases in which surgery is indicated, the procedure is delayed, if conditions allow, until the child has gained adequate size and strength, to minimize operative risk. However, when surgery is elective, it is also preferable, for psychological reasons, to perform it before the child enters school. Thus, the optimal time for operation is viewed as between the ages of four and five. Of course, if the cardiac defect is life-threatening, surgery is performed as indicated, even in newborn infants. In some instances, an operation to provide temporary relief may be carried out in infants too small to undergo complete correction of a defect. The definitive surgical procedure can then be done later, at age four or five.

Transposition of the great arteries. In this disorder, as the name implies, the "great arteries," the aorta and the pulmonary artery, are transposed. Thus the aorta, instead of receiving blood from the left ventricle, receives unoxygenated blood from the right ventricle, and this blood circulates throughout the body. The pulmonary artery normally recycles oxygenated blood back to the lungs. However, in "transposition," the pulmonary artery receives oxygenated blood from the lungs and then needlessly carries this oxygenated blood *back* to the lungs. Babies born with this defect will only survive if they have another defect present, such as a "shunt" that allows the passage of oxygenated blood to the body and unoxygenated blood to the lungs.

Coarctation of the aorta. This means the aorta is narrowed or constricted (this can occur during fetal development). This constriction results in an obstruction of blood flow. In mild cases, this defect may not be detected until adulthood. In more severe cases, it may be treated with drugs, or surgery may be performed to excise (remove) the coarctation area.

Patent ductus arteriosus. This was the first congenital heart defect to be corrected surgically. Today, approximately 15,000 infants per year are born with this condition. In normal babies, the ductus arteriosus, which is a vital structure throughout intrauterine life, closes within the first few hours after birth.

(The ductus connects the pulmonary artery with the aorta in the fetal blood system.) The ductus normally closes shortly after birth as the infant begins to utilize its lungs to take in oxygen. If the ductus remains "patent," or open, oxygenated blood is passed from the aorta to the pulmonary artery and then to the lungs—an abnormal route that results in cardiac and respiratory difficulties and, possibly, death. Fortunately, surgical techniques have vastly improved, and many infants with this type of defect have been saved. But a recent scientific breakthrough has also made it possible to correct this defect by drug therapy, where formerly only surgery was possible. Specifically, indomethicin, a drug which has been used for some time for arthritis, may be given to neonates with a patent ductus to induce closure. The drug is administered via a tube that enters the stomach. In those circumstances in which the physician may *want* the ductus to remain patent to compensate for an associated cardiac defect (obstruction of the aortic arch, for example), prostaglandins (naturally occurring substances in man that cause dilation of the vascular beds) may be given, since this drug can inhibit closure of the ductus. (See Figure 14.1.)

Ventricular septal defect. This common congenital heart lesion is sometimes referred to as a "hole in the heart." In effect, there is an opening in the septum (wall) that separates the left and right ventricles. This creates an abnormal route of blood flow between the ventricles, which can result in congestive heart failure with its symptoms and complications. Small septal defects may close spontaneously; in other instances, palliative and/or corrective surgery is needed.

Atrial septal defect. This opening or "hole in the heart" is located in the tissue separating the two atria and it allows some oxygenated blood to flow from the left atrium into the right atrium, and then to the right ventricle and lungs. Blood that has already been through the lungs is *returned* to the lungs—along with blood from other parts of the body—instead of being pumped through the left ventricle and out the aorta. Thus, the workload of the right side of the heart is increased and there is excessive blood flow to the lungs. Children with this defect may be asymptomatic until adulthood. Surgical correction is carried out in childhood or adulthood, depending on the time of detection, the severity of the lesion, and any complications. Sometimes, the large "holes" are patched with plastic, such as Teflon®. This type of surgery is usually quite effective, the risk is low, and the prognosis excellent!

Pulmonic stenosis. This is caused by a deformed pulmonic valve that does not open sufficiently, causing obstruction to outflow of blood from the right ventricle; ultimately the workload of the right ventricle is increased so much that it can fail and signs of heart failure may develop. Very mild cases may go untreated, but, in others, the valve must be opened surgically. Again, operative risk is very low, and the prognosis is generally excellent.

Figure 14.1: Patent Ductus Arteriosis

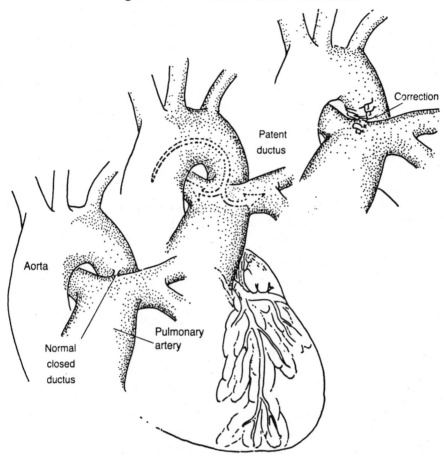

Patent ductus arteriosus resulting from failure of normal closure after birth of fetal connection between the aorta and pulmonary artery.

SOURCE: Illustration adapted from a drawing by Herbert R. Smith, from DeBakey, M., and Gotto, A., The Living Heart, N.Y., David McKay Co., 1977.

Tetralogy of Fallot. The most common form of cyanotic congenital heart disease in children, tetralogy of Fallot, actually consists of four defects: 1) ventricular septal defect, 2) pulmonic stenosis, 3) shunting of unoxygenated blood from the right ventricle to the aorta to the body, 4) an abnormally positioned aorta. Symptoms and signs usually appear in the first few days or weeks and "blue spells" (due to increased amounts of unoxygenated blood flow to the body) can occur. This is the defect for which the term "blue baby" was originally coined. Dr. Helen Taussig gained renown for her work developing the first operations for "blue babies." (See Table 14.1.)

Specifically, physical growth may be retarded and clubbing of the fingers and toes is common. Children with this defect use a "squatting" position to relieve symptoms, because the squatting position reduces the flow of unoxygenated blood to the body.

Rheumatic heart disease. This is *not* a congenital disease; rather rheumatic heart disease results from acute rheumatic fever (ARF), which is caused by a preceding infection by the bacterium, *streptococcus*. The infection is usually of the throat ("strep throat"). Acute rhematic fever generally strikes youngsters between the ages of 5 and 15. (See Table 14.2, page 204.)

A small percentage of these streptococcus infections are followed within two to four weeks by ARF, which is an inflammation of connective tissues throughout the body. The most serious involvement is that of the heart valves which, in a small proportion of patients with ARF, suffer permanent damage and scarring. In some cases the inflammation of a heart valve following acute rheumatic fever may resolve and leave no significant damage. In others, significant damage may progress and result in severe heart disease. Rheumatic fever is a recurrent disease; in other words, it tends to occur again in victims who have had the disease once.

The most important approach to the problem of rheumatic heart disease is prevention or early treatment of the inciting factor in the chain of events leading to it. This consists of preventing or eradicating the streptococcal infection. Thus, antibiotics have played the most important role in the marked reduction of rheumatic heart disease in the U.S. in the past 35 years.

Prevention. Still, some children today continue to fall victim to this disease. Once children develop rheumatic fever, long-term penicillin (or other antibiotic therapy) is indicated, to protect them from streptococcal infections which can result in recurrences of acute rheumatic fever.

To prevent recurrent rheumatic fever, streptococcal infections must be properly diagnosed and treated. A strep throat is identified by a throat culture. Once it has been identified, antibiotics are given (the doctor may start this treatment before lab results are in). Of course, once drugs are prescribed, it is up to the parent to see to it that they are taken according to schedule. The purpose of giving the drugs around-the-clock is to keep a constant level of the antibiotic in your child's bloodstream to destroy the streptococcus. Even missing one dose causes the concentration of antibiotic in the blood to drop; thus, the streptococcus may survive.

Also, parents need to be alert to the signs and symptoms of strep throat, and seek medical help as soon as possible: fever, swollen neck glands, a red, inflamed throat and pus in the throat. A throat culture will determine whether or not the problem is caused by streptoccal infection.

(Text continues from page 202)

Table 14.1. Diagnosis and Treatment of Some Congenital Heart Diseases

Heart Defect	Diagnosis	Presenting Signs	Treatment
Ventricular septal defect	First weeks	Congestive heart failure (CHF)	Spontaneous closure of defect occurs in some patients; surgical closure necessary for large defects
Pulmonic valve stenosis	First weeks	CHF Cyanosis ("blue baby")	Direct surgical correction of severely stenotic valve (artificial valve not necessary)
Patent ductus arteriosus	First weeks	CHF	Surgery or drugs to close the open ductus
Atrial septal defect	Early childhood	Normally none in early childhood; major symptoms usually delayed	Surgical closure of large defect
Tetralogy of Fallot	Birth to 6 months	Cyanosis	Before age two, palliative surgery to reroute maldirected cardiac blood flow; after two years of age, complete repair
Coarctation of the aorta	First weeks	CHF	surgery to excise the area of coarctation
Transposition of the great arteries	First month	Cyanosis	Surgical or nonsurgical palliation (balloon septostomy) to reroute maldirected blood flow within the heart; or definitive surgery to correct the defects

*The ages listed here are applicable when the defects are severe; when the defects are less severe, onset of symptoms and diagnosis may be delayed until considerably later in life.

Although there is no "miracle cure" for rheumatic fever, a great deal can be done to prevent it. And while rheumatic fever *per se* is not contagious, the strep infection is—all the more reason to take your child to a physician as soon as symptoms appear.

A final word—most sore throats are viral, not streptococcal, in origin. Precise diagnosis can only be made by obtaining bacterial cultures.

Innocent Murmurs

Simply stated, "murmur" is a heart sound that is usually produced by abnormal patterns of blood flow in the heart or blood vessels. These are often, but not always, caused by structural abnormalities in the path of blood flow. A physician hears these murmurs with a stethoscope. All murmurs don't indicate a structural defect. Often, "innocent" or harmless heart murmurs occur in children between the ages of three and seven, and usually disappear in adolescence. These murmurs are called "innocent" or functional murmurs—they are not due to any abnormality in the heart and no drugs or restrictions are indicated. Children with functional murmurs can participate in all sports and leisure activities.

An "organic" murmur, on the other hand, requires attention. This means that a cardiac defect is present. However, these represent a minority of the heart murmurs heard in children. Organic and innocent murmurs usually can be distinguished by careful, skillful examination and associated findings the physician will seek from the history, physical exam, ECG, chest X-ray, echogram and other tests, if indicated. If a heart murmur is organic, a specific diagnosis can be established and proper therapy initiated.

High Blood Pressure

Blood pressure is measured in children, usually beginning at birth, just as it is in adults, and the causes of high blood pressure are also as varied (see Chapter 2). The prevalence of this problem is far less in children than in adults, but once detected, it warrants active therapy. To begin, most physicians recommend weight loss if indicated, restriction of salt intake, avoidance of oral contraceptives and other medications that might induce an elevation in blood pressure, and avoidance of smoking.

Treatment is similar to that prescribed for adults, although some drugs may be omitted from the regimen, since they are not indicated for children.

Preventing Heart Disease in Childhood

Today, more and more attention is being focused on the role of diet and other risk factors in childhood in the development of coronary heart disease. In two separate studies in fact, each involving autopsies of men in their twenties, killed in Korea and in Vietnam, a considerable amount of coronary artery atherosclerosis was present, suggesting that this insidious disease process actually begins in childhood.

Although doctors will continue to debate the precise role of diet for some time to come, most agree with the following guidelines:

- help your child maintain normal weight

- don't allow smoking

- reduce the intake of foods high in cholesterol and saturated fats

- encourage daily exercise

- if there is a history of cardiovascular disease in the family (stroke, heart attack, high blood pressure, diabetes, etc.), have your child checked periodically for evidence of coronary risk factors (high cholesterol, high blood pressure) and for signs of developing cardiovascular problems

Living with a Child Who Has Heart Disease

Confronted with a child who has a heart defect or heart disease, virtually every parent subsequently experiences feelings of guilt, overprotectiveness, and considerable concern—not only for the well-being of the sick child, but because of financial questions and siblings who demand their share of parental attention.

To begin with, family relationships often undergo certain changes which can be easier to cope with if you are aware of them. For example, a hospitalized neonate usually results in one or both parents making daily trips to the hospital. This in turn disrupts the daily routine of the other siblings, particularly if one is called upon to babysit for the younger brothers and sisters while you are away. Or, other relatives may be called in to help. This can be useful to you, but in such cases, parents should be alert to the effects these changes in home life have on their own relationship, as well as on their relationship to their other children.

To avoid as much stress as possible in these circumstances, it pays to remain alert to the following:

- signs that a sibling is feeling neglected, guilty (change of behavior in school or at home, sudden withdrawal)

- signs that your husband or wife is having difficulty expressing his or her feelings about a child born with a congenital heart defect (avoidance of the partner, little discussion of the problem, etc.)

Even when a child with an inborn heart defect has been treated successfully, however, some reactions may linger on. For example, feelings of anxiety,

(Text continues on page 205)

Table 14.2. Parents' Guidelines for Preventing and Coping with Rheumatic Fever

Prevention

Be on the alert for:

> Fever
> Swollen neck glands
> Red inflamed throat
> Pus in the throat
> Pain when swallowing

Take your child to a physician for a proper diagnosis if any of these symptoms appear.

Treatment

Always follow directions carefully.
Ten days of antibiotic treatment is typical.
Give the drugs *exactly* as prescribed.
Do not miss even a single dose.
Continue to give the drugs prescribed *even* if your child appears well.

Follow-up

Take your child in for another throat culture *after* treatment is concluded.
Do not send your child back to school until your physician gives his O.K.
Report any rise in temperature to doctor.
Watch for pain, stiffness, or redness in your child's joints (indicates inflammation).
Watch for other signs of illness (rash, sudden nausea, etc.).

(Text continued from page 203)

fear of the child dying, having difficulty disciplining the child as he or she grows older, and overprotectiveness and overindulgence are all common, as is anxiety concerning future children. Similarly, parents of children with organic heart defects or rheumatic heart disease go through these stages. In most cases, your doctor or specialized nurses can counsel you. If you need additional information or help however, your local Heart Association may be able to guide you to parent groups formed for the sole purpose of sharing their experiences of raising children with heart disease.

PART IV
How Your Doctor Detects Heart Disease

See It, Feel It, Hear It

In the past twenty years, medical scientists have made tremendous progress in the development of extremely specialized technological equipment designed to detect all types of heart disease. Now, diagnostic tests run the gamut from a simple electrocardiogram, commonly referred to as an "ECG," to highly sophisticated methods such as cardiac catheterization, cinearteriography, and radioisotope scans.

Fortunately, the heart is structured and functions in such a way that your doctor can literally "go at it" in several ways; for example, he can:

- Feel it (a physical examination).
- Hear it (through a stethoscope).
- See it directly (or with a chest X-ray).
- See it in action (through cardiac catheterization and angiography).
- See it in action indirectly (through printouts such as an ECG, a radioisotope scan, or echocardiogram).
- Analyze it (from blood specimens obtained to detect damage to the heart muscle caused by heart attack).

The tests your doctor selects will depend on several factors, such as your history, age, sex, and symptoms. Also, he may have a good idea of what the problem is based on your descriptions of pain or other symptoms, and those clues often guide him to the selection of a specific technique, say echocardiography.

Some of these tests are highly useful in some cases, but may yield little or no information in others. For example, echocardiography is an excellent tool used to detect mitral valve disease—specifically, *mitral stenosis*, or narrowing of the mitral valve. However, this same technique may provide little information about the presence of coronary artery disease.

Needless to say, very few patients are subjected to the entire battery of available tests. Usually, it's sufficient to have one or two tests performed. We know, however, that the equipment itself often appears intimidating, especially when the test has to be performed within a hospital, where you are apt to become rather anxious about the unknown. Unfortunately, it's also frequently true that, in a busy hospital, even your own doctor may suddenly seem distant to you: dressed in hospital green, mask on, orchestrating other masked individuals whom you've never seen before in a brightly lighted, sterile room, perhaps in preparation for your catheterization. This setting could frighten anyone, and if you do have to undergo a specialized test, chances are you are already anxious enough—to add the fear of a procedure simply because of uncertainty about what is involved is unnecessary. Once you understand what it's all about, you may be able to work with your doctor to care for your heart. Of course, each physician has his or her own pattern of puzzle-solving; our discussion provides a detailed explanation of the types of tests that may be used in their evaluations.

15
A Guide to Diagnostic Tests

Before any tests are ordered, your physician will want to obtain your complete medical history and perform a thorough physical examination. Based on the findings, a number of tests may be indicated. These diagnostic procedures are classified as noninvasive and invasive. In the following chapter, the importance of providing your physician with an accurate and detailed medical history is discussed, along with the indications for these tests, and what is involved with each.

THE BASICS: YOUR MEDICAL HISTORY AND THE PHYSICAL EXAM

Your medical history tells a lot about your health. It is your own personal story and, much like a fingerprint, it can be matched only to you. From the doctor's standpoint, the more detail you can bring to the story, the more he can help you. Here are some examples of the types of questions he will ask:

- Did either of your parents or grandparents, or any of your aunts or uncles, die of heart attack? A stroke?
- Do, or did, any of your relatives have high blood pressure?
- Does anyone in the family have diabetes?
- Do you smoke?

Your doctor may then progress to more personal questions—a social/medical history, so to speak. Some patients resent such intimate questions but, again, remember that it is easier for your doctor to help you once he has the whole picture. In our opinion, if your doctor seems hesitant to raise intimate questions with you, you should direct the interview that way yourself to demonstrate that you are willing to be as cooperative and helpful as possible.

QUESTIONS ASKED IN A MEDICAL/SOCIAL HISTORY

How much alcohol do you drink per day?
Do you have an sexual problems or complaints?
Are you happily married?
Do you enjoy spending time with your children?
Do you like your job and your co-workers?
Do you ever feel anxious or depressed?
Do you have nightmares?
Do you have trouble getting up in the morning?
Do you have trouble sleeping straight through the night?
Do you have difficulty falling asleep?
How is your appetite?
Have you been losing weight without trying?
Do you ever contemplate suicide?
Are you seeing any other physician or counselor right now?

Always inform your doctor when you are under the care of other physicians, including dentists, allergists, ophthalmologists, and psychotherapists. This is particularly important if you are taking any prescribed medications. Also, be sure to alert your physician to any and all drugs that you are taking, including all over-the-counter products such as cold tablets, sleep remedies, and cough medicines. Drugs can interact with foods, liquors, and other drugs and create problems for you, but your doctor can help you avoid hazards *providing* you give him adequate information.

THE IMPORTANCE OF REPORTING SYMPTOMS

A distinguished twentieth-century American cardiologist, Dr. James Herrick, once remarked that:

> The doctor may also learn more about the illness from the way the patient tells the story than from the story itself.

Ideally, you should give your physician an accurate description of all pain or discomfort that you have experienced or that you experience while under his care. If you begin to notice that you have some slight chest pain after eating, don't automatically assume it's indigestion. Indeed, it may be only that, but you should be alert to other symptoms that may be indicative of coronary heart disease. For instance, do you have mild chest pain after climbing stairs?; do you feel short of breath after a moderate walk?, and so on.

If you do have specific symptoms or complaints, your doctor will ask you to detail these thoroughly. How long have you had a certain symptom? What does it feel like? What precipitates it? How long does it last? What, if anything, relieves it? Your answers provide the clues that help your doctor decide whether or not any further investigation is necessary for a diagnosis.

For example, typical anginal pain is often described as a "pressing, squeezing tightness in the chest." However, in a minority of patients, the history does not provide adequate information on which to base a diagnosis of angina. In fact, a motley and confusing array of diseases may cause a person to clutch his chest in pain. Knowing this, your doctor must rule out heartburn, gallstones, disorders in the lungs (such as pulmonary embolism), arthritis of the joints of the breastbone and ribs, to name a few possibilities. Still, your medical history does give your doctor a good idea of your overall health, and your cardiovascular status, in particular. The next step, then, is the physical examination.

WHAT YOUR DOCTOR LEARNS FROM THE PHYSICAL EXAMINATION:

Inspection and Palpation of the Heart

As revealed by direct inspection of the front of the chest over the area of the heart, an abnormal location of the cardiac impulse—the normal movement of the chest wall produced by the heart's activity—may inform the physician that the heart is enlarged. Alteration of the cardiac impulse, as seen (and felt) on the chest, can indicate certain other abnormalities as well.

Your doctor can also use his sense of touch to examine, or palpate, your heart. Palpation of the heart provides information about the size of the left and right ventricles and about their function.

Ausculation of the Heart

If you place your ear against someone's chest, you will hear noises that sound like "lub-dub, lub-dub." These are the normal heart sounds. The "lub" sound marks the closure of the tricuspid and mitral valves. The "dub" sound marks the closure of the aortic and pulmonic valves after ventriclar contraction. The "lub-dub" combination frames the period of ventricular contraction. The ventricles relax in the period of time between one "lub-dub" and another.

A distinct series of "lub-dubs" without associated sounds is good evidence that your heart valves are opening and closing normally to allow blood to flow smoothly through them. A whooshing noise, however, usually indicates a murmur, which suggests the valves are either not opening or not closing properly.

In addition to the normal pattern of two heart sounds, your doctor may listen for a third, or even a fourth, sound. These sounds are lower in pitch than the easily audible "lub-dub." The third sound may be deemed normal in younger people, but both extra sounds may indicate cardiac trouble in adults. These are known as "gallops" because they sound like the pounding of horses' hooves.

The normal "lub-dub" may be altered in a variety of ways, by any one of a number of cardiac maladies which may produce extra sounds and murmurs. The combination of these abnormalities is frequently present in patterns that are characteristic of specific cardic diseases. These patterns help the skilled practitioner reach a diagnostic impression.

THE NONINVASIVE TECHNIQUES

The Conventional X-Ray

Chest X-rays can also provide helpful clues to the presence of some types of heart disease. By examining the shadows and silhouettes on the X-ray, a physician can see whether or not any of the chambers or large blood vessels of your heart are grossly larger or smaller than they should be.

THE ELECTROCARDIOGRAM: BASIC DIAGNOSTIC TOOL

By the time you are 50 years old, your heart has beat approximately two billion times—an impressive work load! This steadfast beating depends on the spread of the wave of "electricity" from the sinoatrial, or SA, node (the heart's "pacemaker") to the ventricles. Not surprisingly, if you could follow and measure the movement of this electrical wave along your heart, you could learn a great deal about how well your heart is functioning. Your body tissues are fairly good conductors of electricity; if they were not, you would not be susceptible to electrical shock. Your doctor can measure the rise and fall of electrical potential in your heart by hooking up a series of electrical sensors to your skin.

The "Resting" Electrocardiogram

The electrocardiogram is the record produced by the electrocardiograph, a machine for which the name is derived from the wedding of three Greek words meaning "writing of heart electricity." Electrocardiography is safe, simple, and painless, despite its complicated appearance. A technician positions the electric sensors against your chest, arms, and legs, using a special paste to complete the connection, and secures the sensors snugly in place with tape. (This is referred to as the "resting" electrocardiogram because you are lying down while the test is done.) These sensors detect the electrical activity of your heart and transmit this information to paper strips called *electrocardiographic strips*. (See Figure 15.1.)

The Sensors. Specifically, a sensor, or lead, on one part of your body picks up

Figure 15.1 Lead Arrangement of the Standard Electrocardiogram

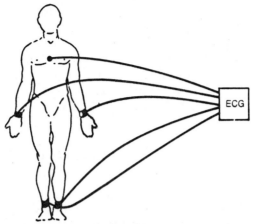

The spread of electrical activity through your heart is traced as a pattern of peaks and valleys on the electrocardiogram (ECG). Each wave corresponds to a different event in the cardiac cycle.

what is going on in one area of your heart; the information it provides differs from the information another sensor on any other part of your body yields. For example, if you worked for a television station and you wanted to get good coverage of a baseball game, you would want to provide coverage of the game from different parts of the playing field. Thus, you might station one cameraman behind home plate, one at each of the bases, and so on. With these various units in place, you would probably ensure your audience a "total" view of the action. In a similar way, the twelve ECG leads provide total coverage of your heart's activity.

All of the electrical impulses from your heart are traced on a narrow strip of paper, the electrocardiogram, that unfolds from inside the electrocardiograph machine. The paper is divided into small squares. The vertical and horizontal lines are one millimeter apart. A rise or fall in the vertical direction represents a rise or fall in the electrical potential of your heart. Movement in a horizontal direction reveals the amount of time it takes the electrical activity to travel through your heart.

The normal electrocardiogram shows five "waves," conveniently labeled P, Q, R, S, and T. The first is the *P wave*, which represents the spread of electrical activity (depolarization) through the atria. The spread of electrical activity through the ventricles is represented by the *Q–R–S complex*. The *T wave*, fifth and last, represents repolarization, or electrical resetting of the ventricles, in preparation for the next wave of electrical activity.

To decipher an electrocardiogram, a doctor evaluates the wave forms and intervals on the tracing. For example, appearance of Q waves where they normally are not present may mean that a previous heart attack has damaged some of the muscle tissue of the ventricles. Abnormalities in the ST segment (that portion of the ECG strip between the end of the Q–R–S complex and the start of the *T wave)* also may suggest that an insufficient amount of blood is reaching the heart muscle, which is the basic problem in coronary arteroschlerotic disease. Similarly, when a myocardial infarction, or heart attack, occurs, the ECG is affected in several ways:

- the *T waves* become inverted, or appear unusually tall;
- the ST segment initially is elevated, and then may become depressed;
- *Q waves* appear where they normally are not present.

  A *Q wave* of sufficient size and in a lead in which it is normally absent strongly suggests necrosis or dead myocardial cells; the ST changes reveal injured muscle, and the inverted *T wave* indicates ischemia (inadequate oxygen supply).

The electrocardiogram can also reveal abnormalities of heart rhythm—arrhythmias. The pattern that appears on the ECG depends on the type of rhythm disturbance present. For instance, ventricular fibrillation, a lethal arrhythmia, produces bizarre, disorganized pattern of ECG waves.

The Stress Test

A resting electrocardiogram may show telltale abnormalities, but it can look perfectly normal even if coronary artery disease is present. For this reason, your doctor may decide to see how your heart functions when it is subjected to extra work. To obtain this information, an electrocardiogram is taken while you are exercising actively, a procedure that is called "stress exercise testing."

The Treadmill Test. Briefly, you start off at a stroll on the treadmill, heading ever so slightly uphill. For ten or fifteen minutes, your doctor gradually steps up the pace of the treadmill (therefore, your pace as well) and makes the tilt of the treadmill a little steeper. By the end of ten minutes, if you can reach this level, you may be trotting along at a speed of five and a half miles per hour. While your cardiovascular system "shifts gears" in response to this stress, and you begin to take in more oxygen, your doctor monitors your pulse and blood pressure, and watches the action on the electrocardiogram. The electrocardiogram is constantly displayed on an oscilloscope, as well as printed out on paper every minute. If you feel short of breath, become tired, or feel any pain, the doctor will stop the test knowing that you have reached your exercise limit.

A stress ECG can provide clues regarding the presence and severity of coronary artery disease. Does ST segment abnormality occur? Is it early in the course of exercising or late in the test? An ST segment that plunges before one builds up much speed on the treadmill may signal extensive heart disease. (See Figure 15.2.) The findings on the stress ECG may relate to the risk of future heart attack. Often, the greater the ECG abnormalities, the greater the risk.

Since the whole point of stress testing is to coax coronary heart disease out into the open, you are probably wondering whether this troubleshooter test, itself, may spark some actual trouble. In other words, do people get heart attacks on the treadmill? Fortunately, this is exceedingly rare. In fact, the safety of the technique is one of the many reasons doctors rely on it to help them establish a diagnosis of coronary heart disease.

Figure 15.2: ECG Pattern for Normal Heart and Heart Attack Victim

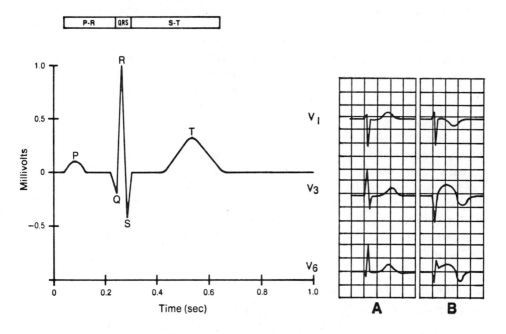

The figure on the left shows a normal ECG pattern. The most prominent features are the P waves, the QRS complex and the T wave. The figure on the right shows (Column A), normal ECG patterns, and Column B shows typical ECG findings of myocardial infarction.

You should be aware that considerable controversy surrounds this test in certain circumstances. In people with clinical evidence of coronary heart disease, the test can provide further objective evidence of the presence and extent of the problem. However, it is far from foolproof and can be normal in patients with coronary artery disease (false negative result) and indicate evidence of coronary artery disease where there is none (false positive result). In patients with known CAD it is basically reliable. False negative results are also a problem. Thus, the exercise test must always be evaluated in light of the patient's complete medical background, and it can be utilized as but one factor in reaching diagnostic conclusions. Both physicians and patients need to remain aware of the possibility of misleading results.

THE TWENTY-FOUR-HOUR ECG: HOLTER MONITORING

The exercise test is a good way to evaluate the heart's response to stress, but there are two obvious drawbacks. One is that the stress is artificial and both the resting and stress ECGs follow only a small fraction of the 150,000 pumping cycles your heart goes through in a single day. Furthermore, you cannot go through twenty-four hours hitched to a cumbersome electrocardiograph machine to learn how your heart functions during a typical day. One solution to this dilemma makes use of an ingenious instrument—the Holter monitor. This device weighs little more than an average camera, and its tiny electrodes can easily be attached to your chest while the boxlike Holter monitor is attached to your belt. The Holter monitor can record a continuous tape of your electrocardiogram twenty-four hours, while you pursue your usual activities, such as walking, working, sex, sports, eating, sleeping, laughing, and crying. Later, the Holter recording is analyzed by means of a special highspeed scanning device to zero in on possible ECG abnormalities. If any abnormalities appear, your doctor will attempt to match these with any symptoms or changes in an activities diary that you keep during the monitoring period.

ECHOCARDIOGRAPHY:

THE USE OF SOUND TO DETECT HEART DISEASE

Imagine for a moment a bat flying through a dark four-chambered cave with narrow, winding passageways and a series of gates that open and close automatically. Luckily, the bat is equipped with its own natural ultrasound system, which emits high-pitched sound waves, inaudible to the human ear, that zoom along until they strike an object, such as the wall of a cave or a gate, from which the sound waves bounce, or echo, directly back to the bat. The strength of the echo and the time it takes to come back tell the bat what lies ahead—the size of the cave chambers, the thickness of the walls, and their distance away. Equipped with this ultrasound system, the "blind" bat is able to navigate through his surroundings rather easily.

Like bats (and dolphins, whales, and porpoises), a physician can use ultrasound to evaluate your cardial status, thereby eliminating some of the guesswork in diagnosis.

Essentially, ultrasound waves give your doctor a direct picture of the size of the heart chambers and valves and the movement of these structures as the heart relaxes, fills, and contracts. Thus, the reporting of heart echoes, *echocardiography*, sizes up both heart form and heart function, which makes it a unique diagnostic tool, indeed. Briefly, here is how it works. (See Figure 15.3.)

At the heart of the echo system is the *transducer*, a two-inch-long metal cylinder which contains a special crystal. Actually, you rely on transducers every day in microphones, speakers, and telephones to convert the sound of your

Figure 15.3: How Echocardiography Works

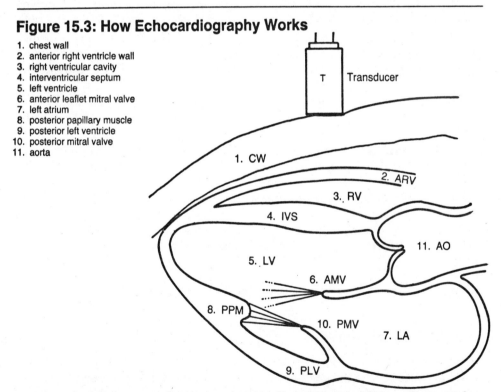

1. chest wall
2. anterior right ventricle wall
3. right ventricular cavity
4. interventricular septum
5. left ventricle
6. anterior leaflet mitral valve
7. left atrium
8. posterior papillary muscle
9. posterior left ventricle
10. posterior mitral valve
11. aorta

The transducer is placed on the chest wall and "catches" the echoes and "translates" them into electrical impulses. These electrical impulses appear as bright "blips" on a screen to which the transducer is connected.

voice into electric signals that travel over a wire and are "changed back" to sound again at the other end. Similarly, when a transducer is placed on your chest to obtain an echocardiogram, one ultrasonic pulse after another is directed at your heart. (This is a harmless, painless procedure.)

As the pulse reaches a layer of tissue, some of the ultrasound energy keeps on going and some bounces, or echoes, back to the transducer. The pattern of the echoes will vary, depending on whether the pulse is passing through a solid substance (like muscle), or a liquid (like blood), or an empty space. For this reason, a single pulse will send back many separate echoes. In between pulses, the special crystal mentioned earlier "catches" the echoes and "translates" them into electrical impulses. These electrical impulses show up as bright blips on the screen to which the transducer is connected. This is an *oscilloscope*. (See Figure 15.4.) Time-motion wave forms related to the structure of the heart are displayed on it. Particular areas of the heart can be examined by directing the transducers at them from one side of the chest.

To begin, the doctor aims the transducer at the space between the patient's ribs on the left side of the breastbone. Echoes appear on the tracing as wave forms made up of small, rounded valleys and hills. The doctor "reads" or interprets these valleys and hills as the movements produced by cardiac chambers and valve activity. The depth of the dark areas reveals the size of the right and left ventricles.

To record the echo signals from other heart structures, the angle of the transducer is shifted. Often, it is focused on the mitral valve because its strong jagged peaks and dips form a clear *M*-shaped landmark on the echocardiogram. The upswings of the *M* indicate that the valve is opening; the downswings reveal that it is closing. Alteration of the characteristic normal pattern may indicate the presence of mitral valve disease. The echocardiogram can also provide a picture of other disorders of the heart involving the valves, muscle, or other structures. Indeed, second to electrocardiography, the echocardiogram is probably the most widely used test in the diagnosis of certain cardiovascular diseases today.

THE INVASIVE TECHNIQUES

Cardiac Catheterization

Cardiac catheterization involves evaluation of the heart by direct measurements made within the cardiac chambers. It is a reconnaissance method; the heart is evaluated from direct data obtained by use of a catheter, a small, soft hollow tube, inserted into an artery or vein, which the physician then directs into any one of the four heart chambers. The catheter is introduced through an

Figure 15.4: Adaptation of the Cathode Ray Oscilloscope to Electrocardiographic Monitoring

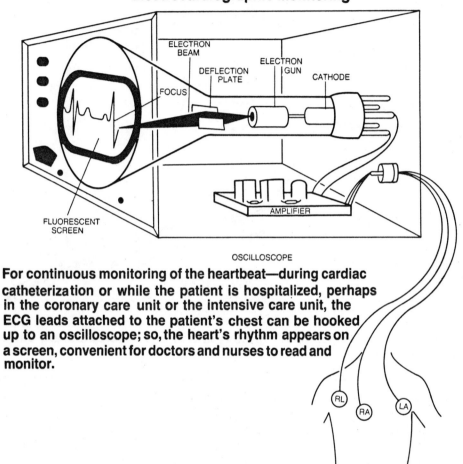

For continuous monitoring of the heartbeat—during cardiac catheterization or while the patient is hospitalized, perhaps in the coronary care unit or the intensive care unit, the ECG leads attached to the patient's chest can be hooked up to an oscilloscope; so, the heart's rhythm appears on a screen, convenient for doctors and nurses to read and monitor.

artery or vein in the leg or the arm and is then manipulated along the course of the vessel directly into the heart.

Catheterization allows a number of procedures to be performed that provide various types of information regarding the anatomy and function of the heart. For example, pressures within the chambers of the heart can be obtained only through direct assessment with a catheter. It is connected to a pressure-measuring device outside the body; thus, it is possible to measure and record pressures inside the heart. These pressure measurements from inside the heart provide important information regarding the function of each chamber. (See Figure 15.5.)

Figure 15.5: Coronary Arteriography

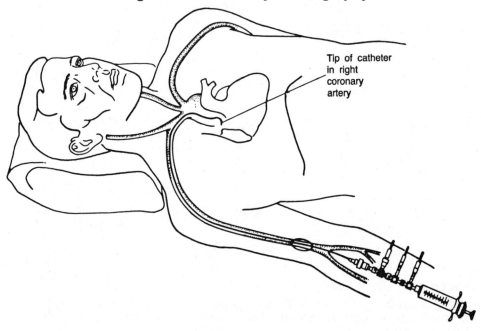

Tip of catheter
in right
coronary
artery

The catheter is inserted through an artery or vein and directed into any one of the heart's chambers.

Chemical substances can also be injected into the heart, and their concentration in the blood, which is pumped out of the heart, can then be measured by sensitive measuring devices. The alteration in concentration is related to the rapidity with which the blood is pumped, thereby providing an accurate measurement of the amount of blood being pumped by the heart per unit of time. In this manner, the cardiac output (liters per minute of blood pumped) can be determined.

When radiopaque dyes are injected into the heart, a record of images produced by the radiopaque dye can be obtained on either separate X-ray films (serial-film angiography) or X-ray motion pictures (cineangiography). To obtain these films, the patient is positioned on a table beneath a large cylinder that holds the X-ray camera and takes X-ray movies of the heart in action. These records provide outlines of the dynamic anatomy of the heart, that is, the changing shape of the heart with each beat; the amount, the degree, and type of movement of heart muscle with each beat; and the course of the blood within the heart during each contraction. Thus, the contractile movements of heart muscle can be assessed in terms of their adequacy, and any abnormalities can be quantitated and localized. Furthermore, abnormal pathways of blood, such as those that occur with congenital "holes in the heart" or leaky valves, can be detected. Data that are obtained from pressure measurements involve the detection of valves that are too tight or stenotic.

The coronary arteries can also be evaluated by directing dye into them via special catheters, which may be positioned at the openings of the coronary arteries. Then, X-ray motion pictures or large separate X-ray films are taken as the dye is injected into the artery. This enables the physician to obtain anatomic records of the patency (openness), or narrowing of the coronary arteries.

Needless to say, every person who complains of a potential cardiac symptom does not undergo cardiac catheterization. This diagnostic test is usually performed for one of the following reasons:

> 1. Cardiac catheterization is used to identify precisely a cardiac abnormality, and quantitate the severity of disease in patients in whom serious and incapacitating heart symptoms are present. Such identification and quantitation of an abnormality is a critical step in determining overall management of the patient. For example, this information will help the physician decide whether or not surgery is needed.

> 2. This test is indicated for some patients who do not necessarily have incapacitating symptoms, but in whom there are clinical signs and symptoms suggestive of the presence of a disorder which, if not treated early, could result in irreversible and life-threatening cardiac damage in the future. Identification of the presence of such a disease by catheterization is frequently an indication for definitive surgical correction prior to the onset of serious symptoms. In other instances, patients require cardiac catheterization because of symptoms such as dizziness and chest pain which, while not typically cardiac, may be related to heart disease and are producing significant impairment of the patient's ability to function. The diagnostic evaluation in these patients may involve cardiac catheterization, which can exclude or include the presence of cardiac disease as part of the patient's problem.

> 3. Cardiac catheterization is performed only after a variety of noninvasive cardiac studies have been performed that do not yield the definitive information required. For many cardiac problems, catheterization is the most precise and definitive method of evaluation. However, some of the newer, noninvasive studies, such as radioisotope scanning and echocardiography, have equaled, or even surpassed, cardiac catheterization for evaluation of certain cardiac problems.

Although cardiac catheterization itself generally only takes between thirty minutes and four hours to perform, (usually less than two hours, depending on the amount of information that is required, and the ease with which it can be obtained), it does require hospitalization. The patient usually comes in one day prior to the procedure, and certain preliminary studies, such as routine laboratory blood tests, are made to ensure that the patient is in a stable condition and has had no acute overt or occult cardiac or systemic illness.

The patient is taken to the catheterization laboratory after having been in the fasting state (no food or water) for eight or more hours prior to the test. A mild tranquilizer or analgesic (pain medication) is given prior to the patient's arrival in the catheterization laboratory, but the patient is conscious throughout the procedure. The patient *must be conscious* because his voluntary cooperation may be required at times during the procedure—for example, he may be asked to take a breath or to cough—and general anesthesia cannot be justified for a procedure such as catheterization. Catheterization generally involves only minor discomfort, frequently considerably less painful than what one experiences during dental work.

The catheterization laboratory is run as efficiently as any operating room. All personnel involved in the procedure wear surgical gowns, caps, masks, and gloves. The procedure is usually performed by two or more physicians, two technicians, and a special nurse. (The personnel present may vary from hospital to hospital, but usually three support staff members are required to assist the two physicians.) The patient is placed on a special table above which is a suspended fluoroscopy unit containing a movie camera. Antiseptic material is applied to the skin in areas where the catheter will be inserted to render them sterile. The patient is then draped, leaving the skin areas involving the procedure exposed. Electrocardiographic electrodes are also placed on the patient, so a continuous record of his electrocardiogram can be obtained on a monitor in full view of the physicians. Finally, an intravenous catheter is placed in the right arm to provide ready access for the administration of any medications or materials required during the procedure, and a special, short catheter is usually placed in an artery in the arm or leg to obtain a continuous record of the patient's blood pressure on a beat-to-beat basis.

Once in position, special chemicals can be injected into a cardiac chamber and blood withdrawn from an artery to measure the changing concentration of the chemical, thereby rendering quantitative information on cardiac output. Radiopaque dye can be injected into any of the chambers or vessels of the heart during simultaneous acquisition of X-ray motion pictures to identify the structures and any abnormalities in them, and determine the adequacy of the contractile motion of the right side of the heart.

Either right or left heart catheterization may be performed. Left heart catheterization provides information regarding the function and structure of the left side of the heart. The same information is obtained on the right side of the heart from the catheterization.

It is important to realize that, throughout this procedure, it is impossible to "feel" the catheter passing through the blood vessels or the heart. In most instances, the patient is lying comfortably on his back, and the physicians communicate with the patient throughout the procedure. In all but exceptional cases, patients on whom cardiac catheterization is performed are able to leave the hospital the day after the test is completed. Complications rarely develop, but any invasive procedure carries some risk. Your physician will explain these in detail to you. However, most patients have only a slight soreness where the catheter was inserted.

Scintigraphy: Radioisotope Scanning

Radioisotope scanning is a new, relatively simple diagnostic method that involves the use of radioisotopes and special equipment. It is used to help detect heart disease in adults and in children. Cardiac scanning is especially useful in detecting "hidden" cases of coronary artery disease, and, as stated earlier, this is significant, since, in approximately one-fifth of all patients with coronary heart disease, sudden death is the first "sign" of coronary heart disease. *Scintigraphy*, or nuclear scanning, (from Greek meaning "writing of sparks") enables a physician to locate tissue damage in the heart and to see just how the damage is affecting the function of the heart. The terms *scintigraphy or scintiscanning* are appropriate, since the images recorded on the screen resemble the patterns made by waving Fourth of July sparklers.

To obtain a *scintigram*, or scintigraphic picture, several simple steps are followed. First, a radioisotope (also called a radioactive tracer because its passage through the body can be traced with an external counter) is injected into a vein in the patient's arm. The radioisotope is carried along in the blood flowing through the heart. The pattern of distribution of the radioisotope in the heart is recorded by a special (scintillation) camera providing the needed diagnostic information.

Blood Tests for Heart Damage

Blood tests can be helpful in detecting the presence and the extent of damage to the heart muscle when the diagnosis of heart attack is considered. Essentially, blood is drawn, and tests are made to measure the level of certain enzymes in the blood. These enzymes are normally present in the blood, but the heart is especially rich in three different types: creatine phosphokinase (CPK), serum glutamic oxaloacetic transaminase (SGOT), and lactic dehydrogenase (LDH). When myocardial tissue is damaged, these three telltale enzymes leak into the bloodstream. Within six hours of a heart attack, the level of CPK in the blood rises, followed by a rise in SGOT. It may take twenty-four hours or more for LDH to rise after myocardial tissue damage due to a heart attack has occurred. Although an elevated level of LDH shows up late, this elevation lingers on, and may help a doctor establish a diagnosis of a heart attack in a person who has put off coming to the hospital following an episode of chest pain or shortness of breath. The degree of rise in these enzymes can correlate roughly with the extent of damage during a heart attack.

However, a rise in the level of these specific enzymes in the blood does not always indicate heart attack, since other organs of the body contain these enzymes, too. For example, damage to the central nervous system may result in release of CPK into the bloodstream. Thus, the results of enzyme levels must be integrated with the total clinical picture.

Is there a way to pinpoint the tissue or organ leaking an enzyme? Medical scientists have developed a means of accomplishing this aim. Although the same enzymes are present in different body tissues, it has been established that the forms of these enzymes vary somewhat from tissue to tissue. These different enzyme forms are isoenzymes—they are all made up of roughly the same chemical building blocks, but the building blocks are arranged in slightly different patterns. We now know that the isoenzyme MB CPK is most highly concentrated in the myocardium; thus, its appearance in the blood is a strong sign of recent damage to myocardial, or heart, tissue. Currently, investigators are trying to determine whether the amount of MB CPK detected in the blood is a reliable quantitative indicator of the actual extent of damage to the heart.

Blue Shield Keeps a Watchful Eye on the Value of Tests and Second Opinions

In 1978, the national Blue Shield Association advised its individual plans to discontinue routine payments for numerous surgical and diagnostic procedures. The new guidelines were issued to ensure that all tests performed on subscribers are "medically necessary" and in keeping with "quality medical care."

In another ruling, Blue Cross/Blue Shield has made it widely known that, before a subscriber undergoes surgery based on the recommendation of one physician alone, he or she may consult another doctor for a second opinion, and the cost of that visit will be covered.

Finally, we suggest that all those who undergo cardiac radioisotope scanning tests check to ascertain if they are eligible for reimbursement, since regulations governing this procedure vary from state to state.

PART V
Treatment for Diseased Hearts

Sorting Out Drug Therapies and Surgical Techniques

In the last twenty-five years, great gains have been made in the development of effective antihypertensive agents. Today, there are over fifty drugs available to treat hypertension. For many hypertensive patients, one pill a day is sufficient to control high blood pressure. In others, however, two or more pills—sometimes a combination of various types of drugs—may be needed to control high blood pressure effectively.

The class of drugs still most commonly used to relieve the pain of angina pectoris is called "nitrates." Whether these agents are taken in the form of a long-acting tablet, used in the form of topical ointment, or taken sublingually, the effect is the same: reduction of the workload of the heart to relieve the imbalance between its oxygen needs and supply. Beta-adrenergic blockers—atenolol, metoprolol, nadolol, pindolol and propranolol—are also used in the management of angina pectoris, and a new class of drugs—calcium antagonists, diltiazem, nifedipine and verapamil are now available to manage angina.

A wide variety of drugs is also available to treat cardiac arrhythmias. Some drugs such as atropine act to increase heart rate, whereas other drugs such as lidocaine act to abolish abnormal, extra heart beats.

Several classes of drugs—diuretics, vasodilators and digitalis—are used to manage another cardiac problem, congestive heart failure.

Finally, antibiotics, which are used to treat many types of infection, are also indicated in the treatment of cardiac infections.

Part V also discusses in detail aspects of the coronary care unit and various types of surgery available for the cardiac patient.

16
Drugs for Cardiovascular Disease

In this chapter, we discuss the drugs most commonly used to treat various cardiovascular diseases and disorders, such as hypertension, angina pectoris, arrhythmias, congestive heart failure, and infections of the myocardium, pericardium, and endocardium. As you will see in the pages that follow, certain classes of drugs, such as diuretics, are used in the treatment of hypertension *and* congestive heart failure. Similarly, propranolol is also used to treat both hypertension and certain arrhythmias. Whatever the case, if you are given medication for *any* problem, it is important for you to adhere to the schedule prescribed. In addition, you should always obtain the information that appears in the box.

Drugs for Hypertension

Once your doctor decides that drug therapy is necessary, you should understand that a lifetime commitment to treatment is necessary. You cannot take antihypertensive medication for several weeks or months and then discontinue it, thinking that your disease is under control. On the contrary, your blood pressure will probably creep up again within days if you stop taking your medication; thus, strict adherence to the regimen prescribed by your doctor is mandatory.

Although the exact cause of high blood pressure remains unknown in about 90 percent of patients, we do know that numerous mechanisms—neural, renal, and so on—are involved. Consequently, several types or classes of drugs have been developed; each group works at a different site to control high blood pressure. For example, the group called diuretics acts on the kidney; certain of these drugs act on *specific* sites within this organ to achieve their unique effects. Vasodilators affect the arteries.

227

In most hypertensive patients, the classic approach is to start off with a diuretic, commonly called the baseline, or "cornerstone," treatment. If, after a few weeks, blood pressure has not returned to normal, other drugs may be added to the diuretic. This is called the "stepped-care" approach to therapy. However, a physician may bypass the diuretic altogether and start a hypertensive patient on a beta blocker. Beta blockers and several other classes of drugs we will discuss here are also used to treat other forms of heart disease, including various arrhythmias and angina.

Essentially, there are four classes of antihypertensive drugs; diuretics, sympatholytics, vasodilators, and converting enzyme inhibitors.

Diuretics. This group may be broken down further; for example, diuretics, which are given to effect *diuresis* (elimination of water), may be mild, extremely potent, or potassium-sparing (they help eliminate sodium and water but "spare" or do not promote potassium loss). Their effects differ somewhat because they act on different sites in the kidney. Reduction of fluid and sodium from within the arterial system reduces the pressure in that system. (See Table 16.1 for a list of diuretics by trade and generic name.)

Sympatholytics. These agents interfere with neurohumoral circulatory control mechanisms; their ultimate action is to reduce the effect of the sympathetic nervous system on the heart and/or blood vessels, which will result in lower cardiac output (less blood pumped by the heart) and/or less constriction of vessels and a decrease in blood pressure. Like diuretics, this group of drugs can also be subdivided. Each subgroup of drugs within this class acts on a specific site within the sympathetic nervous system: central (the brain), peripheral (the ganglia or adrenergic nerve endings); central and peripheral; alpha and beta adrenergic receptors (the sites in end organs through which sympathetic nervous system stimuli are affected). (See Table 16.2.) Generally, these drugs are added to the basic diuretic; in some cases, two or more different types of drugs are selected to provide additive action. Smaller doses of each may be given because of the additive effects.

Vasodilators. These drugs also can be subdivided according to their specific sites of action within the arterial system. Some act in the arterial bed only, while other vasodilators affect the arterial and venous systems. Vasodilators do just that: they dilate or open up the arterioles—the smallest arteries, which account for the major component of resistance in the arterial system. Two drugs, hydralazine and diazoxide, primarily dilate the arterioles, while nitroprusside and prazosin dilate both arterioles and veins. Thus, blood pressure is lowered because the arterioles dilate and resistance to blood flow is reduced. The decreased resistance in the arterial system permits the heart to work at a lower blood pressure. (See Table 16.3.)

Other drugs. Recently, a new type of drug, an angiotensin converting enzyme inhibitor, was approved by the Food and Drug Administration for treatment in certain cases of hypertension. The only available drug in this class is captopril (generic name) or Capoten (the trade name). This drug acts to inhibit the formation of angiotensin, the most potent arterial constrictor produced in the body. The result is a lowering of blood pressure.

Finally, chronic high blood pressure is usually not directly related to "nerves;" as such, sedatives and tranquilizers are rarely used to treat high blood pressure. It is true, however, that emotional stress can aggravate hypertension.

Side effects. Slight side effects such as headache, rash, dry mouth, or diarrhea may occur with the use of antihypertensive drugs, but such mild effects usually pass within a few days. Other side effects, such as dizziness on standing up or interference with sexual function, can be more troublesome. Since there are so many antihypertensive medications available, most patients can be treated effectively with no or minimal adverse effects. Consult your physician for specific information. (See Table 16.4.)

Drugs for Angina Pectoris

Remember the fundamental cause of angina pectoris is an imbalance between the demand of oxygen by the heart muscle and the supply of oxygen that it receives from the blood passing through the coronary arteries, i.e. oxygen supply cannot meet demand because of inadequate blood flow. The most common cause of this inadequate blood supply is atherosclerotic narrowing of the coronary arteries. Treatment of angina is aimed at restoring a more favorable balance between myocardial oxygen supply and demand. This can be achieved (1) medically, by elimination of aggravating factors (strenuous activities, smoking cigarettes, high blood pressure, etc., and the use of a number of effective drugs; (2) surgically, by coronary artery bypass graft surgery; and (3) by percutaneous transluminal coronary angioplasty (PTCA). Drugs act to lower myocardial oxygen demand; surgery and PTCA act to increase oxygen supply.

Treatment of angina pectoris consists of a comprehensive approach, and may include some or all of the following:

- Appropriate activity level (avoidance of strenuous exertion but in some cases a program of mild physical exercise)
- Reduction of aggravating factors (emotional and physical stress, high blood pressure, anemia).
- Discontinuing smoking
- Weight loss, if appropriate
- Drug therapy—nitrates, beta-blockers, calcium antagonists
- Coronary artery bypass graft surgery
- Percutaneous transluminal coronary angioplasty (PTCA)

(Text continues on page 236.)

Table 16.1. A Guide to Oral Diuretics

Types	Names		Remarks
	Trade (Brand)	Generic (Chemical)	
Thiazides	Anhydron	cyclothiazide	All thiazides promote excretion of salt, water, and potassium. Some are long-acting, others are short-acting, and, in equivalent doses, they are about equally effective.
	Aquatag	benzthiazide	
	Aquatensen	methyclothiazide	
	Diucardin	hydroflumethiazide	
	Diuril	chlorothiazide	
	Enduron	methyclothiazide	
	Esidrix	hydrochlorothiazide	
	Exna	benzthiazide	
	HydroDiuril	hydrochlorothiazide	
	Hydromox	quinethazone	
	Metahydrin	trichlormethiazide	
	Naqua	trichlormethiazide	
	Naturetin	bendroflumethiazide	
	Oretic	hydrochlorothiazide	
	Renese	polythiazide	
	Saluron	hydroflumethiazide	
Loop Diuretics	Edecrin	ethacrynic acid	These two diuretics are extremely potent. They act on different sites in the kidney than the thiazides. Ethacrynic acid is generally reserved for patients with congestive heart failure and/or edema.
	Lasix	furosemide	

Potassium-sparing	Aldactone Dyrenium Moduretic	spironolactone triamterene amiloride HCl-hydro-chlorothiazide	These diuretics achieve water loss by leave potassium in the body.
Other	Diulo Hygroton Hydromox Zaroxolyn	metolazone chlorthalidone quinethazone metolazone	Although their chemical structure differs from thiazide agents, their clinical effect is the same.
Combinations	Aldactazide Dyazide	spironolactone and hydrochlorothiazide triamternene and hydro-chlorothiazide	These agents provide the benefits of diuresis and leave potassium in the body. Unlike the single potassium-sparing agents cited above, these are combination tablets; as such, these tablets act at two different sites in the kidney, rather than one.
	Minizide	prazosin hydrochloride polythiazide	Like other combination tablets the antihypertensive effect is more pronounced with the combination than either drug used alone in equivalent doses.

Table 16.2. A Guide to Antihypertensive Sympatholytic Drugs

Types	Names		Remarks
	Trade (Brand)	Generic (Chemical)	
Central acting	Catapres	clonidine	This agent is used to treat moderate hypertension.
Peripheral acting	Ismelin	guanethidine	There are two types in this group. One, ganglionic blockers, are rarely used today. The other is guanethidine. Guanethidine is reserved for severe, resistant cases of hypertension.
Central and peripheral acting	Aldomet Serpasil	methyldopa reserpine	Reserpine was one of the first anti-hypertensive agents used to treat mild hypertension, but its use for mild hypertension has largely been replaced by diuretics and beta blockers.

Alpha-adrenergic blockers	Dibenzyline Minipress Regitine	phenoxybenzamine prazosin phentolamine
Beta-adrenergic blockers	Tenormin Lopressor Corgard Visken Inderal Blocadren	atenolol metoprolol nadolol pindolol propranolol timolol maleate

Phentolamine and phenoxybenzamine are used under special circumstances—when hypertension is due to a tumor on the adrenal gland, called pheochromocytema. These drugs can control blood pressure until the tumor is surgically removed. Prazosin is used as a step-two or step-three drug after diuretics and beta blockers. Side effects are minimal.

The oldest and most commonly used beta-adrenergic blocker is propranolol. Atenolol and nadolol only have to be taken once a day.

Table 16.3. A Guide to Antihypertensive Vasodilators

Types	Names Trade (Brand)	Generic (Chemical)	Remarks
Direct arterial dilators	Apresoline	hydralazine	These drugs are usually added to other drugs, such as diuretics or a beta adrenergic blocker.
	Hyperstat	diazoxide	Reserved for hypertensive emergencies only. Must be given intravenously.
	Nipride	nitroprusside	Reserved for hypertensive emergencies only. Must be given intravenously.
		minoxidil	A very potent antihypertensive agent used to treat severe hypertension.

Table 16.4. Some Common Side Effects of Antihypertensive Drugs

Side Effect	Drug or Drugs
Diuretics	
Hypokalemia (too little potassium in the blood)	all diuretics but potassium-sparing
Hyperuricemia (too much uric acid in the blood)	thiazide diuretics
Hyperglycemia (too much sugar in the blood)	all thiazide diuretics may cause this—not potassium-sparing drugs
Gynecomastia (enlargement of the breasts)	spironolactone
Sympatholytics	
Edema (water retention)	all sympatholytics may cause this
Depression; sleep disturbances	some beta-adrenergic blockers methyldopa reserpine
Diarrhea	beta-adrenergic blockers guanethidine reserpine
Fever	methyldopa
Impotence Lethargy	caused mostly by methyldopa and guanethidine, but all antihypertensives have been implicated
Retrograde ejaculation	guanethidine
Vasodilators	
Tachycardia (rapid heartbeat), palpitation	diazoxide, hydralazine, minoxidil, nitroprusside
Edema	diazoxide, hydralazine, minoxidil
Drug-induced lupus eryuthematosus	hydralazine

(Text continued from page 229)

Drugs for Angina Pectoris

Nitroglycerin is one of a class of compounds known as nitrates. These drugs share many of the properties of nitroglycerin and therefore are commonly used to treat angina. The nitrates differ from each other in their form (tablet, capsule, or ointment) and in the time of onset and duration of their effects.

Their effect is the same: to dilate the arteries and veins of the body, and thereby reduce the workload of the heart by decreasing resistance of outflow of blood from the heart (arterial dilation), and reducing the amount of blood returned to the heart (venous dilation). (See Table 16.5.)

Table 16.5. Nitrate Preparations to Relieve Angina Pectoris

Sublingual nitroglycerin

These tablets are placed under the tongue and rapidly absorbed into the bloodstream to provide relief from the pain of angina pectoris within minutes. Duration of action is twenty to thirty minutes.

Sublingual nitrates of intermediate duration

These tablets are forms of the long-acting nitrates that are taken like sublingual NTG. Their onset of action is almost as rapid as that of nitroglycerin but they are longer-acting—up to two hours.

Cardilate	erthyrityl tetranitrate
Isordil	isosorbide dinitrate
Nitrostat	nitroglycerin
Sorbitrate	isosorbide dinitrate

Long-acting tablets

These preparations take fifteen to twenty minutes to work but they are long-acting (three to five hours). They are chewed prophylactically or swallowed whole and also are used in combination with the former. They don't provide rapid relief of anginal pain, as sublingual nitroglycerin does. A number of these drugs are available in long-acting and sublingual forms.

Trade (brand) Name	*Generic (chemical) Name*
Antora®	pentaerythritol tetranitrate

Cardilate®	erythrityl tetranitrate
Iso-bid Capsules®	isosorbide dinitrate
Isordil Sorbide®	isosorbide dinitrate
Nitro-bid®	nitroglycerin
Nitroban®	nitroglycerin
Nitroglyn®	nitroglycerin
Nitrong®	nitroglycerin
Nitrospan®	nitroglycerin
Pentritol®	pentaerythritol tetranitrate
Peritrate®	pentaerythritol tetranitrate
Sorbitrate®	isosorbide dinitrate

Ointments

These creams are applied to the skin (any area) through which they are absorbed. Some patients find it very effective to use topical nitroglycerin at night before retiring. These preparations do not stain clothes but they may irritate the skin. These preparations have an effect for up to six hours.

Nitro-Bid	nitroglycerin
Nitrol	nitroglycerin

Recently introduced nitrate preparations

Recently introduced nitrate preparations include the following:

Transderm Nitro® (topical)	nitroglycerin
Nitro-Dur® (topical)	nitroglycerin
Susadrin® (topical)	nitroglycerin

Transderm Nitro® and Nitro-Dur® provide 24 hours of nitroglycerin by continuous absorption through the skin from a special adherent patch. Susadrin® is nitroglycerin in tablet form that adheres to the mucuous membrane of the mouth for 3-5 hours. Its onset of action is the same as that of sublingual nitroglycerin (3 minutes), and its duration is 3-5 hours, thus combining rapid onset with prolonged effect.

Store your nitroglycerin tablets in a cool, dry place, out of sunlight *with the lid securely in place.* Always keep some tablets with you, along with a wallet identification card that says you are taking nitroglycerin.

Replace your supply every three to four months, since this drug commonly loses potency after this period of time.

Specifically, the nitrates reduce the heart's workload by lowering blood pressure and decreasing the amount of blood returned to the heart; thus, the volume "load" that the heart must move is reduced. The pressure against which the heart works and the volume of blood it moves are major factors determining its work and thereby its oxygen, or fuel, needs. By lowering these factors (and thereby reducing the oxygen needs of the heart) the imbalance between oxygen supply and demand is diminished, and an episode of angina is relieved or prevented.

Contrary to popular belief, the principal action of the nitrates, including nitroglycerin is not dilation of the coronary arteries and increased coronary blood flow. These arteries are narrowed by fixed obstructions—arteriosclerotic deposits. Nitrates act to dilate the arteries of the body throughout the arterial system into which the heart pumps blood. This dilatory action lowers resistance to blood flow in these arteries and thus lowers blood pressure. Less blood is returned to the heart by the nitrates' actions because they dilate the veins in the body, causing a "pooling" effect of blood in the body away from the heart, and thus the amount of blood returned to the heart is diminished. The dilating or relaxing action of the nitrates on the arteries and veins throughout the body results in a decreased workload on the heart and is the basis of the therapeutic effect. To summarize on nitrates:

Sublingual nitroglycerin. This preparation (a small tablet placed under the tongue) is the most commonly used form and it is the most effective agent for the treatment of angina. It acts in two to five minutes and its effects last for twenty to thirty minutes. Sublingual nitroglycerin may be used indefinitely without adverse effects or decrease in efficacy.

Long-acting nitrates. These include topical ointment preparations and tablets or capsules that are swallowed. It takes fifteen to twenty minutes for these nitrates to act, but depending on the preparation, their effect lasts for from three to 24 hours. Generally, both short- and long-acting forms of nitroglycerin are used, in order to give the patient broad therapeutic coverage. This therapeutic approach can help to curtail acute episodes of angina as well as help reduce the number of episodes that occur.

Beta blockers. These drugs are used to treat other forms of heart disease, as we mentioned in our discussion on antihypertensive drugs, and these agents are also effective in preventing episodes of angina pectoris because they act to reduce the heart's workload. Specifically, beta blockers act to slow the heart rate and the force of myocardial contraction. Heart rate and force of contraction are the two other important factors, in addition to blood pressure and blood volume in the heart that determine the heart's oxygen needs. The effects of propranolol (Inderal®) last eight to twelve hours and it has to be taken two or three times daily. The newer beta-adrenergic blocker nadolol (Corgard®) may also be used. Nadolol has to be taken only once a day.

Calcium antagonists. Three agents are in this class of drugs—nifedipine (Procardia®), verapamil (Calan® and Isoptin®), and a third agent, diltiazem (Cardizem™). Calcium antagonists also are used for the treatment of angina. These drugs are very effective in preventing coronary artery spasm, thought to be a factor in many cases of angina. The calcium antagonists are also beneficial in angina unassociated with coronary artery spasm because they also reduce the work of the heart by decreasing blood pressure and the force of cardiac contractions. These drugs inhibit the actions of calcium in cardiac and smooth muscle cells in all arteries of the body. Calcium plays an important role in contraction of arterial smooth muscle and heart muscle and inhibition of calcium activity can prevent spasm of the coronary arteries, lower blood pressure by relaxing the body's arteries, and reduce cardiac work by decreasing the force of the heart's contraction.

Drugs for Arrhythmias

As you may have already surmised, several antiarrhythmic drugs are available, and the one selected depends on the results desired. You may recall that arrhythmias—abnormal heart rhythms—essentially fall into two categories: the heart either beats too slowly (bradyarrhythmias) or too fast (tachyarrhythmias). If the heart is beating too quickly, one or more drugs will be given to slow the beat. Antiarrhythmic agents can be administered by injection in a hospital setting, either through the muscle (intramuscularly) or through the veins (intravenously). The latter is most common. These drugs may also be given orally. When the problem is urgent and warrants rapid treatment, the intravenous route is used. In less demanding circumstances requiring long-term therapy, oral treatment is prescribed. Frequently, therapy is initiated intravenously and, if continued treatment is necessary, it is switched to the oral route. In many cases, the abnormal rhythm consists of premature or extra beats that occur irregularly and can be very frequent.

Finally, it should also be pointed out that, in addition to heart disease, arrhythmias can be provoked or aggravated by excessive ingestion of stimulant agents such as coffee, tea, certain types of drugs (e.g., weight-reducing medication) and by physiological abnormalities such as fever, reduced oxygen levels in the blood and other acute illnesses (e.g., pneumonia). Noncardiac disease or ingestion of excitatory agents can result in arrhythmias—even in a normal, healthy heart. Thus, when treating patients with arrhythmias in the presence of obvious heart disease or in its absence, careful evaluation is always made to detect the presence of the previously noted factors, i.e., use of drugs (including tobacco), other stimulatory agents, and systemic disease. Elimination or control of these factors may abolish or reduce a cardiac arrhythmia.

Here, we will discuss some commonly used antiarrhythmics, which have been divided into two major categories: drugs that stimulate cardiac electrical activity—in other words, drugs given to accelerate the heartbeat—to treat bradyarrhythmias; and drugs given to depress abnormal (rapid) electrical activity—in other words, drugs given to slow the heartbeat—to treat tachyarrhythmias.

Drugs That Stimulate Cardiac Electrical Activity

These drugs—isoproterenol (Isuprel®), and atropine—are given to increase the heart rate in cases of excessively slow heart rhythms. They are used for temporary treatment—in a hospital setting. These drugs are generally replaced by the use of a temporary, artificial cardiac pacemaker for therapy of more than a few hours. If the condition is chronic, a permanent, artificial pacemaker is inserted.

Drugs that Depress Abnormal (Rapid) Electrical Activity (Tachyarrhythmia or Extra Beats)

Quinidine and Procainamide. Two other drugs, quinidine (which is available under a wide variety of brand names) and procainamide act directly on the cardiac cells to alter cellular activity. Both of these agents may be used to suppress atrial and ventricular tachyarrhythmias such as atrial premature beats, ventricular premature beats, atrial fibrillation, etc. They are usually given orally—quinidine is given primarily to abolish premature beats and to prevent atrial flutter or fibrillation, and procainamide is prescribed primarily to prevent premature ventricular beats and ventricular tachyarrhythmias.

Lidocaine. Among the most frequently used antiarrhythmics, it is used to treat abnormal cardiac rhythms originating in the ventricles, such as premature ventricular beats and ventricular tachycardia. Lidocaine (Zylocaine®) is a fast-acting drug that can only be given intravenously. (It cannot be given orally because of destruction in the GI tract.) This drug is highly efficacious and has a low degree of toxicity.

Disopyramide phosphate (Norpace®). This agent is effective against atrial and ventricular tachyarrhythmias. It is only available in the oral tablet form.

Propranolol (Inderal®). This agent may be given orally or intravenously. Propranolol blocks the effects of the stimulatory hormones epinephrine and norepinephrine on the heart. By blocking the effects of these hormones, extra beats and tachycardia that may originate in either the atria or the ventricles are suppressed. Nadolol acts in a similar way to control arrhythmias. Indirectly it may prevent arrhythmia by anti-ischemic effects.

Phenytoin (Dilantin®). This antiarrhythmic agent, which can be administered intravenously, intramuscularly or by oral tablet, is a so-called second-line antiarrhythmic agent because it is used after the primary agents, such as quinidine, procainamide or lidocaine have been unsuccessful. Dilantin® is usually used in conjunction with these other agents. Initially introduced for the treatment of epilepsy, it suppresses irritable foci in the heart, which generate arrhythmias, just as it suppresses irritable foci in the brain, which generate abnormal discharges, causing convulsions.

Bretylium tosylate (Bretylol®). This agent is available in parenteral (intramuscular, intravenous) form for use in refractory, life-threatening ventricular arrhythmias, such as resistant ventricular extra beats, ventricular tachycardia and ventricular fibrillation.

Verapamil (Calan®, Isoptin®), a calcium antagonist, has gained widespread use for its effectiveness in treatment of tachycardias originating in the atria. Given intravenously, it either converts these arrhythmias to normal rhythm or slows the rate of the abnormal rhythm in a majority of patients.

Digitalis. This agent has been used to treat heart disease for over two hundred years. It is used primarily to treat heart failure; in these cases, digitalis acts primarily to increase the force of myocardial contraction and thereby helps to restore the heart's ability to pump blood. However, digitalis is also important in the treatment of supraventricular tachycardia, atrial flutter and atrial fibrillation.

Specifically, in the treatment of these arrhythmias, use of digitalis results in a depression of conductivity (conduction of impulses) through the atrioventricular node; thus, the number of impulses from the atria that reach the left ventricle is reduced, and this in turn results in a lower, more physiological ventricular rate than is present in untreated superventricular tachyarrhythmias such as atrial fibrillation. With digitalis therapy, the ventricular rate may be controlled to a normal level of 70 to 80 beats/minute, in contrast to a rate of 150 to 200 beats/minute, which is common in the untreated patient. These two uses of digitalis, i.e. for heart failure and for arrhythmias, are separate and distinct. If both of these cardiac problems occur together, then this single drug can be helpful in both. In many instances of superventricular tachyarrhythmias, such as atrial fibrillation, the heart rhythm remains chronically abnormal and the therapeutic effect consists of establishing a reasonable ventricular rate. Digitalis may not convert the arrhythmia to a normal sinus rhythm. However, in certain instances of atrial fibrillation, atrial flutter or atrial tachycardia, the rhythm may convert to normal during the course of therapy.

A special caution should be exercised when taking digitalis, since it can interact with a wide variety of other drugs, including some over-the-counter cold and allergy remedies. Anyone taking this drug must follow directions carefully and advise a physician if he is taking any other drugs. Finally, errors in dosage can produce toxic effects.

The aforementioned drugs are the ones you are most likely to hear mentioned or have prescribed for you. Like all cardiac drugs, the antiarrhythmic agents are potent—their therapeutic action is based on their potency. However, these agents also have a potential for toxicity, which can affect the heart and other organs. When given in excessive dosage, for example, these agents may cause myocardial depression, resulting in heart failure, and they aggravate rhythm disturbances. In addition, noncardiac side effects such as loss of appetite, diarrhea, and skin rashes can occur. Proper utilization of antiarrhythmic agents involves careful evaluation of the underlying condition and selection of the appropriate drug in the proper dosage.

Drugs for the Failing Heart

Remember, "heart failure" doesn't mean the heart has stopped; it simply means that it is unable to pump an adequate amount of blood. This may be because the heart muscle is damaged due to any number of conditions that can affect the heart. Initially, then, the heart tries to compensate for this damage by working harder—beating faster to pump sufficient amounts of blood through the circulatory system. Ultimately, the added strain becomes too much for the heart and it fails. Reduced blood flow also results in decreased urine production; thus, the kidney's ability to remove sodium and water from the blood results in retention of salt and water in the body.

Treatment of congestive heart failure begins with rest—to reduce the heart's overall workload. Diet is also in order. Obese persons must reduce—again, to reduce the heart's workload. In addition, a low sodium diet may be recommended—and it should be followed exactly as prescribed. Digitalis, diuretics and vasodilators are the drugs used to treat heart failure.

Diuretics. These agents are given to enhance the elimination of excessive sodium and water. The more potent diuretics, furosemide and ethyacrinic acid—Lasix® and Edecrin®, respectively—are used frequently, although the thiazide diuretics may be tried initially.

Digitalis. Although we don't understand *exactly* how digitalis works, we do know it is extremely effective in the treatment of congestive heart failure. Because it acts directly on cardiac cells, its use often achieves prompt relief of congestive heart failure by improving the heart muscle's ability to contract. This, in turn, results in a reduction in heart size (to normal or near-normal), improved circulation, and a slower, more efficient rate of heartbeat. Although congestive heart failure is a serious condition, many patients have benefited tremendously from the combined treatment of digitalis, diuretics, proper diet, and reduced activity.

Vasodilators. These drugs relax both the arterial and venous smooth muscle, which results in dilatation of arteries and veins. The latter effect causes a reduction of blood flow from the body back to the heart (venodilating action), thereby reducing excessive blood volume in the lungs (pulmonary congestion) and relieving the associated shortness of breath. The arterial dilating action reduces resistance to outflow of blood from the heart, resulting in increased cardiac output (flow of blood from the heart to the body).

Converting enzyme inhibitor. Captopril (Capoten®) is a new drug that recently became available for the treatment of congestive heart failure. Captopril inhibits the formation of angiotensin, the most potent vasoconstrictor produced by the body. Its primary action in the treatment of congestive heart failure is to increase the amount of blood pumped by the heart (the cardiac output) by lowering the arterial resistance against which the heart pumps.

What You Need to Know About Your Prescription Drugs

- Know the generic (chemical) name of the drug, as well as the trade (brand) name.

- Know the dosage prescribed.

- Know how many times per day you are supposed to take your medication.

- Ask your doctor about storage of the drug. Some medications, such as nitroglycerin, for example, which is often prescribed to relieve the pain of angina, should be stored out of sunlight, preferably in the refrigerator.

- Know if there are special requirements for taking the drug; for example: Should it be taken before or after meals? Should it not be taken with certain foods or alcohol? and so on.

- Ask your doctor about side effects—what kinds of reactions can you expect from taking this drug?

- Ask your doctor about substitution. As you may already know, doctors commonly prescribe a specific pill for you by brand name. However, you may pay more for the brand name than you would if you obtain the drug by its generic or chemical name. Equal units contain equal chemical components, but, with a brand name product, you pay more for the manufacturer's label. In some cases, the brand-name product may be more reliable; your physician can advise you. Your doctor may recommend you use the chemical name, since this is usually cheaper. In fact, in some states, pharmacists are required by law to substitute the less expensive generic drugs. Cost of a drug is a genuine consideration when one is buying medications for a lifelong disease such as hypertension.

- Ask your doctor about special precautions. (Can the drug possibly cause drowsiness—which may mean you shouldn't drive for several hours after taking it?).

- Ask your doctor about contraindications. (Be sure your doctor is thoroughly apprised of your medical history. Certain drugs should not be given to pregnant women, and there are numerous other conditions that may preclude taking specific drugs.)

17

What the Coronary Care Unit Is All About

The nurses at the station are watching closely. In cubicle A, Mr. John R., a 52-year-old insurance broker who was admitted to the hospital three days earlier after having suffered a heart attack, suddenly loses consciousness as the oscilloscope showing his electrocardiogram reveals ventricular tachycardia, a life-threatening arrhythmia. There is an immediate and coordinated mobilization of personnel into a swift, purposeful series of actions to meet the emergency. One nurse dials the "cardiac arrest" code number on the phone—a team of physicians will respond immediately—while two other CCU nurses quickly move the "crash cart" and the defibrillator from its place in the CCU to the patient's bedside and begin to initiate life-saving measures. Within thirty seconds, Mr. R's cardiac rhythm is restored to normal, and a short time thereafter he awakens and wonders what all the fuss is about.

Meanwhile, in cubicle B, Mrs. Jane M. is sitting up in bed and reading, and in cubicle C, Mr. Steve K. is talking to his wife.

Events such as these are common in the "CCU," a short name for coronary or cardiac care unit, where highly trained nurses and very sophisticated equipment are on hand around-the-clock to provide comprehensive care for the cardiac patient. In particular, the nurses assigned to the coronary care unit are ready to manage any cardiac emergency that might arise, and thereby prevent a CCU catastrophe. This chapter will help you understand how the CCU works.

The idea of a specially designed unit equipped to provide care for cardiac patients was introduced in 1960. Today, there are more than 1500 such units in the U.S. and many experts believe that these specialized coronary care units have helped reduce the number of deaths due to a heart attack after the patient reaches the hospital.

The concept of the coronary care unit was an outgrowth of medical advances of the 1950s, when physicians learned to convert the lethal cardiac arrhythmias, ventricular tachycardia and fibrillation, by applying an electrical current to the chest wall. At the same time, the method of cardiopulmonary resuscitation was refined.

The coronary care unit is as much a concept as it is a physical unit. It brings together the patients at risk for sudden cardiac emergencies—chiefly victims who have very recently had a heart attack—with highly trained personnel and specialized equipment for monitoring and treating them. This approach provides for immediate treatment and prevention of catastrophes such as cardiac arrest during the high-risk period—the first few days of hospitalization in the CCU.

HOW THE CORONARY CARE UNIT EVOLVED

On close monitoring of heart attack patients in the first days, it became apparent that "warning arrhythmias" (premature ventricular beats not necessarily serious in themselves) often appear, and that these arrhythmias may precede lethal arrhythmias. Once this was recognized, the emphasis shifted to preventing cardiac arrest by eliminating these warning arrhythmias with a drug, lidocaine, which had just become available for that purpose.

Physicians at the Peter Bent Brigham Hospital in Boston were among the first to report the benefits of this approach. In the first year of operating the coronary care unit there, only 1 patient out of 130 had a cardiac arrest; this incidence was much lower than what was expected with conventional care. According to Dr. Bernard Lown's report (the physician in charge of the CCU there), this was in large part due to the fact that the nurses responsible for monitoring the unit initiated treatment (based on specific orders left by a physician) as soon as any minor arrhythmia developed. Using this approach, Dr. Lown and his colleagues recognized that cardiac arrest did not simply strike like a "bolt from the blue"; rather, it was most typically preceded by less serious cardiac rhythm abnormalities, the abolition of which could in some cases prevent cardiac arrest and "sudden death."

What's in the Coronary Care Unit?

First, there are the patients. For the most part, patients in the coronary care unit are heart attack victims, but they also include patients with any serious, unstable cardiac problem such as arrhythmias due to causes other than heart attack, heart failure of any cause, or patients with what appears to be an acute, serious, but incompletely diagnosed cardiac disorder. This unit provides a setting in which the acutely ill cardiac patient can receive careful, continuous monitoring and immediate treatment during the unstable phase of his illness.

Depending on the size and needs of the hospital, the CCU may be quite large, and contain twenty or more beds, or it may only accommodate four to six patients at any one time. Regardless of size, however, all CCUs have certain features in common. For example, every bedside is equipped with an oscilloscope on which is continually displayed the patient's electrocardiogram and, depending on the sophistication of the equipment, other important information such as blood pressure, heart rate, and related measurements of heart function. (See Figure 17.1.)

An intercom is generally located over the patient's bed, a call button for the nurse is at the bedside, and an oxygen tank and mask are situated close to each bed in case the patient requires them. Each "cubicle," or patient area, is divided from the others by curtains, wall dividers, or glass.

Figure 17.1: Five-bed Coronary Care Unit

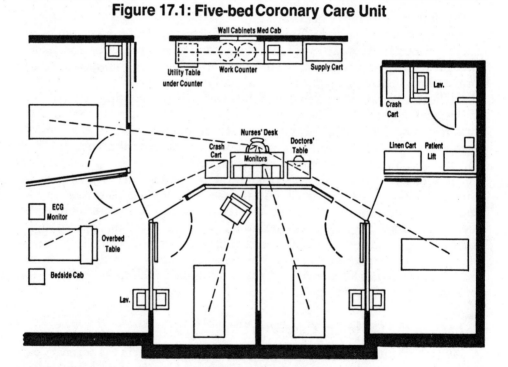

Adapted from *Coronary Care Units*, U.S. Department of Health, Education, and Welfare, Public Health Service Publication No. 1250, March, 1966.

Within the unit, there is a "crash cart" that holds all the necessary medications for cardiac emergencies. A defibrillator is kept on hand to apply electrical shock when needed to control a life-threatening arrhythmia. Finally, there is a central nurses' station, which is equipped with a "slave" oscilloscope that continuously displays all of the patients' heart rates and rhythms. In some cases, compact computers are also used; at the push of a button, the patient's vital signs (pulse, heart rate, etc.) over a 24-hour period are available. (See Figure 17.2 and 17.3.)

Helping the Patient in the CCU

Surprisingly, a number of heart patients actually begin to feel better once they are admitted to the CCU. Here, they know that expert care is literally at their fingertips, and such knowledge provides them with a sense of security. Still, most patients also realize that their condition is serious, and such awareness may make them anxious or depressed. For many, repeated explanations of their disease—and of the healing process—are quite helpful, along with reassuring words that life is far from over. Most victims of heart disease go on to lead normal lives—one need only recall that both Presidents Eisenhower and Johnson continued their work for many years after suffering heart attacks. Finally, a program of gradual ambulation, often combined with physical exercise, is set up for CCU patients that, once begun, helps them to realize that they can continue to enjoy routine activities. In some cases, drugs

Figure 17.2: Electronic ECG Monitoring Equipment

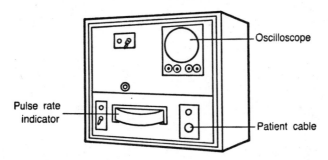

The cardiac monitor provides continuous electrocardiographic signal on oscilloscope at patient's bedside; audiovisual alarm signal in serious rhythm disturbance; and a central monitoring and control panel to transmit data to the nursing station.

Figure 17.3: Special Resuscitation Equipment

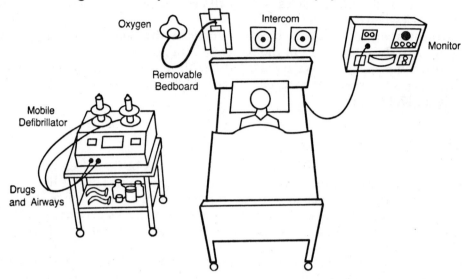

Adapted from *Coronary Care Units*, U.S. Department of Health, Education, and Welfare, Public Health Service Publication No. 1250, March 1966.

such as tranquilizers may be given. No matter what therapeutic program is prescribed, however, family members and friends should help the patient to follow his physician's advice—and should be as supportive as possible in an emotional sense.

18
Advances in Cardiovascular Surgery

The spectacular achievements of modern cardiovascular surgery are numerous, indeed. Headlines were made in 1967, when Dr. Christian Barnard performed the first human heart transplant. Since then, more than 350 heart transplants have been performed. Dramatic as this particular type of cardiovascular surgery is, the results are not nearly as promising as those achieved in other types of cardiovascular surgery, such as valve replacement coronary artery bypass surgery, surgery to implant a pacemaker, and surgery to correct congenital heart defects. (See Chapter 14.) In this chapter, we outline the indications for each type of surgery, and the benefits and risks of each method.

The Heart-Lung Machine

One of the most important developments in modern medicine and a critical factor in making possible modern cardiac surgery is the heart-lung machine. By temporarily taking over the normal functions of the heart and lungs and providing a continuous supply of oxygenated blood to the body while the heart is inactive, this device allows the surgeon to perform complicated, lengthy operations on the heart. Before the availability of this remarkable machine, only the simplest cardiac surgery could be performed, because periods of induced cardiac arrest could not be tolerated due to the damage that the heart and other organs would sustain.

Specifically, complete mechanical takeover of the function of the heart and lungs is achieved by the heart-lung machine or pump oxygenator. It provides circulation of blood to the body during open-heart surgery when the heart is totally at rest. This device consists of a pumping mechanism and a series of membranes which aid the blood to take up oxygen and give off carbon dioxide. The pumping mechanism, to which blood is diverted from the body by a series of tubes inserted into large veins, and returned to the body through tubes inserted into large arteries, maintains the circulation, pumping the blood through the series of membranes and thence back to the body. The membranes perform the functions of the lungs, the blood taking up oxygen and giving off carbon dioxide as it passes through them.

THE BYPASS SURGERY EVERYONE IS TALKING ABOUT

In a busy hospital hallway, a resident physician casually remarks to an intern that the "cabbage" in operating room C went off without a hitch. Two patients standing nearby look at each other quizzically and ask the first nurse they encounter: "What does cabbage mean? And what does anything with a name like that have to do with surgery?"

Quite simply, "cabbage," as it is commonly called, refers to one of the latest types of cardiovascular surgery: Coronary Artery Bypass Graft (CABG—pronounced "cabbage"). With this technique, appropriately selected patients with angina pectoris may undergo surgery to relieve their pain and, hopefully, prolong their lives. To date, more than 500,000 people have had bypass surgery; in fact, in 1980 approximately 104,000 operations of this kind were performed. This operation demands a highly skilled surgical team and generally costs upward of $10,000.

Coronary Artery Bypass Surgery (CABG)

Like other types of medical and surgical treatment, coronary bypass surgery is not indicated for every patient with coronary heart disease. Before any decision regarding the need for this surgery is reached, the patient must undergo numerous diagnostic tests. Careful criteria have been established to help physicians select the patients in whom bypass surgery is likely to be of most benefit. However, differences of opinion regarding the applications of this procedure persist among highly respected physicians, and a patient should feel free to consult another physician for a second opinion. (Actually, Blue Cross/Blue Shield will reimburse patients who seek a second opinion on the need for surgery.) Finally, such surgery, which has proven beneficial for many patients, should only be performed by a surgeon experienced and skilled in the technique. A patient should feel free to ask about the operative risk and likelihood of success of surgery in his case, as well as the surgeon's record, i.e. number of patients he has operated on, frequency of complications of surgery, and success rate. Further, the patient's physician should be thoroughly familiar and satisfied with the personal records of the cardiologist and surgeons to whom he refers his patient.

To begin with, patients who are diagnosed as having angina pectoris are generally treated with nitroglycerin, supplemented by long-acting nitrates and nadolol or propranolol, and/or an exercise program. In some instances, however, this therapeutic program isn't sufficient to relieve the frequent chest pain of angina pectoris. When life-style is significantly impaired by symptoms, it is appropriate to consider coronary artery bypass surgery. Surgery is also considered by many physicians in relatively young patients with angina (less than 50 years old) or in those in whom evaluation indicates severe, extensive coronary artery disease and shortened life expectancy, even if angina is not incapacitating. The goal in the latter groups is to try to prevent heart attack and prolong life, rather than just to alleviate angina. Although not yet unequivocally demonstrated, there is increasing evidence to show that in patients with disease of all three coronary arteries or of the left main coronary artery, this type of surgery can prolong life. Very briefly, here is what to expect in terms of the usual problem that raises the possibility of bypass surgery and the evaluative process that follows:

- There will be frequent angina poorly responsive to maximum medical treatment and/or evaluation will indicate high risk coronary disease, as noted above. However, not every patient with these conditions is eligible for coronary bypass surgery; other factors, such as overall health and age must be evaluated too.

- A resting, and usually, an exercise electrocardiogram will be performed. A radioisotope scan of the heart during exercise may also be performed.

- A number of blood tests (for cholesterol and other factors) will be obtained.

- A coronary arteriogram will be performed. This procedure is part of a cardiac catheterization by which the anatomy and function of the heart can be evaluated.

The angiogram, in which radiopaque dye is injected into the coronary arteries, enables the physician to clearly see on X-ray motion picture or still film the anatomy of the coronary arteries and any obstructions present in them. (You may recall that fatty deposits, known as atherosclerotic "plaques," can build up in the coronary arteries over years and obstruct the flow of oxygen-rich blood through the arteries. Angina is often a symptom indicating such obstruction.) Angina is usually associated with obstruction of 70 percent or more of the arterial diameter and these obstructions are present in two of the three major coronary arteries in about two-thirds or more of patients with angina. However, angina does not always mean coronary artery obstruction. Certain diseases that place a strain on the heart, such as aortic valve stenosis or high blood pressure, may also result in angina, even in the presence of normal coronary indices. However, the great majority (close to 100%) of patients with angina have coronary artery disease. It has also been recently recognized that normal (or diseased) coronary arteries may have transient spasms or constrictions; these spasms cause a temporary decrease in coronary blood flow and produce attacks of angina, even at rest. Spasm of the coronary arteries is poorly understood and its frequency as a cause of angina is uncertain.

If your cardiologist recommends coronary bypass surgery, and you agree to have it, you should learn as much as you can about the procedure, and what to expect postoperatively. Remember, the purpose of the operation is to alleviate pain and prolong life; therefore, although there is considerable discomfort the first few days postoperatively, most patients are back on their feet, and often back to work, within six weeks. Even Jackie Gleason resumed many of his activities in time after he underwent coronary bypass surgery in a Chicago hospital in 1978.

What Happens in CABG?

Essentially, there are two kinds of procedures: one involves the removal of and grafting of the saphenous vein from the leg into the coronary circulation to bypass obstructed coronary arteries, while another technique utilizes the internal mammary artery, a small artery situated along the breastbone. (The former procedure is far more common than the latter, although both require about three or four hours to complete.) Of course, the purpose of such surgery is to implant an unobstructed blood vessel—one that is open and clear and can therefore carry normal amounts of blood to the heart muscle. The obstructed coronary artery is "bypassed"; nothing is done in the course of surgery to remove, alter or clear the obstructions from the diseased arteries. In effect, the newly implanted artery is a "detour" or bypass around the obstructed one. Finally, the "new" vessel or vessels will be implanted to bypass all major obstructions—generally, there are at least two and sometimes four or more areas of obstruction that need to be bypassed. (See Figure 18.1.)

In coronary artery bypass surgery utilizing the saphenous vein method, the vein is removed from the leg and one end is attached to the aorta and the other is grafted to the diseased (obstructed) coronary artery downstream from the obstruction. If the mammary artery is used, it is removed from its connection downstream and sewn to the coronary artery beyond the obstruction.

Results of CABG

Successful surgery consists of the following: (1) the vein graft must remain open; (2) blood flow through the grafted artery must be sufficient in quantity; and (3) that section of the myocardium (heart muscle) which is being resupplied with blood by the grafted artery must be healthy tissue, not scar tissue from a prior heart attack (if it is, it can't benefit from the blood being supplied by the graft).

In an effort to determine the efficacy of coronary artery bypass surgery, a

Figure 18.1: Coronary Artery Grafts

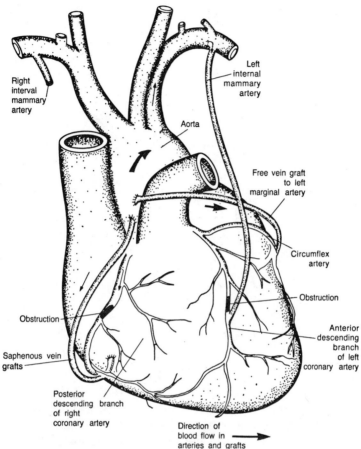

Coronary artery grafts bypass obstructed arteries.

number of studies have been carried out to evaluate medical (treatment with drugs only) against surgical therapy. In one of the most well-known and controversial studies, the Veterans Administration hospitals survey, a select group of coronary disease patients in thirteen VA hospitals were randomly assigned to be treated by either coronary artery bypass surgery or drugs alone. Overall, 596 patients were followed for three years: 310 received medications, while 286 were treated surgically. At the end of three years, the survey showed that surgery was clearly superior to medication therapy in relieving anginal symptoms. However, long-term survival of the medically-treated patients and the surgical group were virtually the same, 87 percent and 88 percent, respectively. These results led some to conclude that surgery was no more effect-

Figure 18.2: Quadruple Coronary Artery Bypass Grafting

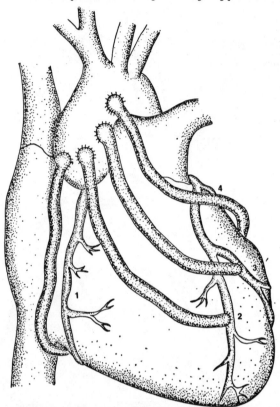

This diagram illustrates coronary artery bypass grafting. There is one bypass to the right coronary artery (1) and three bypasses to the left coronary artery including the left anterior descending branch (2), the diagonal branch (3), and the circumflex branch (4) which wraps around the backside of the heart.

ive than medication therapy in regard to effect on longevity in coronary disease patients. In the eyes of many, however, there were a number of factors that detracted from this study, despite its attempt to carefully compare medical and surgical therapy. Patients who had unstable angina or complicating factors, such as diabetes, were excluded. Further, patients with heart attack within six months were also excluded. The VA study's report of a 5.6 percent death rate due to operation itself has been, perhaps, the most consistent criticism. Today, the mortality rate associated with coronary bypass surgery is below 1 percent in some centers, and a mortality rate of less than 3 percent is commonplace.

Finally, critics of this study have also pointed out that those patients selected had the lowest risk of death from coronary heart disease; i.e., they were a low-risk group in whom surgery would be unlikely to improve longevity, in contrast to patients with a higher risk of dying from coronary artery disease in whom a beneficial effect by surgery would be demonstrable. The VA patients had only 50 percent or more narrowing of coronary artery diameter, whereas the generally accepted criterion is at least 70 percent narrowing.

On the basis of additional data, it has become apparent that certain high-risk subgroups of coronary patients, who have had coronary bypass graft surgery, show improved longevity—a result not yet attainable by medical treatment. The Veterans Administration hospital findings and the more recent European Cooperative Trial on coronary bypass surgery have demonstrated improved survival following surgery in patients with obstruction of the left main coronary artery. In the European Trial, survival also was increased in patients with obstructions in all three major coronary arteries. Both the Veterans Administration Cooperative Study and the European Cooperative Trial were "randomized," controlled trials in which two comparable groups of patients were assessed in each study—one group received medical treatment and the other underwent surgery. The results from the two groups were compared.

Summary

Open-heart surgery has been performed in this country since 1953, but coronary bypass surgery was not initiated until 1967. Overall, most experts agree that coronary artery bypass surgery is very beneficial in the relief of anginal pain and may be very effective where drug therapy fails. In addition, in some patients, such surgery may prolong life. For those in whom surgery is indicated, the benefits can be enormous—relief of pain, return to work, resumption of numerous activities. Each patient, however, must be evaluated individually, and any patient who is scheduled for such surgery should be sure he understands the potential benefits and risks of this procedure.

A Cardiovascular Surgeon Talks about His Own Bypass Surgery

Dr. Albert Starr is Chief of Cardiopulmonary Surgery at the University of Oregon in Portland. He is well known as co-inventor of the Starr-Edwards artificial heart valve, a prosthesis used to replace the valves in patients in whom the natural heart valves are severely damaged. In addition, he is Professor of Surgery at the University of Oregon School of Medicine, where he has helped to train hundreds of cardiovascular surgeons. In 1974, after Dr. Starr recognized symptoms of heart disease in himself and underwent tests, coronary bypass surgery was performed on him by his associates. Here is what he has to say about life after coronary artery bypass surgery:

Seven years ago, my own surgical team performed coronary artery bypass surgery on me at St. Vincent's Hospital in Portland. I was 47 years old at the time—a busy surgeon, and an enthusiastic skier. At first, I only noticed a feeling of pressure in the chest after running up a few flights of stairs in the hospital. When it happened repeatedly, I knew tests were indicated, so I underwent ECGs and a coronary arteriogram. The results suggested that coronary artery bypass surgery was needed.

The operation lasted about four hours, and just about a week later, I became rather depressed. Apparently, this is fairly common—in my case, I think I was upset by the fact that I realized I was no longer "intact"; now, I had had major surgery, and for a man like myself, who was never before ill, that realization came as quite a shock. Shortly thereafter, a physical rehabilitation program was recommended. Within six weeks after the surgery, I was walking quite a bit and, within two years, I was running up to three miles a day. Of course, the exercise is not only good for me from a physical rehabilitation standpoint, but it makes me realize how important it is from an emotional standpoint as well. Once you're exercising, you feel reassured that you are all right, and now that I've been working again for several years, I know that, in particular, many of my patients feel reassured just looking at me and seeing me walking around and working—seven years after my bypass surgery was performed.

REPLACEMENT SURGERY: NEW VALVES FOR OLD

In the last few decades, remarkable advances have been made in cardiovascular surgery. In addition to coronary artery bypass surgery, it is now also possible—indeed, in some hospitals even commonplace—to replace diseased heart valves with artificial ones. In 1978, actor John Wayne underwent such surgery for replacement of the aortic valve at Massachusetts General Hospital in Boston.

Essentially, there are three types of valve operations:

1. The narrowed or "stenotic" valve, in which the cusps are scarred, thickened, and immobile, can be opened by the surgeon's finger or the scalpel. This will permit more blood to flow through the valve.

2. If the valve does not respond to that treatment (or that approach is deemed inadequate), then "replacement" surgery may be indicated. In this procedure, a man-made or animal valve is inserted in place of the malfunctioning one.

3. This type of surgery is performed to correct a "leaking" or stenotic valve. Leaking valves are usually quite difficult to repair; as such, these valves are almost always replaced with artificial valves.

Today, valve replacement surgery is performed to replace any of the cardiac valves if they are malfunctioning. In adults, the aortic and mitral valves are most commonly involved. In some cases, a pig's valve may be substituted; this has been found to be very effective. In other instances, synthetic valves are used. These are made of nylon, Dacron, and Teflon, to name a few materials. Interestingly enough, some patients become alarmed at the idea of a "plastic valve"; yet plastic is actually one of our more durable substances. Replacement valve surgery generally involves hospitalization for two or three days for tests (including catheterization), and usually a stay of less than fourteen days for the procedure and recovery.

Valve Replacement

Several common types of valves inserted to replace the mitral valve are the natural pig valve, adapted to fit the human heart, the "ball valve" and the "toilet seat" valve. The *ball valve* is actually a metal cage with a ball inside of it. (See Figures 18.3 and 18.4.) When blood is pumped, it pushes the ball upward, and the blood flows around it. Then the ball falls backward, thereby closing off the opening and preventing the blood from flowing backward.

The *"toilet seat"* valve was so named because, although it works similarly to the ball valve, its design resembles that of a toilet seat; it is a hinged device that regularly flaps open and shut just as the normal mitral valve does.

The aortic valve may also be replaced surgically. Again, either a pig's valve or synthetic materials may be used. Tricuspid valve replacement can also be easily achieved; pulmonic valve replacement is rarely indicated.

For most patients, life after such surgery is routine. Work and most leisure activities may be pursued without concern about the artificial valve. Remember, the new valve was designed to work for a long time. However, when the artificial valve is made of synthetic materials (as opposed to the use of a pig's valve, which is mammalian tissue), anticoagulant drugs must be taken to prevent clots from forming in the valve. Finally, the ultimate longevity of many of the artificial valves is not yet known and, in some cases, valve failure may require re-operating. However, continued improvements in valve design can be expected to improve their function and prolong their lives.

Surgery of the Aorta

Modern cardiovascular surgery has corrected a number of serious abnormalities involving the "great" vessels—the aorta and the pulmonary artery. Two major conditions that affect the aorta and are amenable to surgery are described here.

Aortic Aneurysm. In this situation, part of the aorta is removed surgically, and

Figure 18.3: A Prosthetic Ball Valve

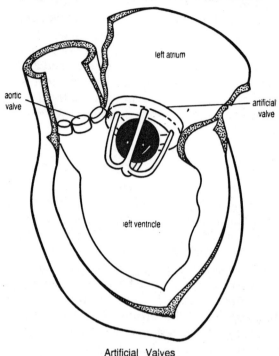

Artificial Valves

An artificial mitral valve of the ball and cage type. The ball drops down when the blood pressure builds in the left atrium and blood flows readily into the ventricle. When the ventricle contracts, the ball is forced upward into the cage and prevents backflow.

Illustration adapted from a drawing by Herbert R. Smith, from DeBakey, M., and Gotto, A., The Living Heart, N.Y., David McKay Co., 1977.

replaced with synthetic grafts, usually Dacron.

Coarctation of the Aorta. This condition, which amounts to localized constriction of the aorta and is usually present at birth, is also treated by removing surgically the constricted segment of the aorta and then sewing the ends together. Sometimes, a graft may be required.

BACK TO A NORMAL BEAT WITH A PACEMAKER

What is a cardiac pacemaker? What does it do? Why do you need one? As the name implies, a pacemaker, which is actually a small round or square transistorized battery, does just that—it helps to pace the rate and rhythm of the heart. Both children and adults may need a pacemaker, simply because their own heart does not have a normal rhythm—usually the problem is an ex-

Figure 18.4: The Function of a Prosthetic Ball

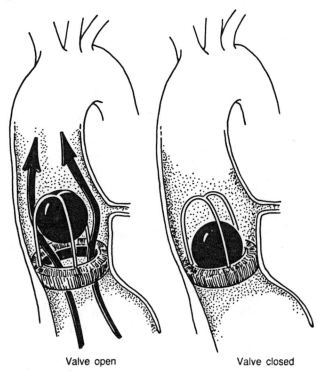

Valve open   Valve closed

Illustration adapted from a drawing by Herbert R. Smith, from DeBakey, M., and Gotto, A., The Living Heart, N.Y., David McKay Co., 1977.

cessively slow rate of beating, and the heart therefore needs to be "paced," or set to beat at a normal rate and rhythm. In order to understand why your doctor might recommend a pacemaker, let's review briefly how the heart works.

Remember, the heart is a pump—it beats rhythmically, twenty-four hours a day, non-stop. To do this, electrical impulses are produced by the heart's "natural pacemaker," normally a small area of tissue located in the right atrium and called the sinus node. From the sinus node, the electrical impulses travel along special pathways and cause the heart muscle to contract, enabling it to pump blood. In the healthy heart, these electrical impulses occur regularly at about 60 to 100 beats/minute. The rate may be lower during sleep or rest and can rise, as necessary, during increased activity. In some people, abnormalities of the normal pacemaker or electrical conducting pathways can reduce the frequency of pacemaker activity or the spread of its electrical impulse, thereby decreasing the heart rate. In such cases, the heart pumps too little blood to the body, and a variety of problems can develop, such as fainting and heart failure. Fortunately, however, a solution for this problem was developed approximately twenty years ago—the artificial cardiac pacemaker.

Birth of the Pacemaker

Interest in pacing the heart by using electrical currents goes back over several decades; however, it wasn't until 1958 that an American physician treated a patient with heart block by using a small transistorized battery-operated external pacemaker. Then, a year later, an implantable cardiac pacemaker was developed. After several years of work to improve this idea, the first total pacemaker implant in this country was performed in 1960. Since then, there's been a steady increase in improvements and use of cardiac pacemakers. For example, the first group of pacemakers were often referred to as "fixed-rate" types, because they paced the heart at a rate that was set or "fixed" by the manufacturer. In some patients, however, problems developed because the patient's own heart occasionally competed with the artificial pacemaker. Later, another model, called the "demand" pacemaker was developed. Quite simply, it works on "standby"; in other words, it paces the patient's heart *only* when the rate falls below the present pacemaker rate.

The first pacemakers were powered by mercury-zinc batteries. The batteries, as well as the electrical apparatus, were embedded in plastic and all of this was then generally covered by rubber. Today, even more sophisticated and capable pacemakers have been developed—in fact, even nuclear-powered pacemakers have been tried, although they are not commonly used. The most typical pacemakers now being inserted today are those that utilize lithium-powered batteries. Pacemakers that rely on nickel-cadmium batteries have also been used with considerable success in the last few years. This latter type of pacemaker can be recharged from outside of the body while the device remains within the body; thus, it's considered "permanent," since subsequent surgery to implant a new model is not necessary.

How a Pacemaker Works

Quite simply it works as your heart's natural pacemaker is supposed to work. (See Figure 18.5.) The "demand" pacemakers take over automatically, as soon as the patient's heart rate drops below a certain level. Thus, the patient can continue his activities even when his "natural" heart rate drops. Today, more than 250,000 Americans have pacemakers, and projections indicate that number will increase annually by 20 percent.

A pacemaker is implanted surgically, although this procedure does not involve major surgery. The generator component of the pacemaker which is about the size of a cigarette pack, is usually implanted beneath the skin of the

Figure 18.5: How an Artificial Pacemaker Works

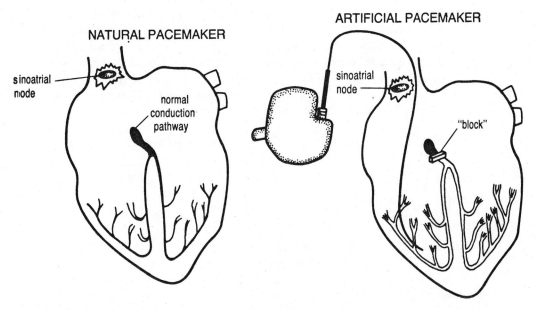

The heart's natural pacemaker (left) is the sinoatrial node. When the electrical conduction system pathway is blocked (right), a pacemaker may be needed to restore an adequate cardiac rate.

axilla (armpit) and the wires leading from it are connected to the heart. This is done either by sewing the wires directly to the surface of the heart or placing a singled lead containing the wire into the inside of the right ventricle, through a large vein in the neck. All components of the pacemaker and its wires are beneath the skin. The latter procedure is normally used since it is simpler and does not require opening of the chest, which the former does. Once implanted, most patients can't feel the pacemaker and aren't in any way troubled by its presence. Since the pacemaker is a piece of equipment, some parts may have to be replaced occasionally. Once you have a pacemaker, the important thing is to know what its pulse rate should be; variations should be reported to your doctor. Similarly, symptoms such as dizziness, chest pain, and shortness of breath should be reported. Finally, a patient with a pacemaker should follow all of the physician's instructions: take all medications according to directions, and follow diet and exercise plans as specified.

What Is Life with a Pacemaker Like?

For most patients, this is *the* crucial question. Thanks to modern technology, pacemakers may be implanted in both children and adults to treat severely reduced heart rates. Today, thousands of people have pacemakers and continue to work and enjoy numerous leisure activities. Those in doubt should speak with someone who is using a pacemaker. In fact, we did just that in October 1978, when the late Henry Fonda, who was then 73 years old and had a pacemaker, was in New York to star in a Broadway play, *First Monday in October.* Here is what he had to say about life with a pacemaker.

An Interview with Henry Fonda on "Living with a Pacemaker"

Holmes:	Mr. Fonda, how long have you had a pacemaker?
Fonda:	Just three years.
Holmes:	What signs or symptoms did you have ?
Fonda:	I began to notice shortness of breath, so I decided to see my doctor here in New York.
Holmes:	What was his diagnosis?
Fonda:	Well, after a checkup in his office, he decided to hospitalize me for further tests. I went into the hospital right away and underwent numerous diagnostic procedures—blood tests, an electrocardiogram, and for about a week I was, in effect, "hooked up" to a pacemaker; in other words, a temporary pacemaker was inserted while my doctor monitored my heart rate and rhythm. After monitoring me for several days in the hospital, my physician recommended a permanent pacemaker to correct the abnormal rhythm and rate of my heart.
Holmes:	Were you worried about having a heart attack?
Fonda:	No, because my physician explained very clearly to me that my shortness of breath wasn't due to any type of heart attack or heart muscle failure.*
Holmes:	Did you remain in the hospital at that time ?
Fonda:	Yes I did, and I was released from the hospital just a few days after the operation.

Holmes: What preparation did you undergo for this?

Fonda: Actually, I was rather surprised to learn that a pacemaker—which is about the size of a pack of cigarettes—could be inserted under a local anesthetic. In other words, I was able to talk to the doctors throughout the procedure, since I wasn't unconscious.

Holmes: Do you still have the same pacemaker that was implanted three years ago?

Fonda: No I don't. The first one I had needed to be recharged fairly often and about two years after implantation, it just stopped working, for no apparent reason.

Holmes: When was that pacemaker removed and another one implanted?

Fonda: My doctor in California discovered in the course of a routine checkup that my pacemaker had just stopped functioning, so I went into a hospital in California and had the first pacemaker removed and another one implanted.

Holmes: Have you found that living with a pacemaker impairs your function in any way?

Fonda: To the contrary. The pacemaker doesn't interfere with my ability to function or perform in any significant way; in fact, if it weren't for the pacemaker, I probably wouldn't be able to take long walks, which I enjoy, or perform for two hours every evening on Broadway, which I've now been doing for a month.

Holmes: What type of exercise do you engage in?

Fonda: Well, I prefer long walks—I don't play golf, although I certainly could if I wanted to—and I don't jog or run. Nevertheless, I'm a very active man—I continue to travel and work, and my hours are often long and tedious. Again, I don't think I could do all of these things, if it weren't for the pacemaker.

Holmes: Did your physician restrict any of your activities?

Fonda: No, not really. I have been told, however, that I am not supposed to lift heavy objects or strain myself physically in any other way.

Holmes: Do you often think about the fact that you have a pacemaker—are you aware of it?

Fonda: No, I'm not aware of its presence at all. It was a very simple surgical procedure to undergo, and it's made my life easier. Now I can perform, take long walks, et cetera, without becoming short of breath.

Holmes: What thoughts would you like to share with others who may have to face surgery for a pacemaker implant soon?

Fonda: First, I think it should be emphasized that implantation of a pacemaker is a minor operation; there's nothing to fear. Second, anyone who is going to have a pacemaker should keep in mind that this is a *corrective* device. It's meant to help a heart beating too slowly get back on track, so to speak. Generally speaking, in fact, I think most people with pacemakers would probably say that their lives improved somewhat as a result of this surgery. After all, the rhythm problem in the heart resolves itself once the pacemaker is implanted, and this usually results in a relief of symptoms, such as shortness of breath or dizziness.

Holmes: Any additional points?

Fonda: Yes. I'd like to say that except for an occasional conversation like this, I rarely think about my pacemaker, but when I do, I actually feel good about it because I know it's keeping my heart beating, at a consistent seventy beats per minute. Believe me, I feel secure in knowing the pacemaker is there to do what my heart wasn't up to doing any longer. Of course, if your doctor recommends a pacemaker for you, you should feel free—as I did—to ask questions, et cetera. I can only hope that anyone who has to undergo this procedure will benefit as much as I have from it.

What Henry Fonda said is right.* Life with a pacemaker doesn't have to be difficult**. Still, it's understandable for anyone who is about to have a pacemaker implanted to be concerned. For additional information on living with a pacemaker, contact the following organizations:

International Association of Pacemaker Patients
P.O. Box 54305
Atlanta, Georgia 30308

This organization was established to help pacemaker patients understand the use and purpose of pacemakers and to better educate and inform the patient and his family. This organization also publishes a trimonthly informative magazine, *Pulse;* a glossary of pacemaker terms appears in each issue.

Pacemakers Unlimited, Ltd.
P.O. Box 5481
Fort Lauderdale, Florida 33310
(305–772–4950)
The purpose of this group is to keep pre- and postoperative pacemaker patients, their families, and their friends informed.

Your local chapter also probably has booklets on pacemakers.

---

*Author's Note: Fonda was experiencing symptoms of congestive heart failure, but they were not caused by inadequate function of cardiac muscle, but rather by a severe reduction in heart rate, which is caused by degenerative disease of the electrical conduction system of the heart, exclusive of any problems in the heart muscle itself.

**Fonda lived with a pacemaker for eight years and followed a rigorous work schedule until the last 18 months of his life, which ended on August 12, 1982. A few months earlier he was awarded an Oscar for his performance in the 1981 film *On Golden Pond*.

WHAT'S HAPPENED TO HEART TRANSPLANTATION?

Overnight, the name of Dr. Christiaan Barnard, a South African cardiovascular surgeon, became a household word. On December 3, 1967, in Cape Town, a human heart from one patient was transplanted into the chest of another. As a result, in the following year 64 medical teams in 22 countries raced to duplicate this seemingly impossible feat. Since the first heart transplant, more than 350 such operations have been performed in over 50 medical centers. In fact, at the Stanford University Medical Center, 204 heart transplants had been performed as of February, 1981, and of those, 75 patients were still alive. At present, the five-year survival rate there is approximately Dr. Denton Cooley of the Texas Heart Institute have also performed a number of successful heart transplants, but they concede that this is a "last resort."

Over the years, both physicians and patients have learned that the technical aspects of heart transplanation—removing a fatally diseased heart and replacing it with a healthier one—is the easiest part of the entire surgical procedure. In fact, the real challenge lay in getting the recipient patient's body to accept the "foreign" or donor's heart. In most cases, however, the "foreign" organ is not accepted, and rejection sets in within days. Thus, most of the earlier heart transplant recipients died within a few weeks after surgery.

Today, experts agree that this approach is certainly not the solution to treatment of severe heart disease. Not only is it difficult for the patient's body to accept the foreign tissue, but this procedure is also hampered because compatible donors are not readily available, surgical teams skilled in this procedure are few, and the cost is very high, but there have been success stories.

Research has gone on for more than twenty years to develop an artificial heart that could be implanted in humans. Investigators at the University of Utah's College of Medicine have developed an artificial heart made of aluminum and plastic for use in humans.* Experiments in animals showed that a calf lived more than 250 days with an artificial heart. However, the first known at tempt to use an artificial heart to save a patient's life was made by Dr. Denton Cooley in 1969. The artificial heart pump kept the patient alive for nearly three days, until a heart transplant could be performed. The patient died 32 hours later, due to pneumonia.

Until methods are developed to improve the rate of patient acceptance of heart transplants, no physician would advocate this procedure—at least not until all other therapeutic possibilities have been exhausted. For the few in whom the transplanted heart has worked effectively, however, the procedure has certainly been worthwhile.

---

*Barney Clark, a 62-year-old dentist, survived more than three months with an artificial heart. Physicians at The University of Utah Medical Center performed the operation.

PTCA AND STREPTOKINASE FOR TREATMENT OF CHD

Percutaneous transluminal coronary angioplasty (PTCA)

This is a new technique that is currently under clinical investigation. Early results suggest that this mode of treatment may have an important therapeutic role in selected coronary patients, such as those with stable angina, but considerably more data are required before any conclusions can be drawn.

The application of percutaneous transluminal angioplasty is not limited to the coronary arteries. In fact, it has also been successfully applied to the iliac (artery in the upper leg) and renal arteries. This procedure can significantly reduce the stenosis (narrowing) and increase the patency (openness) of an atherosclerotic artery. The use of PTCA does not usually result in the normalization of the caliber of the arterial lumen but, typically, reduces the severity of a stenosis so that it is no longer hemodynamically significant. A major advantage of this method is that it involves several of the techniques of cardiac catheterization. It takes several hours in-hospital and the patient can be discharged on the following day, provided there are no associated complications. There is no convalescence period after angioplasty.

Percutaneous transluminal angioplasty involves catheterization of the coronary artery in the usual manner, but a special balloon catheter is used. Patients are selected on the basis of the presence of appropriate coronary lesions, identified from the preceding diagnostic coronary angiogram. Angioplasty is then scheduled; this is a separate procedure and is usually performed within a few days or a week or two of the diagnostic study.

Patient selection

Criteria for the procedure are the presence of a significant, discrete, proximal, noncalcified coronary lesion in a patient with symptomatology that would qualify him/her for coronary artery bypass surgery. Ideally, the lesions should be no longer than one centimeter, and they must be accessible to the dilating catheter. The vessel should have no other significant stenoses.

On the basis of the foregoing criteria, it appears that the use of percutaneous transluminal coronary angioplasty would be indicated in 20 percent—and perhaps less than 10 percent—of coronary patients. Of course, criteria may change as experience with this technique increases, but it is likely that the patients who qualify for this will remain in the minority of coronary patients.

Rationale of balloon angioplasty

The concept underlying this procedure is based on the fact that it is known that much of the material that makes up atherosclerotic plaques is relatively soft and compressible; as such, investigators believed that the plaque could be flattened and spread beneath adjacent endothelium, thereby reducing the stenosis and enlarging the vessel lumen. Experimental and clinical data have demonstrated the feasibility of balloon angioplasty; calcification precludes angioplasty.

Methodology

On identification of an appropriate coronary lesion for dilatation (on the basis of coronary angiography performed in a properly selected patient fulfilling the criteria enumerated here), percutaneous transluminal coronary angioplasty is scheduled. A large-diameter guiding catheter is placed percutaneously (through the skin) into the femoral artery (the chief artery in the thigh) and advanced into the ascending aorta and then into the orifice of the coronary artery to be dilated. Through this guiding catheter, the smaller, special balloon catheter is fed into the coronary artery to the site of the stenosis. Transient inflation of the balloon compresses the atherosclerotic plaque, resulting in enlargement of the vessel lumen. Techniques vary, but in general the small balloon is inflated for fifteen to thirty seconds at several atmospheres of pressure.

Patients receive anticoagulant and antithrombotic therapy before and during angioplasty. This consists of aspirin and/or dipyridamole and heparin. Anticoagulant therapy is then continued for a variable period after the procedure.

Results

Based on coronary angiography performed before and immediately after PTCA, results show that balloon dilatation can reduce coronary artery stenoses of 80 percent or greater in lumen diameter to less than 40 percent of lumen diameter, and pressure gradients of 50 mm Hg or more have been decreased to about 20 mm Hg. Thus, significant lesions can be reduced to nonsignificant lesions—from a hemodynamic viewpoint. In association with these anatomic results, anginal symptoms are reduced or abolished, as is objective evidence of myocardial ischemia determined by pre- and post-dilation exercise electrocardiography and myocardial perfusion stress scintigraphy.

Approximately 10 percent of coronary patients are currently candidates for percutaneous coronary angioplasty. Of these, the dilating catheter can be passed to the area of the lesion and successful results achieved in the majority. The total clinical experience with PTCA in this country is being carefully collected and analyzed through the cooperative effort of the cardiologists using it and the National Heart, Lung and Blood Institute at Bethesda, Maryland.

Complications

The risks of percutaneous transluminal coronary angioplasty include laceration of a coronary artery, rupture of a plaque with subintimal hemorrhage, arrhythmias, angina, myocardial infarction and death. Major complications occur in less than 5 percent of the total documented experience, which is still limited. Thus, only patients who are candidates for coronary artery bypass surgery on the basis of symptoms and understand that the procedure may result in an emergency complication that requires urgent surgery should undergo it.

Summary

Percutaneous transluminal coronary angioplasty is a nonsurgical method for reducing the degree of coronary artery stenosis. Lesions for which this method can be utilized are proximal, discrete and noncalcified. Although still being tried, it appears that this procedure will be applicable in a small proportion of patients with coronary artery disease. Potential complications involve the spectrum of clinical coronary syndromes. The role of percutaneous coronary angioplasty in the treatment of coronary artery disease will be determined by investigations currently in progress.

Use of Streptokinase to Help Heart Attack Victims

It has become apparent from angiographic studies of the coronary arteries of patients in the early hours of acute myocardial infarction that an important factor in the production of myocardial infarction is the formation of a thrombus (clot) at the point of preexistent atherosclerotic narrowing in the artery. Remember, atherosclerotic narrowing is a chronic, degenerative process, and a clot can be superimposed upon it. Although this set of circumstances is not the only mechanism by which myocardial infarction may occur, it appears to be a very frequent, if not the most frequent, cause. The myocardial infarction results from the sudden, severe reduction in blood supply to the area of myocardium (heart muscle) supplied by the diseased coronary artery. Other mechanisms by which blood flow in coronary arteries may be reduced severely enough to produce myocardial infarction include spasm (transient constriction) of the artery due to unknown causes, very advanced atherosclerotic narrowing and obliteration of the coronary lumen, and obstruction of the lumen by hemorrhage within the wall of the artery, resulting in expansion of the wall into the inner canal of the artery.

Recognition that coronary artery thrombosis is an important factor in many cases of myocardial infarction has resulted in interest in methods of removing or dissolving the thrombus, and thereby restoring blood flow to its pre-thrombotic level in the coronary artery in hopes of interrupting the infarction process in its early stages, thereby minimizing or limiting the extent of myocardial damage. This goal is an extremely important one for physicians, since the mortality and complications of myocardial infarction are largely related to the extent of myocardial damage.

Clinical trials to evaluate methods of restoring blood flow through coronary arteries in the early stages of acute myocardial infarction have recently begun in a number of medical centers in Europe and in the United States. The techniques used are in their early stages and are preliminary in nature. However, a number of interesting and important observations have thus far been noted.

Methods utilized to date to restore blood flow in obstructed coronary arteries in the early stages of acute myocardial infarction include "recanalization" of the artery by passage of a thin, soft guide wire into the artery and through a thrombus, if present; administration of nitroglycerin to relieve spasm of the coronary artery if this is the mechanism of obstruction in a given patient; and administration of streptokinase, an enzyme which promotes the formation *in vivo* of plasmin, an enzyme that degrades clots by breaking down the fibrin component of the clot. (Fibrin is a protein that is an important component of clots.) The breakdown of fibrin results in dissolution of a clot that has already formed. All three of the foregoing methods have resulted in recanalization of the coronary artery to some degree in some patients in the early stages of myocardial infarction, but streptokinase has had by far the most success. This latter finding is consistent with data indicating that thrombosis in a diseased coronary artery is the most common cause of acute myocardial infarction. If thrombolytic therapy with streptokinase is shown to be effective in patients with acute myocardial infarction, this form of therapy will have major advantages in that it can be given intravenously and does not require the invasive procedure of cardiac catheterization and coronary angiography. At present, investigations include these latter procedures, since the therapeutic method is still in its initial stages and angiography allows documentation of whether or not thrombi in the coronary arteries can truly be lysed (dissolved). However, a recent large study, the European Cooperative Streptokinase Trial, did show reduced mortality following myocardial infarction in patients given intravenous streptokinase, compared to placebo controls. Only mortality was assessed; no angiography was done. If it is established that this therapy is effective in this regard, it can be given to large numbers of patients in most hospitals, since intravenous administration of any medication is a routine, standard procedure employed universally. In fact, therapy would be carried out as it was in the early study of the European Cooperative Trial, in which intravenous streptokinase was administered without invasive catheterization or angiography and the patients' mortality was evaluated. As indicated here, the patients receiving streptokinase showed a significantly lower mortality following myocardial infarction. Trials now underway are being carried out to further assess the effect of streptokinase immediately on the mortality rate and to assess the actual mechanism by which the drug acts to decrease mortality in acute myocardial infarction. This is an acute procedure; efficiency depends on implementation in the earliest hours after a myocardial infarction. Finally, it should be noted that although the foregoing results are impressive, they are early and the therapeutic role of streptokinase in myocardial infarction can only be determined by futher investigation.

The Intraaortic Balloon Pump

A device that can be inserted very simply and assists the failing heart, but does not take over its function, is the intraaortic balloon pump. This device can be utilized in certain critically ill patients in intensive care units. It consists of a balloon of 30-40 cc mounted on the end of a catheter attached to a console that houses a pump and instruments for programming the mechanical activity of the pump. The pump controls the movement of gas, such as carbon dioxide or helium, into and out of the balloon to make it expand and collapse. The balloon is positioned in the aorta in the chest by insertion through a large leg artery. The device is programmed to cause balloon expansion and collapse in coordination with the heart beat so that during diastole, the rest period between ventricular contractions, gas is moved into the balloon so that it expands, forcing blood backward in the aorta toward the heart and increasing coronary blood flow and nutrition of the myocardium. Just before the left ventricle contracts, gas is withdrawn from the balloon and it collapses, reducing the resistance in the aorta to ventricular outflow and allowing the impaired left ventricle to contract against a lowered resistance. By this phasic expansion and collapse of the balloon at the appropriate times, the diseased, failing left ventricle receives increased nutrition through augmented coronary blood flow, and is able to provide the same or greater amounts of outflow of blood to the body with reduced work by the heart. These results are accomplished because of the expansion of the balloon in diastole, which increases nutritional coronary blood flow, and by collapse of the balloon in ventricular systole, reducing resistance against which the failing left ventricle must pump.

The intraaortic balloon pump is chiefly applicable to patients with myocardial infarction complicated by shock, a dire situation in which the function of the left ventricle is marginally compatible with maintenance of life, and in the immediate postoperative period in patients who have had open heart surgery and whose heart function is sluggish and slow to recover. Intraaortic balloon pumping is usually carried out for a few hours or days, but has been maintained for several weeks in some patients. It is indicated in situations in which there is a potentially reversible defect of the heart which can heal or improve within a relatively short time, while the intraaortic balloon temporarily aids in maintaining adequate circulation. It is not indicated when there is permanent, extensive, irreversible heart damage.

PART VI
Living with Heart Disease

How to Live a Full Life
After Heart Disease Is Diagnosed

These days, life after a heart attack, coronary artery bypass surgery, cardiac valve replacement, or insertion of a cardiac pacemaker is not necessarily restricted or dreary. In some cases, a patient may decide to retire early—but not to withdraw from life and its pleasures. Quite the contrary, after recovering from cardiac problems or heart surgery, many people begin to travel extensively; others pursue hobbies; and still others "retire" from one job to start a brand new career. For example, Mr. Peter J. was a successful lawyer who always had a heavy caseload. His favorite pastime, however, since he was a young man, had been carpentry. He enjoyed the hours working alone in his tool shack, which he himself had constructed; but as he grew more successful in his legal work, he had less and less time for it. After his heart attack, he decided to "retire" early—but only from the practice of law. He soon began to make cabinets, bookcases, and other items in which his neighbors and friends began to take a considerable interest. Within a year, Mr. J. was selling many of his handcrafted pieces to local stores, and, at last report, he was enjoying himself tremendously and was able to decline offers to build furniture for two department stores!

Today, more than three-fourths of those who have heart disease return to work, drive cars, and so on. Many, in fact, even report certain improvements; for example, they see more of their children and play with them; they relax more, and take advantage of the things for which they have often worked so hard but had such little time to enjoy.

Of course, no one would deny that the initial shock of a heart attack or other serious cardiac problem is traumatic, both for the victim and the family. Typi-

273

cally, it is not just the victim's life that is altered, but the lives of all those around him. Consider the following case:

> Mr. Steve L. suffered a heart attack at 51. He was vice-president of a major corporation and the father of seven children. After he was released from the hospital, he was given certain instructions, such as to lose weight, to stop cigarette smoking, and to reduce his long hours in the office. His wife responded appropriately, and did all that she could to help him with his diet, but he continued to "sneak" foods, and his weight did not decrease. He also couldn't give up smoking.
>
> Unfortunately, three of the older children were adversely affected by all of this. They knew what their father was *supposed* to be doing; now, they couldn't understand why he wasn't doing it. About two years later, Mr. L. suffered a second heart attack. The oldest child was so angered by this (after all, he argued with his mother, what did his father expect—he hadn't followed any of the doctor's orders) that he flatly refused to speak with his father for nearly two months. The second oldest child, who rarely missed school, suddenly started missing days, with various vague complaints. The third child, who had been thoroughly enjoying his second year in a boarding school, pleaded to come home. With only six weeks left until school was out, his mother advised him to stay and assured him that his father was going to be fine. Despite this, the boy left school without authorization and hitchhiked more than three hundred miles home.

It's very important to realize that when any member of a family is hospitalized, the effects can reverberate. Often, a wife is so concerned about her husband that neither he nor she is aware of what is happening to the children, and the physician is usually not aware of their problems, either. In situations such as these, children, too, can be brought to the physician's office to learn—in terms that they will understand—just what the problems are and what can be done to correct them. More than ever, this is a time that family members and relatives need to communicate with each other, and share fears and anxieties. Most important of all, it is not a good idea to seek advice from well-meaning, but frequently uninformed, neighbors. Every heart attack, for example, is not the same, nor is every patient. Each case is unique, and the rules that apply to one may not necessarily apply to another.

In most situations, of course, the person making the most adjustments is the patient himself. As soon as he discovers that he is in the coronary care unit and can speak, the questions begin: Can I go back to work? Can I have sex? Do I have to stop smoking? Will I have to give up all of my favorite foods? I hate the idea of jogging—do I have to run? Can I drive a car? Will I be an invalid for the rest of my life? Fortunately, many patients will have relatively few restrictions. However, in every case, cigarette smoking is absolutely out; in fact, doctors have recently coined a new phrase, "passive smoking," because studies show that persons with heart conditions who sit in a room filled with smokers will experience a rise in blood pressure and pulse from the smoke in the room.

Other than that, however, limitations are ordinarily few. Your doctor will work with you to help ease you back into life's mainstream. For example, the majority of patients can go back to work, but most are advised to start with half-days, and nap in the afternoon as is needed. Similarly, if the patient is overweight and has a high serum cholesterol level, the doctor will prescribe an appropriate diet—but this doesn't mean starvation, nor does it mean being deprived of favorite foods. Instead, the recovery program he will outline will be one of moderation, not deprivation, and, thanks to the many food substitutes now available, such as diet margarines and egg and bacon substitutes, one can enjoy the taste of many of the foods one likes. Once the weight is normal, the doctor will probably allow some foods that may have been strictly limited back into the patient's diet, but he will probably advise moderation.

And, even if a person must remain on a low-salt or low-cholesterol diet for life, the number of fine cookbooks that specialize in the preparation of foods meeting these requirements make it easier to adhere to restrictions. *The American Heart Association Cookbook* is a classic work in this respect. For additional information, you can consult your physician, the hospital dietitian, your local Heart Association, or the local library.

Despite the gains that have been made, signs and symptoms of anxiety and depression frequently do develop after a heart attack. It is best to share these feelings with your doctor and/or supportive members of your family in order to resolve them. It is important to try to overcome these feelings, especially since studies show that patients who are depressed immediately after a heart attack, and remain depressed for a year thereafter, have a higher hospital readmission rate, frequently fail to remain at work, and often fail to function sexually. Your best bet is to accept what has happened and decide to do everything that will enhance the chances of significant improvement.

In order to help you through these periods, it is advisable to take advantage of the services now offered to recovering cardiac patients. Many doctors have discovered that most of their patients, regardless of their education, know little about how the heart actually functions and what a heart attack actually means.

Moreover, many people are unwilling to admit their lack of knowledge, and may harbor such misconceptions as: a heart attack causes a hole in the heart or, the occurrence of one heart attack automatically dooms the victim to another within a few years. These people should be reminded of the many people who have had heart attacks and continue to lead busy, prosperous lives. Some patients are particularly reassured upon learning that many physicians have also had heart attacks and returned to their work. Dr. Irvine Page, Professor Emeritus at the Cleveland Clinic Foundation, is one whom we have mentioned, as well as Dr. Albert Starr, Professor of Surgery at the Oregon Health Sciences Center, and Dr. William Nolen, the well-known surgeon-author. Even more reassuring is the news that eight of the runners who competed in the 1973 Boston Marathon were persons who had recovered from a heart attack. (Of course, this isn't recommended for every heart attack victim, and all exercise programs must be approved by your doctor.)

The point is, life after a heart attack, as well as after other types of heart disease and heart surgery, can be normal—and sometimes even better than before, depending on what the patient makes of the situation. But if you don't really believe us, listen to what some of the victims themselves had to say when we talked with them about their heart disease:

> I've always believed that stress and tension are at the root of many illnesses. As a victim of heart disease myself, I know how important it is to try and avoid stresses and aggravation—it's just not worth it.
>
> My advice to those who have to live with someone who has heart disease is simple: be loving and compassionate, but treat the person as a human being—*not* as a heart cripple. Don't just give them your shoulder to cry on—that's the easy way out—give them your continued support. In other words, give them your heart, and your love, as my family did for me, and that will help any victim of heart disease stay on the road to recovery. God knows, it worked for me.
>
> Pearl Bailey

> I entered Massachusetts General Hospital in the summer of 1975, and on July 11, I underwent what doctors call a "double cabbage"— from the abbreviation CABG—a double coronary artery bypass graft. In my operation, one vein graft was used to connect the aorta to the circumflex coronary artery, and a second was used to connect the aorta to the left anterior descending coronary artery. The whole operation took about four hours. The first two postoperative days were painful and unpleasant—but the doctors had me back on my feet by the third day, and after just eight weeks, I was running a mile a day, generally in half- or quarter-mile portions. By the early fall—in September to be exact—I was back in the OR in the Litchfield Clinic—*performing* surgery once again. Since then, I've performed numerous operations, and I continue to travel, jog, play tennis and racquetball. I've even made some television appearances—including Johnny Carson's *Tonight Show.*
>
> Of course, not everyone who has coronary artery disease is eligible for this type of surgery, but for those in whom it is indicated, the results can be excellent—in my case, for example, it put me back into the mainstream of life.
>
> William A. Nolen, M.D.

> One day, I felt a tightness in my chest while walking, but it went away when I rested. After a while, I became concerned about this, and went to see my doctor. He told me that I had angina and high blood pressure. I began to take medications for both, and I felt better. Because I was approaching retirement age, however, I decided to retire from my job as a

field manager with John Hancock Life Insurance Company early, and live a little.

In the last eight years, my wife and I have traveled extensively; we've been to Europe more than ten times, and I've had the opportunity to enjoy some of the things that have always interested me, but I never seemed to have the time for before.

Mr. Aldo Luciani
Newark, New Jersey

These stories, and thousands like them, from celebrities, physicians, businessmen—people from all walks of life—should be ample evidence that a full and prosperous life can be yours despite heart disease. Read on, to discover a world of programs and services designed to help you.

19

A Heart Patient's Diet Is a Healthy Diet

If your health is impaired in any way, be it by heart disease or other medical problems, it is, obviously, especially important for you to do all that you can to attain and maintain good health; in other words, to "keep in shape." Then, if heart disease and its complications develop, all other factors will be favorable, and your fine physical condition might be just the difference that places the odds in your favor.

It is especially important to stay trim if you have heart disease. Extra pounds put an extra burden on the heart, and no damaged heart should be subjected to this added strain. This chapter outlines which diets are appropriate for cardiac patients.

Although some patients who have angina or who have had heart attacks are physically fit, the majority of victims have had a weight problem at some time, and many are overweight when angina or heart attack first strikes. For these patients, weight loss is mandatory, and maintenance of normal weight is equally important. (In some cases, such as Dr. William Nolen's, the patient had avoided cigarette smoking and maintained a healthy diet all his life, which facilitated his recovery.)

Frequently, the physician recommends a low-calorie diet for the hospitalized patient. In this setting, compliance is usually forced. However, long-term compliance is often a problem once the patient is released and returns to his own home and work. Then, the old habits can creep back in.

On the one hand, the knowledge that weight gain is a real threat to life is often so frightening that some cardiac patients may be inclined to make dieting their own personal project. Since many have had experience with popular diets such as Dr. Atkins' Diet or the Stillman Diet, they think they know which regimens seem to work best for them. They want to get weight off in a hurry, assuming that this is the best course.

278

Unfortunately, this assumption is far from the truth. As we indicated earlier, "fad" diets may get you started, and the rapid initial weight loss will be gratifying, but not only are the results rarely long-lasting, some of these diets can also be harmful. This is especially true if you already have some form of heart disease—coronary heart disease, in particular. Under no circumstances should a patient with coronary heart disease attempt to diet without specific consultation with his or her physician. Despite our admonitions, however, you may be inclined to take three or four weeks on one of the more popular diets just to get rid of those pounds you gained, perhaps, since you left the hospital. To discourage fad dieting, we will review the "essentials" of some of these diets, and then outline very clearly for you the reasons why patients with heart disease, and particularly coronary heart disease, must avoid certain diets.

Rather than plunge into a popular "fad" diet, we have recommended some of the better cookbooks published to help the cardiac patient continue to enjoy eating and dining out, while sticking to his or her low-cholesterol and/or low-salt diet. Once you peruse one or more of these cookbooks, you will quickly see that the meal plans are varied and that the menus are organized so that these meals can be prepared for the entire family. Today, a heart patient's diet often just comes down to sensible eating . . . the whole family can and should participate. Because you are trying to establish a better eating pattern for life, we don't consider the menus and suggestions offered here a "diet" in the real sense of that word. Only your doctor can place you on a diet. Rather, we view the guidelines here as recommendations that can pave the way for healthy eating patterns, and carry you through for the rest of your life.

Dr. Atkins' Diet

This diet, which swept the country several years ago, supposedly "revolutionized" dieting. For many, it seemed ideal, since it offered the best of both worlds: eat as much as you want of certain foods (including tasty, normally restricted foods such as steaks and even heavy cream) and still lose weight.

In the early weeks of the diet, intake of carbohydrates is severely restricted; little, if any, fruits or vegetables, and certainly no pastas, rice, or potatoes are allowed. Otherwise, you are free to eat as much as you want of eggs, marbled (fatty) beef, cream, butter, oil (both in cooking and in salad dressings), mayonnaise, bacon, and filled meats (sausages, hot dogs, and so on).

Despite many of these high-fat, high-calorie foods, the dieter loses weight, because, as Dr. Atkins says, your body secretes a "fat mobilizing hormone." In fact, this very low-carbohydrate diet causes ketosis (without a sufficient intake of carbohydrates, ketones build up in the blood and urine in excessive amounts and become a burden on the kidneys). What's worse, however, is that achieving ketosis is actually one of the primary objectives of this diet—you are even encouraged to buy "ketostix" from the drug store—small sticks with treated paper that can be passed through the urine stream to test for ketones in the urine. If the paper turns purple, you are in ketosis. According to Dr. Atkins, this is most desirable—but few physicians would agree!

Besides this obvious drawback, the diet is particularly inadvisable for the cardiac patient, because it is generally a high-fat, high-cholesterol diet and places an extra burden on the kidneys. True, egg substitutes, lean meats, and bacon substitutes can be eaten, but this seems to encourage a rather large intake of synthetic products; in addition, a diet virtually void of carbohydrates will not help you "retrain" your eating habits and, when they are reintroduced, the diet essentially remains high in fats.

The Stillman Diet

This regimen is frequently referred to as the "water diet" because you are required to drink eight or more glasses of water per day, in addition to tea, coffee, and diet beverages. You are allowed to eat as much lean meat and low-fat cheese as you like, but nothing else. This diet has pitfalls, as does the Atkins Diet. It is not balanced; it won't help you learn to improve your poor eating habits; and it's monotonous!

The "Save-Your-Life" Diet

This diet followed on the heels of the Stillman and Atkins diets, and reigned as *the* diet for about a year. According to Dr. David Reuben, who introduced it, putting fiber back into the typical low-fiber American diet can "save your life." Certainly, a daily moderate amount of fiber is good for you. You can get it by eating fruits with skins, potato skins, vegetables such as celery and tomatoes, whole wheat and other unprocessed breads and cereals, and so on. But no one foodstuff can be responsible for saving your life.

Although the claim is extravagant, this diet has some good points. It is balanced; it emphasizes the importance of eating fresh foods and unrefined products as well as eating lots of fresh fish, poultry, and lean meats. Your doctor may approve of this diet for you, or he may make some modifications because of your specific requirements to reduce cholesterol intake or to decrease your salt intake. Still, this diet provides a nutritious framework from which you and your physician can work, (and a family can accept this diet, too).

The Scarsdale Diet

This is a later diet craze, and virtually all fad dieters who have been on it swear by it.

It's called the Scarsdale Diet because the physician who outlined the plan practiced in Scarsdale, N.Y. The diet is very strict; no deviations whatsoever are allowed. There is a list of "forbidden" foods, which includes alcoholic beverages (not allowed on the Atkins' or Stillman diets, either), mayonnaise, and oils. An exact menu plan is provided for fourteen days; initially, no one was supposed to stay on it longer than that, but longer-range Scarsdale Diet plans are now available. No substitutions are allowed (you can't change meals around, nor can you eat more at lunch if you omit some items at breakfast). You are instructed to eat exactly what is outlined for you, in the *order* in which the food items are listed.

This diet has more going for it in the way of balanced nutrition than the Atkins' or Stillman diets. It has the advantage of carbohydrates (fruits, protein bread, and some vegetables). However, Dr. Herman Tarnower, who was credited with developing it, specifically attached a disclaimer: "This diet is *not* for cardiacs. If you have a heart condition or other health problem, do not go on this diet without your doctor's supervision."

Because several of the weekly dinners consist of steak (as much as you want), lamb chops, eggs, and so on, this diet has a cholesterol content that could be considered excessive for cardiac patients. In addition, since many cardiac patients are on low-salt or salt-free diets, this diet is inappropriate for them because many of the foods allowed have a fairly high salt content.

Since Dr. Tarnower himself directed cardiac patients to avoid this diet (unless their physicians give approval), we hope that you will heed his precautions.

The Pritikin Program

The Pritikin Diet, a dietary program developed by Nathan Pritikin, consists of four different diet plans of varying caloric levels (the range is 850 to 1,200 calories per day). Dr. Pritikin claims a good success rate—he opened his first Pritikin Center in 1976, and 7,000 people have been through his program since.

Essentially, his diets include the natural, whole carbohydrate foods and reduce drastically the intake of other foods. Regimens are stringent—*regardless* of the dietary program selected. Lots of high-fiber vegetables and fruits are permitted, along with whole wheat breads; but there is very little in the way of fish and chicken—and no beef. Herb teas and carbonated mineral waters are the preferred beverages—even diet colas, plain tea and black coffee are not allowed.

Pritikin claims his diet and exercise program, which is taught at all of his centers, is very beneficial for cardiac patients, as well as others. However, we believe it is very difficult to turn Pritikin's diet and exercise regimen into a lifelong habit—it is simply too rigid for most individuals. Also, for cardic patients in particular, assessment by your physician is *mandatory* before you attempt this diet.

The Ultimate Diet: Fasting

Many physicians have severely criticized this method of weight control; even individuals whose laboratory test results are normal, and who appear to be in reasonably good health except for their obesity, frequently suffer consequences ranging from remedial problems such as hypotension (dizziness on standing) to more damaging complications such as kidney disorders and gout. Even deaths have been attributed to this diet.

Once a person begins to fast, the body starts to utilize its excess weight for energy. This works out for a short period, but soon the body also begins to break down muscle mass—remember, the heart is a muscle, too. To prevent this, a protein-sparing supplement is given with the diet—a very low-calorie liquid mixture high in protein.

For the cardiac patient, a fasting diet—even a fasting program supplement—is absolutely prohibited. Besides the burden it places on every organ in the body, such a diet is even more hazardous when medications are being taken. In addition, the blood chemistry can change profoundly; for example, the level of potassium drops, while uric acid concentration in the blood can rise appreciably, perhaps even enough for gout to develop. No one, least of all a cardiac patient, should subject himself to these stresses. In fact, it is inadvisable for a cardiac patient who takes medications routinely (and most do), to even go a day without food—it is an added burden, and all stress should be avoided.

Forget the "Fad" Diets: Here's the Way to Fitness

To begin with, most people don't realize that fad diets are very effective because they all feature a reduction in total daily caloric intake. For example, a five-foot, five-inch woman who is reasonably active might need an average daily caloric intake of 1,500 to 1,800 calories to maintain her weight of 120 pounds. If she weighed 180 pounds, however, her total daily caloric intake to maintain this weight would soar to about 2,500 calories or more.

Now, if this woman goes on Dr. Atkins' Diet, for example, she could have two strips of bacon and two scrambled eggs (with butter) for breakfast, a piece of cold chicken for lunch, with a diet soda, and a good portion of steak and a salad made with oil and vinegar for dinner. By average standards, this might be considered a lot to eat, but for this woman, it is actually a reduction in total caloric intake—probably amounting to not more than 1,500 or 1,600 calories for the day, instead of the usual maintenance of 2,500 calories for 180 pounds.

For this individual, that's a drop of about 1,000 calories per day, and since 3,500 calories are equivalent to a pound, she loses weight. The Scarsdale Diet is also a low-calorie, essentially low-fat, diet. For instance, even though the "Scarsdale" dieters are permitted steak and lamb chops, they are advised to eat lean portions.

These diets are also generally effective initially because the individual is highly motivated and wants to try the new diet that everyone seems to be raving about. Thus, most "yo-yo" dieters stick to a diet for the first few weeks, or even months—it's the lifelong maintenance that presents the challenge.

Cardiac patients should follow the diets given to them by their family physician or cardiologist. Many physicians will recommend one of the sensible approaches outlined by Weight Watchers, etc. (See Chapter 6 for a list of diet organizations—your physician might find one that has a program suitable for you.) Fortunately, with so many substitute products available and so many dependable cookbooks on the shelves, it is relatively easy to prepare tasty nutritious meals that will not only meet the cardiac patient's special needs, but are also suitable for the entire family.

If you have to stick to low-salt and/or low-cholesterol diets, you can begin to learn how to revise some of your favorite recipes by checking *The American Heart Association's Cookbook*. In it, you will find hundreds of recipes for meat and game dishes, salad dressings, and even desserts, as well as holiday menu plans, so you never have to deviate from your "healthy eating" program. Your local library probably has a copy of this book, and you can contact your local Heart Association to obtain your own copy. Worthwhile cookbooks for the health-wise dieter are:

The American Heart Association Cookbook
David McKay Company, Inc., New York, 1973.

Cooking Without Your Salt Shaker
published by The American Heart
Association, Northeast Ohio Affiliate, in
cooperation with the Cleveland Dietetic Association, 1978.

Nutrition Labeling: How It Can Work for You
The National Nutrition Consortium, Inc.
24 3rd St., N.E.
Washington, D.C.
(202-547-4819)
Explains the nutritional labeling on food products.

Finally, to help you keep your eye on your cholesterol intake, refer to the chart on page 31. A more complete list appears in the AHA Cookbook.

The cholesterol content of over five hundred food items is also included in *Composition of Foods*, a thorough manual on nutrition information published by the Department of Agriculture. You can obtain a copy by contacting the Department of Agriculture.

DIETARY CONSIDERATIONS FOR THE CARDIAC PATIENT

Alcohol

Most physicians will permit some consumption, but excessive alcohol intake is to be avoided. Since most cardiac patients are taking one or more types of medications, it is especially important for them to query their physicians about potential drug and alcohol interactions. Various types of foods, as well as common over-the-counter medicinal products, can interact with alcohol and more potent medications, so be sure to advise your physician of your total dietary and medicinal regimen (and that includes "harmless" medications purchased without a prescription).

Coffee, Tea, and Other Products Containing Caffeine

Is caffeinated coffee a risk factor for coronary heart disease? Reports vary, but it is generally felt that drinking caffeinated coffee in moderation is permissible (about two cups per day). Again, however, it is important to let your physician know if you also intend to drink tea along with diet cola (which also contains caffeine). Similarly, some common over-the-counter medications contain caffeine, so you and your physician will have to determine your caffeine limit.

20
Exercise to Help the Diseased Heart

Benefits of Exercise in Patients with Coronary Heart Disease

Exercise has had demonstrable benefits in certain patients with angina pectoris and in rehabilitation after myocardial infarction. These patients must be carefully selected since exercise can be deleterious if the diseased heart cannot tolerate the increased stress. Thus, such patients must have stable cardiac conditions, including uncomplicated myocardial infarction and angina that is well controlled by medication. The principles of an exercise program for cardiac patients are similar to those presented previously, but with these patients the intensity of exercise is usually modest, and activities are performed in groups supervised on site by medical or paramedical personnel. All patients in this type of program have exercise tests as part of the evaluation of their suitability for the program.

The benefits of exercise for patients are a direct result of the physiological changes previously discussed. In patients with coronary artery disease and resultant angina pectoris, the symptom of chest pain typically occurs with effort that raises cardiac activity, i.e. heart rate and blood pressure. In the presence of obstructed coronary arteries, insufficient increase in coronary blood flow (and therefore cardiac oxygen supply) results, providing support for the increased activity of the heart muscle, and angina occurs. Since exercise training produces a lower heart rate and blood pressure for a given level of submaximal activity (see above), angina can be averted in many instances by this form of therapy. It may even allow a reduction in dosage of antianginal medication. For example, if a patient's heart rate rises to 130 beats/minute on climbing a flight of stairs, and angina occurs, this abnormality can be eliminated by an exercise program which reduces the rise in heart rate, for example, to only 115 beats/minute while climbing the same flight of stairs.

The post-myocardial infarction patient can be aided by an exercise program which will improve his physical capacity and allow earlier return to

285

work and maintenance of occupational and recreational activity. In many post-infarction patients, diminished physical capacity is related at least partially to excessive restriction of activity by physician and patient, out of fear and overprotectiveness. The inactivity contributes to a "deconditioning" effect, with true reduction of physical capacity, resulting in depression, further inactivity, and greater impairment of performance. Fatigue and weakness may occur, and a vicious cycle is set up. In properly selected patients who have demonstrated adequate recovery from the infarction after discharge from the hospital, a careful, progressive program of exercise can produce improvement in physical capacity, alleviate depression, and allow a return to some level of work and recreation.

Patients with coronary heart disease also obtain the favorable effects of exercise on weight, blood chemistry, and emotional well-being previously described. However, because a patient's exercise is less intense than a healthy person's, all of the physiological changes will be less marked. Further, most of the improvement in exertional capacity is a result of the changes in the trained skeletal muscles, rather than from direct changes in the heart itself, i.e., the heart is not "strengthened," although the patient can perform higher levels of activity without cardiac symptoms. Finally, there is no evidence that these exercise programs reduce the likelihood of a second myocardial infarction or prolong life in survivors of myocardial infarction. However, earlier return to work and improved quality of life have been demonstrated with exercise programs after myocardial infarction. (See Chapter 5 for a complete discussion of exercise.)

21
Sex After a Heart Attack

It is now recognized that, even for the patient who has had a heart attack, sexual intercourse is safe, and can be beneficial to rehabilitation. Patients with virtually any form of cardiac disease are usually concerned about the effect of sexual intercourse on their hearts and whether it will be detrimental to their health. In particular, patients who have suffered heart attacks are eager to know if and when they can resume sexual activity. We hope this chapter helps to allay any fears you may have about this.

Thanks to several studies, doctors now know that it is safe for more than 80 percent of those patients who have had heart attacks to resume coitus, generally within six weeks to three months after the event has occurred.

This news is usually welcomed by coronary patients. However, many postcoronary patients do not raise this subject with their doctors, and often spend months living in fear that sexual intercourse may result in another heart attack. Further, until recently, some physicians have also been reticent about discussing this issue because of their own discomfort with the topic. In fact, coitus often involves no more physical expenditure than climbing two flights of stairs, or taking a brisk walk, and fortunately, most post-MI (heart attack) patients can safely resume exertion to this degree at some point after a heart attack.

Still, it is natural to have some questions and concerns; for example: what to do if pain, particularly anginal pain, develops during sexual relations; how to cope with impotence; and *when* to resume sex after a heart attack. In order to derive as much satisfaction from your sex life as possible, you should not hesitate to discuss such concerns with your physician, and your partner should be present. Your spouse will probably share some of these concerns. He or she may have other questions, too, and should be given the opportunity to ask them. In this way, unfounded myths can be dispelled, and any questions that either of you have can be resolved.

287

To counsel you effectively, your doctor needs to know about your sexual drive and performance prior to your heart attack, and how your partner has responded to your having a heart attack. Once these matters are out in the open, your doctor can tell you what to anticipate. Here are some of the points he will probably cover in counseling you:

- Try positions that put as little strain on you as possible. Lying on your sides, for example, or the female-superior position, may take pressure off the male.

- Avoid sexual intercourse when you are tense, have just had an argument, etc. If your heart is already being taxed, you don't want to add to the burden. Similarly, you should not attempt coitus soon after any program of exercise.

- Don't engage in coitus if you feel fatigued.

- Avoid having sexual intercourse in rooms that are very hot or very cold.

- Avoid having sexual intercourse shortly after eating a heavy meal.

- If impotence is a problem, talk this over with your doctor. It may be that one of the medications you are taking is interfering with your ability, in which case your physician may be able to adjust the dosage of the drug or switch you to another agent. Be open and candid with your partner. Both of you should feel free to express your concerns and feelings.

- Your doctor will probably advise you to keep nitroglycerin handy; in the event that chest pain develops, these pills can relieve the pain. In addition, if chest pain occurs regularly with intercourse, your physician may recommend nitroglycerin several minutes beforehand. This prophylactic use of nitroglycerin frequently prevents the occurrence of angina from exertion.

Finally, it is important to note that some surveys indicate illicit sex is more stressful (from a cardiovascular viewpoint) than sex with your regular partner. This may be due to a combination of factors; for example, the possible guilt associated with the act and the romantic excitement frequently associated with illicit sex. Also, more taxing techniques may be employed in illicit sex; all these factors may combine to produce more stress—and therefore a greater burden on the heart—than occurs during sex with one's regular partner.

If your doctor does not bring up the subject of sex with you, you should raise it with him. If for any reason he seems reluctant to discuss these matters with you, you should feel free to consult another physician.

In this area in particular, it is important to keep the lines of communication open—not only between you and your physician, but between your partner and yourself as well. The following is an all too common—and unfortunate—case: A male patient who had suffered a mild heart attack was, upon leaving the hospital, simply told by his physician to "relax and take it easy" and "not to rush too much." He had no idea *exactly* what that meant, particularly since he had already been advised when he could go back to work, etc. He spoke to his physician for months without bringing up the subject of sex with his doctor, nor did his wife question him. She, too, had heard these departing words of advice and assumed her husband was probably just following through on his doctor's orders. When they were counseled a year later, she explained that she had been "terrified" to show any sexual interest in her husband, since she assumed such activity was prohibited. Unfortunately her husband had assumed the same. The result of this was a rather dreadful year for both of them, in which there was considerable marital strain that could have been avoided by proper counseling.

Your physician will probably tell you that in some cases, postcoronary patients do experience angina with sex, but that it does not affect everyone. The problem can usually be avoided by less exertional sex and/or by using nitroglycerin. Also, remember that pulse rate and blood pressure increase for *everyone* engaged in coitus; this is normal and nothing to be worried about. However, because of your concerns about your heart, you may be more aware of these changes.

It is quite likely you have every reason to think that you can resume a satisfying sex life, provided you consult your physician, and see him if any special problems develop.

PART VII
Resources:
Where to Go for Help

What You Can Do to Help Yourself

Living with heart disease does not have to be difficult, as we intend to show in this section. Once you learn to use all of the helpful information available, you may find living with heart disease considerably easier.

Many people, for example, including a fair number of those with heart disease, are under the erroneous impression that life automatically has to be more complicated for them. For example, patients with heart disease (angina, a history of multiple coronaries, etc.) often believe that it is extremely difficult—if not impossible—to obtain disability and life insurance. On the contrary, however, a good number of insurance companies will give such individuals the opportunity to purchase disability and life insurance—one simply has to know what companies will consider such persons.

Similarly, victims of heart disease—especially those with a history of angina pectoris and heart attack—often feel quite apprehensive about traveling. However, as most of us know all too well, vacations away from our daily routines, and even business trips, can be very enjoyable experiences, and it is a shame to think that anyone with cardiovascular disease might be avoiding travel due to fear alone. Of course, a patient with any cardiovascular problem should consult his or her physician before setting out on a trip. In most cases, however, patients find that their physicians will approve such activities in all but the most unusual circumstances. To help you feel at ease, especially while traveling abroad, we have included in this section the names of several organizations that can easily provide you with a list of physicians in foreign countries, a small guide book of medical phrases translated into several languages,

291

etc. These and other materials can help you line up any assistance you may need if you become ill while traveling abroad, and just having these items with you can help to take the edge off any anxiety you may feel about being away from your local hospital and physician.

We have also learned that many patients with heart disease and their families are very eager to have specific information about their disorder—whether it is a congenital heart defect in a newborn, or high blood pressure, angina, or whatever. In particular, spouses and other relatives of victims of heart attack and angina pectoris often experience a wide range of anxieties and have many questions. For example: What is it like for the individual with heart disease to return to work? How should you discuss this with your children? What happens if the individual has another heart attack, or another episode of angina? How should you act around friends or work associates? Although your physician can answer these and other questions for you, most patients and their families are reluctant to call their physicians, and even if they do, it often takes a few hours for the physician to return a call. In the interim, a slight fear can swell into a very troublesome bout of anxiety. Fortunately, in many communities, there is a very effective alternative available. In addition to contacting your local Heart Association, which has many leaflets and films available on a wide range of topics (high blood pressure, stroke, angina, heart attack, and so on—a selected list of these films and pamphlets is provided in Chapter 27), you can also ask them if there is a Coronary Club established in your area (and if there isn't, your local Heart Association can tell you how to start one!). Specifically, these clubs, whose members consist of men and women with heart disease (usually angina and/or a history of heart attack), meet weekly or monthly to discuss the day-to-day problems in living that the coronary patient must routinely confront. These meetings provide a wonderful opportunity for victims of coronary heart disease and members of their families to discuss problems and share their experiences. Most members have found such organizations quite helpful, and you might too.

Chapter 23 ("Heart Attack on the Job: What Are the Legal Issues?") outlines some legal options for your consideration, should you have a heart attack in the course of conducting business. This chapter also includes a review of two cases of medical malpractice in which one of us (EAA) testified. In one, I believed the defendant (the physician) to be right and, in the other, he felt the plaintiff was justified in filing the claim.

Finally, we have included in this section two unique and important lists: one provides guidelines for selecting a physician and a medical center for treatment of cardiovascular disease, and the other lists medical centers that specialize in the treatment of cardiovascular disease in children. For the anxious patient with cardiovascular disease—especially if cardiovascular surgery is required—this list may prove to be helpful. Similarly, for the parent of any child with heart disease, the list of medical institutions that specialize in their treatment can serve as a guide to selecting the most appropriate medical center.

Overall, we believe this section to be a most unusual—and rather useful guide. It does not contain all the answers, of course, but we think it goes a long way in helping point you in the right direction. We certainly hope that you find it as valuable as we intended it to be.

22
Yes, You Can Get Life and Disability Insurance

DISABILITY AND LIFE INSURANCE

In one way, purchasing insurance is just like buying clothes or food. The cardinal rule is, if you want the most for your money, you have to shop around. For example, Albert A. Kramer, former Director of the Federal Trade Commission's Bureau of Consumer Protection, reported that cost variations of more than 100 percent for virtually the same coverage are not uncommon. This is a problem that every consumer must face, but particularly the cardiac patient, the diabetic, or the hypertensive patient, since disability and life insurance often appear to be totally beyond their grasp. Fortunately, within the last several years, more and more companies have relaxed the criteria for applicants with medical problems to obtain insurance. For example, twenty years ago, life insurance was almost inaccessible to a hypertensive patient—even if the individual could pay high premiums. Today, however, any person with high blood pressure who takes appropriate drugs and can show (by their medical records) that they have had their blood pressure under control for a year or so is usually eligible for life insurance—frequently, at average rates.

Since rates do vary considerably from company to company, it is important to check with several major insurance companies before you make any final decisions, or to investigate all possibilities with your insurance broker. Some companies, for example, will not accept new applications from persons with significant medical problems unless the policy is of a minimum amount, for example, $50,000 or more. Other companies have less stringent regulations.

Finally, it is important to keep in mind that disability insurance differs from life insurance in two major respects. First, disability claims are under the control of the insured to a much greater degree than life claims. While the will to survive is among man's strongest desires, the temptation to file a disability claim and, subsequently, receive unearned income, is also a strong one.

294

Second, when an individual attempts to purchase life insurance, the company is concerned with how long the person will live; whereas, in any evaluation of an application for disability insurance, the company's primary concern is morbidity—what are the chances of the applicant becoming disabled? Some medical problems that are less significant in terms of eligibility for life insurance, such as diabetes, are of major consequence in disability coverage because numerous complications of the disease can develop.

Information on disability and life insurance for patients with cardiovascular disorders may be obtained from your local insurance broker or bureau of consumer affairs. You can also write to the following sourcs for information:

> The National Underwriter Company
> 420 East Fourth Street
> Cincinnati, Ohio 45202

> American Council of Life Insurance
> 1850 K St., N.W.
> Washington, D.C. 20006
> (202-862-4380)

> Consumer News, Inc.
> 502 National Press Building
> Washington, D.C. 20045
> (202-737-1190)

> Consumer News, Inc. publishes an annual volume, *The Helper's Almanac. Who Writes What in Life and Health Insurance* is used by many insurance agents. Other helpful publications include *Best's Insurance Guide* and *Best's Insurance Reports*. Also informative is *Sylvia Porter's Money Book* (New York: Doubleday & Co., 1975). Most of the major insurance companies will send you some informative booklets if you write and request them.

Insurance After Heart Disease Develops

Can you get disability and life insurance if you develop heart disease? The answer is *yes*.

Within the scope of our presentation, it is not possible to discuss the types of life insurance one can purchase (whole life, term, and so on), nor is it practical to review the pros and cons of each type of policy available, or to define basic

terms. For this information, consult one of the guides listed earlier in this
chapter. In general, many of the major companies will sell life insurance to
applicants with various types of cardiovascular disease. Disability insurance,
on the other hand, is more difficult to obtain, for the reasons given above.

If you have a heart attack and subsequently wish to purchase life insurance,
complete medical records must be supplied. Then, a careful review is made
and you may be rated. Some companies will decline an application for life insurance in the first year after a heart attack but will offer it to you thereafter.
Once you have had a heart attack, however, you must be prepared to pay a
higher than average premium. For example, if you are a 45-year-old man
without any diseases or risk factors, the standard premium for a whole life
policy might be in the neighborhood of $600 annually. For a victim of a coro-
nary who is the same age, the rate can jump even more. Still, whole life insurance is a good investment for such individuals, since it provides the beneficia-
ries with an "immediate" estate upon death, and, unlike returns from other
assets, death payments are generally not subject to federal income taxes for
the beneficiary. Finally, you may be eligible for a rate reduction. Specifically,
life insurance is almost always available to the diabetic, often at only slightly
higher premiums, but disability insurance can be a bit more difficult to obtain. For the latter, age of onset is an important factor—the older you are
when the disability is initially detected, the better.

Similarly, persons with elevated serum cholesterol levels can alter their
diets, hopefully reduce their cholesterol levels to normal, and then reapply.
They may obtain life insurance immediately, but the rate often depends on the
level of your serum cholesterol, so it is more economical to alleviate the condition before taking out a policy.

23
Heart Attack on the Job: What Are the Legal Issues?

Many individuals are surprised to learn that numerous litigations involving heart disease arise each year. However, this is not extraordinary when you consider the statistics. To begin with, coronary heart disease afflicts nearly one million people per year. Of those who have heart attacks and survive, many feel that they are entitled to their retirement benefits, particularly if they believe they can demonstrate that the occurrence of the heart attack was, in some way, a result of their employment. In such cases, claims for redress may be filed before pension and insurance commissions, as well as before industrial boards.

In another situation, the "felony murder rule" might apply. According to a statute that has been enacted in many states, the law states that if, in the course of committing a felony (such as robbery), a victim or bystander is harmed as a result of the felonious act (such as the robbery victim subsequently suffering a fatal heart attack), all the felons involved could be tried for homicide.

Finally, malpractice suits have been undertaken by individuals who believed their medical management was inappropriate and detrimental to them. This chapter discusses some of the legal rights of victims of heart attack, and we also consider how legal cases involving other types of heart disease may develop.

Interestingly enough, more than fifteen states currently have laws on the books stating that compensation can be paid for "occupational" cardiovascular disease. Among those who might be eligible to file a claim under this law are certain civil service workers, including policemen and firemen.

Employees of other organizations might also be eligible. For example, an

297

air-traffic controller might be able to collect compensation under this law if he suffers a stroke (providing he lives in a state where it has been enacted). For evidence, his attorney could claim that some medical studies show that air-traffic controllers tend to have higher blood pressure than their peers; thus, the attorney could argue that his client's blood pressure was "stress-induced" as a result of the job. Next, the attorney would show, by referring to additional medical studies, that high blood pressure is an established risk factor for stroke; as such, he could argue, his client had a stroke as a result of the high blood pressure that developed as a result of his employment. Of course, there is no way of determining from this brief description whether or not an award would be made on this claim, but it clearly demonstrates that questions involving "the heart and the law" can be most difficult to resolve.

Nevertheless, we do know of a case in which the widow of a man who suffered a fatal heart attack was awarded a judgment under the Workmen's Compensation Act. In this case, the man was rushing to meet his boss at a private (plane) hangar so that both of them could fly off on a hurried business trip to Chicago. At the hearing, the referee stated that death was due to a "work-related injury." According to the testimony given, during the course of a busy afternoon the victim was summoned to meet his supervisor at the airport as fast as possible with all appropriate papers. The victim quickly filled his briefcase, rushed home to pack for the trip, and then raced to the airport. When he arrived there, no porters were available to assist him. He, therefore, carried his own baggage (which the lawyer showed weighed 45 pounds) the length of the terminal and, as he ran to board the plane in the heat of the summer sun, collapsed from a heart attack and died.

One could say that an award in a case such as this one is inappropriate; after all, this man may have had undetected coronary artery disease for years, and at any given moment might have suffered a fatal myocardial infarction. True, but a number of claims such as this one are filed each year, and in some, awards are made.

There are myriad problems associated with these claims, however. For one thing, few physicians agree on the *precise* role of emotional stress or pressure in the development of coronary heart disease and provocation of its clinical manifestations. Add to that the fact that no lawyer, judge, or physician is willing to say with certainty whether a heart attack or any cardiovascular disorder has resulted from job-related tensions or whether it has been caused by a number of risk factors, the nature of the victim's personality, the pressures of the job—or a combination of all three.

Despite the "gray" areas, however, we can tell you that, in general, it is rare for a court to rule favorably for the plaintiff when the claim is based solely on the effects of work-related tension, pressures, and stress. Yet, when a single precipitating factor can be identified, as in the case described above, the odds for a judgment in favor of the plaintiff increase.

It will be some time before the courts, insurance companies, lawyers, and physicians define eligibility for compensation due to victims of a heart attack or the other cardiovascular disorders that can occur in the normal course of employment; the reasons for this vagueness are numerous. For example, besides the considerable difficulties encountered in attempting to decide which of the accidents (including heart attack) that occur on the job might be attributed to stress, ruling bodies also have to resolve what constitutes "normal job activity." This sounds simple enough, but take a look at this hypothetical case and you'll see how complex the matter can become:

> A fireman is specifically hired by local government to extinguish fires. Obviously, working in the midst of smoke, high heat, etc., is an integral part of his job. One day, fireman John M., age 47, goes out with his company on a routine call and suffers a fatal heart attack in the course of performing his normal duty: firefighting. The question is, can his widow collect Workmen's Compensation on the grounds that her husband's death was an accident resulting from his job? What would you say?

Unfortunately, there is no definitive answer, and both sides could be argued persuasively. For example, a lawyer arguing for compensation could say that although firefighting was part of this man's routine duties, "undue exertion" at the scene of the fire was directly responsible for precipitating the fatal coronary. On the other hand, a lawyer representing the insurance company might argue that firemen are *supposed* to be prepared for strenuous work—that is the nature of their job.

Frequently, in cases such as these brought before the courts or before industrial commissions, compensation is awarded in so far as there is a reasonable degree of evidence to show that the long- or short-term effects of the exertion may have aggravated or precipitated the cardiovascular event, even though it is known that the job at times involves considerable exertion.

Obviously, so many variables must be considered in each case that it is impossible to give you specific guidelines regarding your eligibility for Workmen's Compensation. If you should suffer heart attack or some other cardiovascular event during employment, specific questions about this are best resolved by consulting a lawyer.

Malpractice

Another area involving your heart and the law—but not your job—is malpractice. The number of physicians sued each year grows annually: in 1974, for example, more than 20,000 malpractice suits against physicians were filed. Consequently, from 1972 to 1975, insurance premiums for physicians climbed an average of nearly 170 percent. In most of these cases, settlements were made out of court, or the suit was thrown out or withdrawn. In others, however, awards were made, sometimes justifiably and sometimes not. Consider the following cases:

Case 1—For the Plaintiff

In 1978, I (EAA) was called to testify as a witness in cardiology for the plaintiff, a widow of a man who died of a dissecting aortic aneurysm. This is a disease in which the wall of the aorta splits lengthwise without rupturing, as its inner layers separate from each other and occlude the blood flow to vital organs. The patient was hospitalized, and the physician who examined him detected a loss of pulse in the femoral artery (a major artery in the leg). Because of this, the physician suspected a blood clot in the femoral artery, so surgery was performed to remove it. However, no clot was found, and the patient died before diagnostic studies were instituted. Dissecting aneurysm of the aorta had not been considered.

Unfortunately, although the diagnosis of dissecting aortic aneurysm can be elusive, it is possible to detect it early enough to do something about it, *providing* the physician maintains a high index of suspicion. In this particular case, the loss of pulse in the femoral artery was indicative of a dissecting aortic aneurysm—*not* a clot—although a clot can also produce loss of pulse in an artery. Awareness of all possible causes of a patient's condition will promote early application of appropriate tests and specific treatment, increasing the rate of therapeutic success.

Case 2—For the Defendant

Another case in which I (EAA) was also a witness involved a widow who sued a physician because her husband, who had had a history of angina pectoris, died prior to scheduled hospital admission for cardiac catheterization.

The man had gone to his physician complaining of tightness in his chest, which was subsequently diagnosed correctly as angina pectoris. The patient was given appropriate drug treatment (nitroglycerin and long-acting nitrates) and instructions, and told to return for a checkup within a short period. Instead, the patient returned eight months later—only because his symptoms had worsened. At that point, his physician prescribed additional drug therapy, propranolol, and scheduled a check-up soon thereafter. After two weeks he did not show any noticeable improvement. His evaluation indicated the need for further measures, but not on an emergency basis. The physician scheduled the patient for a cardiac catheterization in two weeks. The patient died several days prior to the scheduled hospitalization. His widow claimed that if catheterization had been performed when the patient first came to the physician months earlier, coronary bypass surgery could have been performed, and her husband would have lived longer. The jury awarded her a judgment.

In this case I believed the physician's course of action was within the range of acceptable medical practice. He had been presented with a classic case of angina pectoris, and apparently the patient responded to the initial therapy quite well. When he did not respond to the added drug, the physician took an appropriate course of action and ordered catheterization. Unfortunately, autopsy findings were skimpy and inadequate where we needed them most; for example, it was never established one way or the other whether or not this man had single-, double-, or triple-vessel coronary artery disease; or, what the specific conditions of his coronary arteries were, as well as other information necessary to determine whether or not a patient is even eligible for bypass surgery. That opinion, though, was irrelevant to the primary question: did the physician's "delay" in ordering catheterization result in this patient's early demise? Again, I felt his approach was within the range of acceptable medical practice. There was no reason to suspect that this patient needed emergency catheterization; over the years, we have seen many patients with similar histories, and all of them have certainly lived until the catheterization (generally a week or two after the physician reviews all of the patient's complaints and tests). In certain instances of an "unstable" condition, emergency diagnosis and treatment are indicated and should be performed. This patient's condition was not of this type.

Obviously, the issue of malpractice is extremely complicated. Too often, for example, juries act on sentiment rather than an objective evaluation of the hard evidence. In addition, it has become increasingly difficult to say where one should draw the line. In the case history just presented, for instance, the patient, as was explained at the trial, represented a classic case; as such, did his physician have any reason to "rush" the patient, on an emergency basis, to the hospital for catheterization? A great amount of experience indicates the answer is no. In many cases, however, the physician is caught in a Catch–22 situation. If he doesn't do a certain test at a certain time, he might regret it. On the other hand, if he subjects the patient to a battery of costly, time-consuming, and sometimes traumatic tests, the physician can also end up in the throes of a malpractice suit, particularly if one of the tests, such as a catheterization, itself results in a complication, and the jurors decide that the test was not needed in the first place. The root of the issue involves the best judgment of the physician in deciding which test or treatment is indicated for a particular patient at a particular time. Of course, all physicians adhere to some general guidelines for ordering diagnostic tests and prescribing treatments, but the problems mount as the diagnostic capabilities and therapeutic armamentaria expand. On the other hand, most physicians also support compensation of some kind when a physician's error is clearly identified as such, and causes harm to a patient. The dilemma that remains to be resolved is, what happens when a truly good physician, because he is human, makes an error that results in injury to his patient? To date, there is no answer to this; "no-fault" insurance is one possibility, but it will take some time before medical associations, the courts, and the public agree on what constitutes a legitimate malpractice suit.

24
Traveling with a Damaged Heart

Just twenty years ago, many physicians were reluctant to let their heart patients travel freely, but today a growing number of people with various types of heart disease are traveling regularly—for business or pleasure—by boat, plane, train, bus, and car across the United States, to Europe, and even to more exotic lands.

Whether or not you can pack up and go off will depend on several factors, each of which your physician will evaluate; decisions regarding travel for cardiac patients must be made on an individual basis.

General Considerations for Travel

Regardless of the type of heart disease you may have, your physician will take into consideration the following:

- Your overall health status.

- The climate and altitude of the areas you will visit.

- The type and number of medications you take.

- The proximity of your foreign residence to medical facilities.

- The range of medical facilities available to you during your journey. (Will there be a laboratory equipped to do the appropriate tests?)

- Your ability to replace lost and/or stolen medications where you are going. (Is a pharmacy nearby?)

303

Your physician may ask you to investigate the latter three questions and report to him before he reaches a final decision about your trip and destination.

On the one hand, many physicians and family members, as well as the heart disease victim, are often eager to explore the possibilities of a relaxing foreign vacation, or the resumption of business travel. Still, it is natural to experience some anxiety about the potential hazards of being away from home—and your regular physician. Should hospitalization be required in the course of a trip, some patients might fare worse than they would at home, where language is not a problem and the environment is familiar to them. One patient who had coronary heart disease and angina suffered a very mild heart attack while on a business trip to New York City. Although he had visited there many times before, the fear of being hospitalized in a strange facility and cared for by impersonal doctors so upset this 45-year-old executive that he quickly arranged for a private "flying ambulance" to transport him home for treatment.

Of course, this is a highly unusual procedure. For one thing, few patients could bear the expense. Furthermore, most physicians would be reluctant to go along with it; in this case, however, the New York cardiologist reported to the man's personal physician that while the heart attack was rather mild, the patient only seemed to calm down—despite fairly high doses of sedatives—when he was assured that a "flying ambulance" could be arranged for him to go home to more familiar care.

Whether a heart disease patient is planning a trip for business or pleasure, the following guidelines should be of use in the preparations:

Avoid climates with extremes of temperatures.

If you have coronary heart disease and will be traveling at high altitudes, your physician may recommend a portable oxygen unit. Discuss this with him.

If flying makes you nervous, let your doctor know before you depart. He may feel a sedative is appropriate, or he might suggest you drive, or take a train or boat, instead.

Travel by Car

If you are traveling by car, you may wish to avoid driving altogether and have a companion drive for you. Take periodic breaks, which will benefit you and the driver. Getting out of your car and walking about stimulates circulation of the blood and helps to deter formation of clots in the legs. Such clots could travel to the lungs, with serious consequences (pulmonary embolism). Check the route carefully, particularly if you are traveling a considerable distance. You should arrange for the following:

- Select hotels or motels along the way that provide for 24-hour medical service (many now have physicians on call).

- Once you know what hotels or motels you will visit, find out how far the nearest hospital is from it. In some cases, two or more hospitals might be nearby, so you should investigate a little more. Does one of them have a CCU? A hospital pharmacy? et cetera.

- As always, be certain your car is in good condition and contains the necessary emergency equipment—including a spare tire, jack, and warning flasher—before you leave.

- Make sure you have your automobile club membership card with you—it is useful in all emergencies.

- If the weather is hot, and your car is not air-conditioned, drive in the early morning or early evening.

- Take your physician's name, address, and office and home telephone numbers with you; be sure to check with him before you leave, to ascertain whether he will be in his office while you are away. If he spends considerable time in surgery, ask him for the name of a backup physician, one whom you might call for advice if necessary.

- If you are traveling by ship, inquire about the medical facilities on board.

- If you are flying, you may want to check with the airline that you select to determine whether or not the pilots and/or flight attendants have been trained in Cardiopulmonary Resuscitation (CPR).

Before You Go

1. Pack a complete and adequate supply of all necessary medication in your "carry-on" luggage. A backup, duplicate supply should be packed in your suitcase. Each bottle of pills should be labeled clearly with the following information:

Name of your physician

Telephone number of the drug store

Address of the drug store

Generic (chemical) name of drug

Manufacturer of drug

Trade (popular) name of drug

Date prescription was filled

Instructions on how and when the drug is to be taken

The prescription number, particularly if refillable

Be sure you know the generic name and manufacturer, since trade names can vary from country to country.

2. Obtain the name of a physician in the area that you will visit. If you are traveling overseas, this might require additional effort, but it is not difficult to locate the names of foreign physicians, particularly English-speaking physicians, who can help you. If your personal physician cannot help you, contact the International Association for Medical Assistance to Travelers (IAMAT), 350 Fifth Avenue, New York, N.Y. 10001; the telephone number is (212) 279-6465. They will provide a list of English-speaking physicians, free of charge—but they encourage contributions since they are a nonprofit organization. (Physicians are not grouped by specialties.) Once you arrive at your destination, it is advisable to contact one of the physicians to be sure that appropriate assistance will be available if needed.

Another organization, Intermedic, Inc., provides a directory of English-speaking physicians with specified rates for the first office visit or call at a hotel. An individual membership is $6; family membership is $10. Additional information may be obtained by writing to 777 Third Avenue, New York, N.Y. 10017; their telephone number is (212) 486-8974.

3. If you are visiting a foreign country, be sure you find out where the nearest hospital is to your residence and what services are available. Locate the nearest pharmacy when you arrive.

4. If you do not speak the local language fluently, take appropriate dictionaries with you. In fact, it is a good idea to have several key phrases jotted down in the native language, such as "I have a history of a heart attack," "I am taking (name of medication)," and so on. A more detailed guide, entitled "A Foreign Language Guide to Health Care," may be obtained by writing to the Blue Cross Association, 840 North Lake Shore Drive, Chicago, Illinois 60611. A list of phrases to use when you go to the doctor's office, hospital, drug store, dentist, and optometrist are offered in English, French, German, Italian, and

Spanish. Responses that the doctor or dentist may use are also provided.

5. If special meals are required (e.g., low-fat, low-salt, diabetic), notify the airlines at least twenty-four hours in advance. Almost every carrier will provide special dietary meals if you give them sufficient notice. (The same is often true on cruise ships.)

6. If your diet and/or activities are fairly restricted, but you still wish to take some sort of vacation, consider renting an apartment—perhaps on a "holiday" island off-season. This is not as expensive as you might think, and it can be most enjoyable, since you will not have to worry about eating out in restaurants, and so on.

7. Prior to your departure, be *sure* you allow enough time for passenger check-in, be it on bus, train, boat, or plane. The number of people traveling is increasing steadily, and the airlines, in particular, may have lengthy check-in lines since all passengers must pass through security.

8. Have someone accompany you to the point of departure—in the event that you cannot locate a porter, your companion should be able to manage your heavy luggage.

9. Do not hesitate to request a wheelchair, particularly if it is some distance from the check-in point to the carrier. You can also request to be boarded first or early to avoid the strain of standing in lines, and so on. Remember, this does *not* mean that you are an invalid, but it does mean that you have common sense, that you recognize your medical condition, and that you know how to take care of yourself.

10. Cardiac patients should *insist* on being seated in a "no smoking" compartment.

11. Patients who have heart attacks should try to plan trips with a spouse or companion who is trained in CPR.

12. Patients with pacemakers should have the device checked prior to departure. To be on the very safe side, you can request a hand search, rather than pass through the airport security systems; however, most experts agree that these do not pose any hazard to a pacemaker.

13. Prepare to take along a variety of "common" remedies, since colds, headaches, or diarrhea can afflict anyone. However, when a cardiac patient

becomes ill from any ailment, considerable anxiety and cardiac stress might ensue; therefore, it is best to be prepared to handle these common problems.

14. If you wear glasses or contact lenses, pack an extra pair.

15. Wear a Medic-Alert bracelet or necklace. This indicates to any medical person who treats you that you have special needs. To date, more than one million Americans wear this tag, which lists your name, condition, and your medications. A toll-free number is also listed, enabling a doctor anywhere in the world to call and retrieve your complete medical record. Additional information may be obtained by writing to the Medic Alert Foundation International, 777 U.N. Plaza, New York, N.Y. 10017, or calling (212) 697-7470 or (800) 344-3226. Other offices are located in Chicago: (312) 280-6366 and Turlock, California: (209) 668-3333. This service is available for a $15 tax deductible contribution.

If you are traveling to a foreign country and you are concerned about language problems, for a nominal fee you can have a tag made up in the language of the country you are visiting. A language teacher can translate the appropriate information for you, and your local jewelry repair shop, locksmith, or hardware store can make a tag for you.

16. If you can, take a copy of your electrocardiogram (ECG) with you. Your physician will be glad to provide you with this record, which will be of value to any new physician involved in your case should you experience a cardiac problem away from home. Comparison with an old ECG is very helpful in determining the presence and extent of any new cardiac involvement.

Payment Abroad

In some countries, such as the United Kingdom, medical care is free to all who seek it. In others, you may simply have to pay the cost of a short office or hospital visit in cash or with a traveler's check. Similarly, medications may be paid for in cash or with a traveler's check. For more prolonged medical care, bills can be substantial. In these cases, you should obtain complete bills and records, and submit them to your insurance company. Regrettably, it may take months to process these forms, since every bill submitted from a foreign country has to be computed in terms of foreign exchange rates, but many companies will ultimately reimburse you. One exception to this is Medicare—subscribers are not covered outside the United States, although the hospital indemnity policies may provide coverage for reimbursement of medical bills incurred abroad. Finally, some insurance companies offer coverage especially for travelers, including evacuation costs, if needed. A few companies to contact include the following: HOME (Help in Overseas Medical Emergencies), a service established by the International Travelers Association, Box 400632, Dallas, Texas, 75240, (214-661-1420); NEAR (Nationwide-Worldwide Emergency Ambulance Return), 1900 MacArthur Blvd., Suite 210, Oklahoma City, Okla. 73127, (405-949-2500 or toll-free 800-654-6700). Other agencies, such as International SOS Assistance, 1420 Walnut St., Philadelphia, Pa., 19102, (215-732-9091) and the Assist-Card Corp. of America, 745 Fifth Ave., New York, N.Y. 10022 (212-752-2788 or toll-free 800-221-4564) may be able to help too.

Two Final Tips

If any other additional questions or problems arise, you can contact your American Express Office or the American Embassy in a foreign country for guidance. Finally, should you travel by boat or fly on a special fare, such as a charter flight, be sure you purchase cancellation insurance in advance. Then, should it become necessary for you to change your plans, you can obtain another ticket and get a refund for your original fare.

25

Is There a Coronary Club in Your Community?

Frequently, both the heart patient and his family are so frightened by the diagnosis of angina, valve disease, heart attack, need for bypass surgery, or the like that they direct all their energies into riding out the acute problem and leaving the hospital, while giving little thought to the long-term aspects of their problem. As we've pointed out, however, what happens after the initial appearance of the problem can make a considerable difference in the life of the patient; family and friends are also affected by the aftermath.

For example, we know of one farmer living in the Midwest who developed angina, had a heart attack a few years later, and promptly retired—not only from farming, but from life itself. To this day, he continues to treat himself like an invalid, despite the fact that his physician has told him repeatedly that this inactivity isn't necessary. Unfortunately, this man's behavior has caused considerable marital strain, since his wife now feels confined to the house to care for him. His children are also very uneasy around him, so much so that they are afraid to bring their friends home.

Another example of a much more constructive approach involved a 33-year-old pediatrician, father of five, who suffered a heart attack. His whole family immediately got involved in his rehabilitation program. His wife mastered creative low-salt, low-fat cooking in a matter of weeks—and her children never noticed the difference. Their oldest son, then nine, prodded his father into a routine exercise program—long walks each morning. All five children learned about coronary heart disease—and heart attack—from both parents, who carefully explained what had happened and what steps were being taken in response to the disease.

This man was a physician; nevertheless, it gave his family no particular advantage in learning exactly how to help him. Like thousands of others, his wife contacted a Coronary Club, an organization founded to help victims of heart disease and their families. At the Club, she and her physician husband learned in detail about the role of diet, exercise, and stress in heart disease, received tips on employment and insurance, and discussed other related topics. Today, his wife says she wouldn't have made it through those first few weeks so smoothly without the guidance of the Coronary Club members.

Unfortunately, although more than 900,000 deaths (52 percent of all deaths) are attributed to cardiovascular disease annually, and there are more than four million people alive today with a history of heart attack and angina pectoris, many victims and their families are uncertain about what facilities and resources are available for counseling and help. Yet, most agree that they could benefit tremendously from a group that shared their concerns about the mode of life after heart attack, bypass surgery, and so on. In short, there is much to gain by talking with others who have had similar experiences. People who know what you are going through can often help you get over any anxieties you and your family may have.

The following is a selected guide to groups and organizations devoted to aiding victims of cardiovascular disease. In many cases, special programs have also been established for spouses, families, and friends. There follows a sampling of some of the groups with which we have become familiar and recommend.

Your Physician or Local Hospital

Ask your doctor to tell you about any organizations, groups, or clubs for heart disease victims and their families in your locale. Often, hospitals sponsor short programs to counsel heart patients and their families.

The American Heart Association
7320 Greenville Avenue
Dallas, Texas 75231

If you have any difficulty contacting your local affiliate of the AHA, write to their national office, listed above. They can guide you to appropriate sources of information and help in your area. In addition, the AHA has a wide variety of leaflets and pamphlets available on subjects such as diet, exercise, cigarette smoking, and so on. Films may also be rented upon request.

The Coronary Club, Inc.
3659 Green Road, Room 200
Cleveland, Ohio 44122
(216-292-7120)

Anyone can join this organization, whose stated objective is to provide information to give you and any member of your family peace of mind "about one of the most important subjects in the world—your own heart."

The Coronary Club was founded in 1968 by Dr. Irvine A. Page, who was well aware that about thirty million Americans have some form of heart disease. Honorary board members include victims of heart attack and other types of cardiac disease, such as Walter Matthau and Pearl Bailey.

As of September 1978, The Coronary Club was established in ten states (several branches may be present in each state) with a total membership exceeding 9,000. Members receive *The Coronary Club Bulletin*, a bimonthly newsletter containing several features, and numerous booklets.

Other selected features on drugs and surgery are also included, as well as articles on the family's responsibilities when a heart attack occurs.

Chapters hold meetings at which common problems are discussed, recipes exchanged, outings planned, and so on.

Furthermore, the Club publishes booklets on various aspects of heart disease, such as bypass surgery, the role of exercise and importance of diet, and so on, authored by leading cardiologists. In these booklets, victims of heart disease sometimes recount their personal stories. Surprisingly enough, a number of booklets are authored by physicians—heart attack victims themselves. One booklet, for example, is entitled "The Good Life, Three Years Later," by Dr. Walter C. Bomemeier, (past) President of the American Medical Association; in another, "My Anniversary—I Think," Dr. John A. Spittel, Professor of Medicine and Consultant, Internal Medicine and Cardiovascular Diseases, The Mayo Clinic, describes the long trip he made so he could participate in the wedding of his oldest son. After arriving, Dr. Spittell had to leave the rehearsal dinner and go to the hospital to check out the chest pains that had occurred during the afternoon rehearsal. Although he knew he might miss the wedding, he entered a hospital and overcame the most common obstacle to getting help in time—denial of his own symptoms.

Dr. Donald Frederickson, former Director, National Institute of General Medical Services at the National Institutes of Health in Bethesda, Maryland, has described his personal experience of a heart attack in a booklet called "The Toxicity of T.L.C." (tender loving care).

Other patients tell their stories too. Jane Rosenthal, a former travel editor of *Bon Appetit*, tells of her own operation in "Open-Heart Surgery: A Patient's Chronicle," and Walter Matthau recalls being seated next to Elizabeth Taylor at a dinner party and then suffering a heart attack later that same evening in "It Happened One Night." These are a few examples of the brochures available, each providing empathy, understanding, encouragement, and support.

The Coronary Club welcomes victims of heart disease, as well as their families and friends, as members. If you don't have a Club in your area, you can contact the National Office (Cleveland), and they will tell you how to get a Club started.

Mended Hearts, Inc.
721 Huntington Avenue
Roxbury, Massachusetts 02115
(617-732-5609 or 617-244-4179)

"It's great to be alive, and to help others." So states the motto of Mended Hearts, Inc., launched in 1951 by four post-surgery heart patients who were all hospitalized at the same time in Boston.

The Organization has these objectives:

- To visit and encourage, with the approval of the physician, persons anticipating or recovering from heart surgery.

- To distribute information of specific educational value to Mended Hearts and potential heart surgery patients.

- To provide advice and services, when possible, to families of patients undergoing heart surgery.

- To establish a program of assistance to surgeons, physicians, and hospitals in their work with heart patients.

- To cooperate with other organizations which engage in educational and research activities pertaining to heart illnesses.

- To assist established rehabilitation programs for Mended Hearts and their families.

- To plan and conduct a suitable program of social and educational events.

Like the Coronary Clubs, everyone is invited to join. Those who actually have heart surgery are designated "Active Members," while others are called "Associate Members." In either case, privileges are the same. Membership dues are tax deductible and are used to cover the printing and postage costs of a newsletter, *Heartbeat*, as well as overhead expenses. Contact Mended Hearts, Inc. for information on current dues, etc.

Heartbeat is published quarterly; news from other chapters is reported, as well as pertinent, newsworthy items. Besides *Heartbeat*, leaflets on significant topics are published by Mended Hearts. In addition, audio cassettes of the 26th Annual Convention (1978) are available. Other topics on tape include "Children's Surgery," "Surgical Trends," "Research-Arteriosclerosis,"

"Diet," and "Heart Surgery Over the Past Twenty-Five Years." All of these lectures were delivered by physicians, nurses, or nutritionists.

To date, 110 chapters have been established in the United States. The Summer, 1978 issue of *Heartbeat* reported that approximately 100,000 heart operations were performed in 1977, and members of Mended Hearts, Inc., contacted 22,000 of these patients. Each year, new chapters open and new members are recruited. Actually, 1977–1978 was the first year in which it was possible for them to hold six Regional Workshops, all well-attended. These workshops are now an integral part of the annual program.

Many doctors support the work of Mended Hearts and agree that patient empathy can facilitate recovery—sometimes, a former patient is more effective in getting a disgruntled or depressed patient back on his feet than his physician. Mended Hearts has no official relationship with the American Heart Association, but members are encouraged to cooperate with the AHA.

Membership applications may be obtained by writing to the address cited above. National Headquarters can also send you a chapter registry, which lists branch chapters.

If there is no Mended Hearts chapter in your area, you might be able to get one started. Begin by asking the National Organization to help you locate other individuals in your community who are members of Mended Hearts, Inc. If this fails, work with your physician or your local hospital to see if you can contact other patients who have had heart surgery and who might be willing to join. Once you have ten or more Active or Associate members of Mended Hearts assembled, you can petition the Executive Committee for recognition as a chapter.

In addition to The Coronary Club, Inc. and Mended Hearts, Inc., numerous other clubs and groups have been established by victims of heart disease, their families, and friends, each with the same general objective: to provide information, encouragement, and support for the patient with heart disease. Again, it is impossible to list all these organizations, but we do want to mention a few of the groups with which we have become familiar in order to give you some idea of the number and type of services being provided.

Identification Tags

Several organizations prepare visible alerting devices such as identification tags, bracelets, necklaces, and wallet cards. These can put you and family members at ease; in the event that any problem develops, your pertinent medical data is readily available to anyone who needs it to assist you. Chapter 24, "Traveling with a Damaged Heart," lists most of this information.

26
Guidelines for Selecting a Physician and a Medical Center

Selection of a medical center that can best meet your needs for highly specialized cardiac diagnostic studies, treatment and surgery can be more simple than you may think. A number of guidelines or criteria will provide you with a sound basis for judging the general quality of an institution, but you must remember that certain factors relating to the specific personal and therapeutic success of a particular physician with a patient may be impossible to predict and assess. Thus, in some cases, the most well-known center may not necessarily be "the best," while in other instances, a large center with special techniques and facilities might, in fact, provide the most effective therapy. These are questions that you should explore with your general physician on the basis of your medical needs. In addition, there are ways that you can obtain information yourself about hospitals and physicians. This chapter outlines some points you should consider in your selection of a physician and a medical center.

Certain considerations can aid you in assessing the general quality of a medical institution, but they may not, in themselves, provide a definitive answer. For example, factors that reflect the standards of a medical institution and its capacity to provide a high quality of care, especially excellent cardiac care, include:

- the proportion of board-certified physicians and cardiologists on its staff

- an active cardiac surgery team to respond to emergencies that may develop during cardiac catheterization

315

- a minimal complication rate associated with cardiac catheterization and cardiac surgery

- presence of a house staff (interns and residents) to provide twenty-four-hour in-house physician coverage

- affiliation of the institution with a medical school

- activity by staff physicians in teaching, research and medical scientific organizations

Even when a physician or institution rates highly in terms of the above criteria, however, the care provided may not necessarily be excellent. In some cases, for example, a very "big name physician" at a large, well-known medical center may be so involved in the administrative aspects of his position supervising a large staff, attending many medical meetings, monitoring budgets, and overseeing applications for grants to do research and build new facilities that he or she may have little time for patients. Thus, you might be better off in a less widely-acclaimed institution in which the care provided may equal or exceed that provided by the "name" facility.

If your physician refers you to a cardiologist, feel free to ask your physician as many questions as you like about the consultant until you are satisfied. For example, you may want to know where he received his medical education and further training, and whether or not he is board certified. Again, however, do not decide that if he isn't a graduate of one of the best-known medical schools he is not qualified to treat you. Some of the best physicians in the country have graduated from lesser-known schools or from medical schools abroad, while less qualified physicians may have been trained at some of the best-known facilities.

Furthermore, publication of important research may be a mark of excellence, although it does not necessarily mean a physician is skilled in the clinical care of patients. Private, non-university hospitals in which none of the staff teaches or does research may have fine records of efficacy, safety, and patient satisfaction. We recommend that, with your physician, you examine the information available to him regarding the hospital you are considering.

If you are apprehensive about selecting a cardiologist and want more information than your physician can provide, or if you have recently moved to a new area, you could refer to the following sources for some guidance:

- Contact the American Medical Association, Chicago, for guidance.

- Go to your local medical library and look through *The Directory of Medical Specialists*, which lists physicians by state and specialty and provides biographical information (where each physician went to medical school, did internship and residency, etc.). This can provide you with some help ful background information, but, again, keep in mind that excellent clinicians may have attended lesser-known medical schools, while less clinically-oriented physicians may have obtained their medical degree at a renowned institution.

- Your local medical library will also have a copy of a publication called *The American Journal of Cardiology.* The March 1980 issue, Volume 45, lists all of the Adult Cardiovascular Training Programs in the United States (in other words, all of the medical centers associated with medical schools that have been evaluated and accredited by the Subspecialty Board in Cardiology of the American Board of Internal Medicine to train young physicians specifically in the practice of cardiology, and have active programs in the treatment of heart disease by staffs of experienced cardiologists). Your physician may obtain a reprint of this list or the 1981 list for you by writing: American College of Cardiology, 9111 Old Georgetown Road, Bethesda, Maryland 20014.

- Consult your local office of the American Heart Association.

- One useful book, entitled *How to Choose and Use Your Doctor,* by Dr. Marvin Belsky and Leonard Gross (Fawcett World, 1976), provides valuable suggestions to assist you in selecting a physician.

But the most important thing for you to do is to try and get a total picture. How will you and your new physician get along on a long-term basis? Does he seem appropriately interested in you as an individual—e.g., what type of job you have, how many children you have? Is he generally available, or does he travel extensively for prolonged periods? It is far better to find a qualified physician with whom you can have a good rapport than it is to go running off in search of *"the best"* doctor or *"the best"* hospital, where in fact, you may get excellent but less personalized care, which can affect your overall disposition and outcome.

We also encourage you to keep in mind that, in general, the medicine practiced in the United States is the best in the world; physicians here are rigorously trained for years, and not one is licensed unil he passes a series of demanding examinations. In addition, new programs are being implemented in many institutions to weed out the very few physicians who might be considered incompetent.

Finally, it should be pointed out that to date, more than 500 hospitals have been licensed to perform various types of open-heart surgery, but, in this area, most experts agree that the more skill the surgeon has (based on the type, number and percentage of operations performed successfully), the better off you are. The number of coronary bypass operations being performed annually now exceeds 100,000, so more and more cardiovascular surgeons are becoming skilled in this procedure. It bears repeating that there are thousands of excellent cardiologists and community hospitals that provide very extensive and competent cardiac care all over the country. Be advised that a facility which may have a superb surgeon on staff to perform coronary bypass surgery may not be especially strong in another area such as pediatric cardiology. For this reason, you should check carefully before reaching any final decision.

Expert Care in Pediatric Cardiology

Coronary bypass operations, insertion of pacemakers, and certain types of valve replacement surgery are becoming somewhat common surgical procedures and, therefore, may be performed successfully in some community hospitals. However, more than 85 percent of all pediatric cardiovascular surgery occurs in university centers. For this type of surgery, these centers have on-staff experts in pediatric radiology, cardiology, surgery, even anesthesiology.

A list of the centers that have accredited pediatric cardiology residency programs (by definition, this means they are university-affiliated hospitals) appears in the March 1978 issue of *The American Journal of Cardiology*. Such hospitals are accredited for teaching purposes only after a comprehensive review of their facilities and teaching staffs. The centers in the list have been accredited by the American Medical Association's Liaison Committee on Graduate Medical Education.

Leaflets and Pamphlets

The following is a selected list of available leaflets and pamphlets excerpted from the American Heart Association's 1981 Master Catalog. Single copies of these publications, as well as some Spanish versions, may also be obtained by writing to your local Heart Association. In requesting any item, be sure to refer to the title and code number. Additional information may be obtained by contacting your local Heart Association office.

Title	Code Number	Description
American Heart Association Cookbook, 3rd ed. New York: David McKay Co.	#53-001A	Cookbook. Over 500 recipes and variations for low-fat and low-cholesterol foods. Includes calorie counts for each recipe, meatless recipes and shopping tips. Recipes collected with "good eating and health" in mind. 574 pp.
Fact Sheet on Heart Attack, Stroke and Risk Factors	#51-024E	Four-page comprehensive information on heart attack, stroke, and risk factors. Includes materials on prevention, detection, and rehabilitation.
Facts About Strokes (Spanish version: 51-00813)	#51-008A	Explains a stroke—how it occurs, what can be done to prevent occurrence or reoccurrence, how treated, and the keys to successful rehabilitation.
Heart Attack	#51-010B	A clear explanation of a heart attack, angina pectoris, and coronary atherosclerosis. General rules for heart patient and what to do in case of heart attack.
1981 Heart Facts	#55-005E	Gives latest facts and figures about heart and circulatory diseases. 25 pp.

Living with Angina	#50-013B	Explains angina and how to live most comfortably with it. 16 pp.
What Every Woman Should Know About High Blood Pressure. Reprint.	#52-004B	Gives basic information on high blood pressure, geared toward women. Includes facts on high blood pressure and contraceptives, pregnancy, and menopause.
After a Heart Attack	#50-001B	For patient who has had a heart attack. Revised and expanded in content to answer questions that may trouble persons who have had a heart attack; useful for patients as a reference piece, a reminder of doctor's instructions; and suggests questions to ask on the next visit to physician's office. 20 pp.
Living with Your Pacemaker	#50-016B	For patient with permanently-implanted pacemaker. Explains purpose and function of device in simple terms and instructs patient in self-care. Tear-off page for individualized medical instructions, and emergency identification card. 23 pp.

FILMS

The list of films, which are available from the American Heart Association, were selected from the *1981 Master Catalog*. Some of them were produced and prepared by the AHA; others were created by independent production companies and organizations. Information regarding rental fees, the length of the film, whether the film is black and white or in color, and so forth, may be obtained by contacting your local AHA office.

Title	Code Number	Description
Can You Avoid a Heart Attack?	#24-0544	Correspondent M. Wallace states that one of every five American men will have a heart attack before age 60. Causes for rise in number of heart attack victims is discussed. Drs. W. Kannel, J. Stamler, D.T. Fredridkson, and others discuss effects of smoking and diet.
High Blood Pressure: What It Is, What It Can Do to You	#24-0608	Explains briefly facts about high blood pressure. Narrator makes it clear that only a doctor can tell if high blood pressure is a serious condition, and what treatment, if any, is required.
It's Your Heart	#24-0603	Five heart attack victims are involved in an innovative exercise program for cardiacs at Hackensack, N.J. Hospital. They tell of their heart attacks, the warning signs, the outcome, and their participation in the exercise program. Risk factors are stressed.
Work of the Heart	#24-0469	Unusual photography illustrates how heart and circulatory system function. Explanation of heartbeat. Shows replacement of heart valve in open-heart operation using the heart-lung machine. B&W version for sale: $130.

GLOSSARY

Aneurysm A sac-like bulge in the wall of a vein, artery or cardiac chamber (usually the left ventricle), which occurs due to weakening of the wall by disease or congenital abnormality.

Angina pectoris This literally means pain in the chest. It results from an inadequate blood supply to the heart muscle, usually, but not always, due to atherosclerotic narrowing of the coronary arteries. The pain may involve the chest and often the arms and neck; it typically is provoked by effort or emotional stress but can occur spontaneously.

Angiocardiography A technique that is used to examine the inside of the heart and large blood vessels by x-rays obtained during injection of a radiopaque material into the area of the body to be studied.

Antihypertensive agents These drugs are used to lower blood pressure. There are a large number and many types of such agents, which may act on the blood vessels, heart, kidneys or brain to produce therapeutic reduction of elevated blood pressure.

Aorta The largest artery of the body, the aorta originates at the base of the heart and terminates in the lower abdomen. The aorta receives blood from the left ventricle and distributes it to the body through the many lesser arteries that branch from it.

Aortic insufficiency This condition, in which the aortic valve cannot close properly, results in leakage of blood from the aorta backward into the left ventricle. This is also referred to as aortic regurgitation.

Arrhythmia This term is used to describe an abnormal cardiac rhythm. It may be slower or faster than normal and may also be irregular, with either extra beats or skipped beats. Some arrhythmias, such as ventricular tachycardia, are life-threatening while others, such as rare extra beats, may not require therapy.

Arterioles The smallest arteries.

Artery A blood vessel that carries blood away from the heart to the lungs or other organs of the body. The left ventricle pumps blood into the aorta (the largest artery in the body) and the right ventricle pumps blood into the pulmonary artery. These large arteries subdivide into smaller branches which terminate in capillaries.

Atherosclerosis A degenerative process that consists of deposition of fatty deposits and other material on the inner lining of arteries to form atherosclerotic plaques. These plaques can narrow the channel through which blood flows within the artery, thereby preventing normal blood flow. Atherosclerosis of the coronary arteries is the chief cause of coronary heart disease and its complications.

Atrial fibrillation A cardiac arrhythmia in which the atria contract at a very rapid and irregular rate (375 beats/min or more), resulting in a rapid, irregular ventricular rate of contraction. The ventricular rate is rapid and irregular, but because of the normal, limiting effect of the atrial ventricular node on the number of electrical impulses that can pass from atria to ventricles, the ventricular rate is usually 150-180 beats/min in the absence of treatment.

Atrial septum A thin wall of cardiac muscle that separates the right and left atria. It is also referred to as the interatrial septum.

Atrioventricular bundle Also called the bundle of His, common atrioventricular bundle and common bundle. (See Bundle of His.)

Atrioventricular node A specialized group of cells, located at the junction between the atria and ventricles, in which a normal delay occurs in the conduction of electrical impulses from the atria to the ventricles. This normally limits the number of impulses that are conveyed from atria to ventricles, thereby protecting the ventricles from the excessive atrial rates that occur in some cardiac arrhythmias. The atrioventricular node usually limits the number of electrical impulses that pass from atria to ventricles to 160–200 beats/min, whereas the atrial rate can exceed 500 beats/min in some arrhythmias.

Atrioventricular valves The valves between the right atrium and the right ventricle (tricuspid valve) and between the left atrium and the left ventricle (mitral valve).

Atrium One of the two chambers of the heart that receive blood and convey it to the respective ventricle. The right atrium receives deoxygenated blood from the body and the left atrium receives oxygenated blood from the lungs.

Auscultation Detecting and evaluating sounds emanating from within the body—for example, heart sounds, breath sounds, gastrointestinal sounds—with a stethoscope.

Autonomic nervous system (ANS) Also known as the involuntary nervous system, the ANS consists of the sympathetic and parasympathetic nervous systems. It regulates the functions of organs not under voluntary control, such as heart rate and force of cardiac contraction. The sympathetic and parasympathetic systems act together to produce a balanced control of vital functions.

Bacterial endocarditis Inflammation of the inner lining (endocardium) of the heart, usually caused by bacteria or fungi. This usually affects the cardiac valves and may result in serious damage and impairment of their function.

Beta adrenergic blocking drugs Drugs that are used in the treatment of a variety of cardiac and other diseases. They act by reducing beta adrenergic stimulation to a number of systems in the body through blockade of the specific beta receptor sites on these organs through which the stimuli are mediated.

Blood pressure The pressure produced in the arteries by the flow of blood. The blood pressure is expressed by two numbers, an upper (systolic) and lower (diastolic) value. The systolic pressure is the highest value measured during each heart beat and the diastolic is the lowest value (e.g., 120/80 mm Hg [millimeters of mercury]).

"Blue baby" A baby whose skin has a bluish hue due to excessive deoxygenated blood pumped from the left side of the heart to the body. This is commonly due to shunting of deoxygenated blood from the right side of the heart directly to the left side, without passing through the lungs. This occurs via a defect or "hole" in a wall separating the left and right heart chambers.

Bradycardia Abnormally slow heart beat, usually less than 60 beats per minute. However, conditioned athletes may have a normal "training" bradycardia.

Bundle of His Also called atrioventricular bundle, common atrioventricular bundle and common bundle, this area of specialized tissue (the atria and ventricles) conducts electrical impulses from pathways through which all electrical impulses from the atria normally reach the ventricles.

Capillaries The microscopic blood vessels into which the smallest arteries divide and which themselves are in direct communication with the smallest veins. The passage of oxygen and other nutrients from blood to body tissues and of waste products from the latter to blood occurs through the capillaries.

Cardiac Pertaining to the heart.

Cardiac cycle A complete heart beat, including the active, contracting phase (systole) and the inactive, relaxing phase (diastole). This process normally takes 0.6–1.0 second.

Cardiac output The volume of blood pumped by the heart each minute; and is usually measured in liters per minute.

Cardiomyopathy This term refers to a group of diseases of varying etiology that directly affect the myocardium. Cardiomyopathy is usually characterized by cardiac envelopment, cardiac failure and arrhythmias.

Catheterization The procedure of inserting a catheter into an artery or vein for diagnostic purposes.

Cholesterol A fat-like chemical substance that is an important constituent of all animal fats and oils and all cells of the body. It is also important in a number of the body's metabolic processes. Cholesterol is produced in the liver from dietary substances. It is an important component of atherosclerotic plaques. Excessive plasma levels of cholesterol are associated with an increased risk of coronary artery atherosclerosis and myocardial infarction.

Coagulation Process of clotting of the blood.

Coarctation of the aorta A congenital abnormality, in which a severe narrowing of the aorta occurs.

Collateral circulation Circulation of blood through arteries that develop in response to blocks or occlusion in the original or native arteries.

Congenital anomaly An anatomic abnormality present at birth.

Congestive heart failure The condition produced by the inability of the heart to pump an adequate supply of blood to meet the needs of the body. It can result in shortness of breath, due to congestion of blood in the lungs, and fatigue and weakness, due to inadequate blood supply to the body's organs.

Constrictive pericarditis Thickening and tightening of the pericardium resulting from chronic inflammation and scarring. This in turn prevents the normal filling and functioning of the heart.

Coronary arteries These two arteries, one left and one right, arise directly from the aorta, and their branches supply blood to the heart muscle.

Coronary artery bypass graft surgery A surgical procedure that is utilized to treat coronary artery disease. It consists of removing a vein from the patient's leg and grafting one end of it to the aorta and the other end of it to a site on the coronary artery beyond the area of obstruction, to provide increased blood flow to the myocardium. In some cases, the internal mammary artery, instead of a vein, may be grafted to the coronary artery beyond the site of obstruction.

Coronary artery spasm The spontaneous, transient constriction of a coronary artery, resulting in the reduction of coronary blood flow and resultant myocardial ischemia. Coronary artery spasm can thus produce angina, arrhythmias, myocardial infarction and sudden death. Identified as a principal cause of Prinzmetal (variant) angina, it has received increasing recognition recently. Spasm may affect a discrete segment of an artery or may involve the major portion of the length of the artery. The cause is unknown.

Cyanosis This bluish tinge of skin is due to an excessive amount of deoxygenated blood in the arterial system. It is present in a number of conditions. Anatomic defects allow shunting of some deoxygenated blood to the lungs, where it is normally oxygenated and loses its bluish hue.

Defibrillator This device delivers an electrical charge to the heart, usually through electrodes placed on the outside of the chest, to convert fibrillation of the atria or ventricles to a normal cardiac rhythm.

Depolarization The electrochemical process by which cells convey an electrical impulse. It consists of a rapid exchange of important chemical elements into and out of the cell. These elements are primarily sodium and potassium.

Digitalis A drug extracted from the foxglove plant that increases the vigor of contraction of cardiac muscle and slows excessively rapid heart rates in certain arrhythmias such as atrial fibrillation. Digitalis is also used to treat heart failure.

Dilated Enlargement of the heart or blood vessels.

Diuresis Process of increased excretion of urine

Diuretic A drug that promotes increased excretion of salt and water by the kidney.

Ductus arteriosus A small connection between the pulmonary artery and aorta that permits a normal relationship between the maternal and fetal circulations. It closes spontaneously in the first moments after birth to permit normal independent function of the newborn's circulation. If it does not close postnatally, a congenital cardiac defect, known as patent ductus arteriosus exists. (See Patent ductus arteriosus.)

Dyspenea The sensation of shortness of breath.

ECG see electrocardiogram.

Echocardiography A method of examining the heart by the use of ultrasound waves. These high frequency sound waves are directed at the heart and their reflections can be visualized as graphic data, which convey information on the structure and function of the heart. It is a non-invasive, relatively inexpensive method that is highly accurate and is now widely applied in cardiac diagnosis.

Edema Accumulation of excessive body fluid that can be detected by external examination because of the swelling it causes in the legs or abdomen. It may be due to heart failure, among other causes.

EKG See electrocardiogram.

Electrocardiogram A graphic record of the electrical activity of the heart that is obtained by electrodes placed externally on the extremities and the chest. It is used to determine heart rate and rhythm, presence of enlargement of the heart, evidence of damage to cardiac muscle and signs of other functional and anatomic abnormalities of the heart.

Embolism Occlusion (obstruction) of a blood vessel by a blood clot or other substance at a site remote from its origin from which it was carried by the blood.

Embolus A substance producing an embolism.

Endocarditis Inflammation of the endocardium, the inner lining of the heart.

Endocardium The smooth membrane lining the inside of the chambers of the heart.

Endothelium The smooth, thin inner lining of blood vessels.

Enzyme A protein produced by the body that "triggers" or enhances certain biochemical reactions. Enzymes are abundant in cardiac muscle and abnormal increases of the concentrations of these enzymes in the blood is one means of detecting cardiac damage.

Epicardium The outer layer of cardiac muscle.

Epinephrine Also termed adrenalin, this hormone is produced by the adrenal glands. It can also be produced synthetically. It stimulates the cardiovascular system by increasing the frequency and force of the heart contractions, augmenting the quantity of blood pumped, and it constricts the small arteries, thereby raising the blood pressure.

Essential hypertension Also called primary or idiopathic hypertension, this term is used to describe chronic elevation of the blood pressure not related to any detectable cause.

Fibrillation Disorganized, chaotic, ineffective cardiac contractions. Ventricular fibrillation is fatal within several minutes if not reversed. Atrial fibrillation is a common arrhythmia that is compatible with adequate, albeit not normal, cardiac function. If it is properly treated, usually with digitalis, the heart rate slows.

Fluoroscope This instrument utilizes x-rays to visualize internal structures of the body by display on a fluorescent screen.

Gallop rhythm An extra heart sound which, depending on the circumstances, may be normal or may signify cardiac distress.

Heart block A condition in which some or all of the electrical impulses of the normal cardiac pacemaker are not conducted to the ventricles due to dysfunction of the specialized conducting tissues. A reduction of heart rate usually results.

Hemodynamics Study and measurement of blood flow and pressures.

Hemoglobin Oxygen-carrying chemical of the red blood cell. It is bright red when combined with oxygen, as after the blood has passed through the lungs, and it has a purple color when unassociated with oxygen, as after the blood gives up its oxygen to the tissues of the body. The blood of the systemic arteries is bright red because it is saturated with oxygen and the blood of the systemic veins and pulmonary arteries is purple due to reduced content of oxygen.

Heparin A chemical that inhibits blood clotting. It is used therapeutically as an anticoagulant and can only be given intravenously.

Holter monitoring Named after its developer, Norman Holter, this is a method that utilizes a small, portable electromagnetic tape recorder, connected directly to several electrocardiographic leads placed on a patient, to continuously record his or her electrocardiogram during normal, daily activities. The recorder and electrocardiographic leads are worn by the subject for up to 24 hours or more to provide a continuous electrocardiographic record during this period. The tape can be evaluated on an electronic scanner at 1/60 or less of the actual time period it contains (e.g., 24 hours of tape data can be examined in 24 minutes). Holter monitoring is utilized to detect cardiac arrhythmias, which may occur intermittently, and to correlate symptoms, such as chest pain, with objective evidence of electrocardiographic abnormalities.

Hypertension Elevation of blood pressure above the normal range. High blood pressure is one of the most important risk factors associated with development of heart attack, stroke, heart failure and kidney damage and failure.

Hypertrophy Low blood pressure that usually occurs in association with specific clinical conditions such as severe hemorrhage or massive heart attack.

Hypoxia State of inadequate oxygen availability to the body's tissues. It can result from decreased oxygen content in the air, such as at high altitudes, or from obstruction of the blood supply to an organ by occlusion of an artery. If severe and prolonged, hypoxia can cause organ damage such as occurs in heart attack or stroke.

Incidence The frequency of occurrence of new cases of a disease. Incidence is usually calculated on an annual basis.

Infarction Death of tissue due to inadequate oxygen supply because of decreased blood flow (e.g., myocardial infarction).

Interatrial septum The thin wall separating the left and right atria.

Interventricular septum The muscular wall separating the left and right ventricles.

Intima The thin, smooth inner lining of blood vessels.

Intraaortic balloon counterpulsation A therapeutic procedure giving temporary assistance to the heart and circulation by the pumping action of a balloon located on the end of a catheter that has been inserted into the upper aorta. The expansion and contraction of the balloon (usually 30-40 cc in volume) is coordinated with the heart beat so that it aids in the pumping function of the heart and produces greater blood flow in the coronary arteries. This device is generally restricted to critically ill cardiac patients who have suffered shock or severe congestive heart failure from myocardial infarction. It is also used in some patients immediately following cardiac surgery to aid in the heart's recovery of normal function during the postoperative period.

Invasive diagnostic method In cardiology, a method used to examine the heart by direct, internal access to this organ. It usually involves insertion of an instrument, such as a catheter, into an artery or vein. The instrument is then passed into the heart's chambers, where it can be utilized to measure pressure or to inject substances used to determine heart function or to visualize internal cardiac anatomy by x-ray images. Cardiac catheterization is an invasive diagnostic method. (See Non-invasive diagnostic method.)

Ischemia Inadequate supply of oxygen to an area of the body due to reduced blood flow, usually the result of obstruction of an artery.

Isotope Refers to different forms of a chemical element that are chemically identical but differ in a characteristic such as possession or absence of radioactivity. Radioactive isotopes are important tools in the study of body function and in treatment of certain diseases.

Jugular veins Large veins in the neck through which blood passes from the head and neck into the superior vena cava and thence returns to the heart.

Lipid Any of the chemical substances in the group of fats.

Lipoprotein A complex of protein with the principal fats, such as cholesterol and triglycerides, in the blood plasma. Fats circulate in the blood in the form of lipoprotein complexes. The lipoproteins are classified on the basis of their chemical and physical characteristics and their protein and fat content. There are two major classes of lipoproteins, low density lipoproteins and high density lipoproteins. The density (weight) of the lipoproteins increases with increasing protein content and reduced fat content. Thus, the high density lipoproteins contain a greater proportion of protein and a lower proportion of fat than the low density lipoproteins, for which the reverse is true.

Low-density lipoprotein cholesterol Also referred to as LDL cholesterol. It is the fraction of blood cholesterol that, in combination with its carrier protein, constitutes one of the lighter lipoproteins in the blood. LDL cholesterol normally accounts for 60-75% of total plasma cholesterol. Increased levels of LDL cholesterol are associated with elevated risk of myocardial infarction.

Lumen Usually refers to the open space or hollow area inside a blood vessel.

Malignant hypertension Severe acute hypertension, associated with rapidly evolving acute complications due to organ damage, including stroke (brain), cardiac failure (heart), renal failure (kidney) and retinal damage (eye).

Mitral insufficiency A condition in which the mitral valve does not close properly and results in leakage of blood from the left ventricle backward into the left atrium.

Mitral valvulotomy A surgical procedure performed on the mitral valve. Stenosis (inability to fully open) of this valve is relieved by enlargement of its opening.

Mortality The ratio of deaths to total number of individuals in a given population during a specific time period, such as a year. This term is commonly used in reference to specific causes (e.g., mortality from coronary heart disease to total number of individuals in a given population during a specific time period).

Murmur An abnormal heart sound that may be caused by dysfunction of a heart valve or may be of "innocent" origin (i.e., unassociated with any cardiac abnormality).

Myocardial infarction The technical term for heart attack. Damage or death of heart muscle (myocardium) due to inadequate blood supply. It is usually caused by obstruction of a coronary artery; therefore, the heart muscle is deprived (partially or totally) of its oxygen supply.

Myocarditis Inflammation of the myocardium (heart muscle).

Myocardium The muscular tissue of the heart.

Nitroglycerin A drug used to relieve the pain of angina pectoris. It acts by reducing the work of the heart because it lowers blood pressure and helps to decrease heart size through its dilating effect on the arteries and veins of the body.

Non-invasive diagnostic method In cardiology, a method used to evaluate heart function that does not require direct access to the inside of the heart and blood vessels and can thus be performed without insertion of instruments into the patient. Non-Invasive diagnostic methods are usually of lower risk, expense and discomfort than invasive methods. Electrocardiography, echocardiography and many nuclear cardiology techniques are non-invasive. (See Invasive diagnostic method.)

Nuclear cardiology The application of radioisotopes and special equipment to measure radioactivity in order to evaluate cardiac function and diagnose abnormalities of the heart. Nuclear cardiology involves measurement of the behavior of injected isotopes as they pass through the heart and circulatory system to detect cardiac abnormalities.

Open heart surgery This surgical procedure involves opening the chest and exposing the heart. During this type of surgery, heart function ceases and blood is circulated to the body by an artificial pump oxygenator (heart-lung machine), which performs the normal functions of the heart and lungs.

Pacemaker These specialized cells (the sinoatrial node) in the right atrium initiate the electrical impulses that produce each cardiac beat. Other areas of the heart can assume pacemaker function when the normal pacemaker is nonfunctional.

Pacemaker (artificial) This refers to artificial electrical devices that can be applied to the inside or outside wall of the heart, temporarily or permanently, to "pace" or regulate the heart rhythm in the absence of normal pacemaker function.

Palpitation This term describes the sensation of an irregular or rapid heart beat. Often only a heightened awareness of the normal heart beat is perceived subjectively as abnormal.

Papillary muscles These two small muscle bundles are in each ventricle and extend from the inner ventricular walls (to which are attached the chordae tendineae) that are, in turn, connected to the atrioventricular valve cusps. Proper function of the papillary muscles maintains closure of the mitral and tricuspid valves during contraction of the ventricles.

Paroxysmal arrhythmia This abnormal heart rhythm (e.g., paroxysmal tachycardia) has an abrupt onset and termination.

Patent ductus arteriosus This congenital heart defect consists of persistent patency (openness) of the fetal connection between the aorta and pulmonary artery. The ductus normally closes soon after birth. Patency after birth results in shunting of oxygenated blood from the aorta into the pulmonary artery, producing overload of blood flow to the lungs. This was the first congenital heart defect to undergo successful surgical correction, and now drugs alone may be used to correct the problem.

Pathogenesis The succession of factors that results in the development of a disease.

Pathology The study of disease and the resulting structural and functional changes.

Percutaneous transluminal coronary angioplasty A therapeutic procedure that consists of increasing the lumen of arteries narrowed by atherosclerosis. The procedure is carried out with a special catheter, on the tip of which is a small balloon. The catheter is passed into the narrowed artery so the balloon is at the point of the constriction. The balloon is expanded, resulting in compression of the soft, fatty components of the obstruction, with consequent increase in the channel of the artery. This technique has been recently developed, and experience with it is still limited. Results in improving or correcting arterial narrowings in the coronary arteries, renal arteries and arteries of the legs have been encouraging thus far.

Pericarditis Inflammation of the pericardium, the membrane that covers the outside of the heart.

Pericardium The membrane that covers the outside of the heart.

Peripheral vascular resistance This term describes the resistance to blood flow in the small arteries. It is determined by the degree of constriction or dilation of the blood vessels, which is variable and regulated by a number of physiological factors. Increased peripheral resistance causes a rise in blood pressure and augments the work of the heart.

Pharmacology The study of all aspects of drugs, including their sources, chemistry and biological effects.

Phlebitis Inflammation of a vein.

Procainamide This drug is used to treat cardiac arrhythmias.

Prophylaxis Preventive therapy.

Pulmonary artery The large artery that carries deoxygenated blood from the right ventricle to the lungs.

Pulmonary circulation The course of blood flow through the lungs initiated in the right ventricle to the pulmonary artery, pulmonary capillaries and thence to the pulmonary veins, from which blood flows into the left atrium. Deoxygenated blood is carried by the pulmonary artery, oxygenation takes place in the capillaries and oxygenated blood is conveyed by the pulmonary veins to the left atrium.

Pulmonary veins The blood vessels that convey oxygenated blood from the lungs to the left atrium.

Pulmonic valve The valve, consisting of three cusps, at the junction of the pulmonary artery and the right ventricle, which prevents backflow of blood from the artery to the ventricle.

Pulse The expansion of an artery produced by blood flow with each heart beat. The pulse of certain arteries may be felt at specific points of the body.

Purkinje fibers The specialized fibers in the ventricles which are responsible for rapid conduction of electrical impulses throughout the ventricular muscle.

Quinidine A commonly used drug to treat abnormalities of cardiac rhythm.

Regurgitation Backward flow of blood through a cardiac valve, resulting from disease of the valve.

Rheumatic heart disease Disease of the heart following rheumatic fever that may be associated with an inflammatory process, particularly affecting the heart valves, and causing stenosis and/ or insufficiency.

Scintigraphy The process of producing a scintigram, or display of the pattern of radioactivity within the body, through the use of injected isotopes. Cardiac scintigraphy provides data on the distribution of a radioisotope within the myocardium or the cardiac chambers and can be used to detect abnormalities of the heart.

Secondary hypertension Hypertension due to known, specific disease entities, in contrast with essential hypertension, the cause of which has not been clarified.

Semilunar valves The aortic and pulmonic valves, so termed because their cusps are shaped like half-moons.

Serum The liquid component of the blood devoid of cellular constituents (e.g., red and white blood cells) and fibrinogen. The clear fluid remaining after blood has clotted.

Shunt An abnormal anatomic passage, usually due to a congenital defect in the circulatory system, allowing blood to flow directly between two areas that have no normal direct connection (e.g., a defect in the ventricular septum that allows direct flow of blood between the ventricles).

Sign Objective evidence apparent to an observer of disease, in contrast with a symptom, which is a subjectively experienced phenomenon. A heart murmur is a sign.

Sinoatrial node An area of specialized cells in the right atrium that produce spontaneous electrical discharges that determine the rate of the heart beat. The sinoatrial node functions as the natural pacemaker of the heart, controlling its rate of contraction.

Sphygmomanometer The instrument used to measure arterial blood pressure by external means.

Stenosis Inadequate opening of a passage or valve. Arteries and valves may be stenotic due to disease.

Stethoscope An instrument used to listen to internal body sounds.

Streptokinase An enzyme that is produced by the streptococcus bacteria. It interacts with components of human blood to produce another enyzme, plasmin, which can dissolve blood clots already formed. It does this by degrading the protein (fibrin) which is an important component of clots. Streptokinase has recently been utilized in the treatment of pulmonary emboli and acute myocardial infarction. Its use in the latter condition is investigational.

Stroke Damage to brain tissue, most commonly caused by inadequate blood flow because of arterial occlusion or hemmorhage.

Sympathetic nervous system One of the two major divisions of the autonomic nervous system (the other is the parasympathetic nervous system). The sympathetic nervous system exerts automatic, involuntary effects over many organ systems that are outside of voluntary control. It plays an important role in determining the heart rate, the force of cardiac contraction and the tone of the blood vessels as well as the function of other organ systems.

Symptom A subjective feeling or experience of a disease or clinical condition (e.g., pain). (See Sign.)

Syncope Fainting.

Syndrome A set of associated clinical findings that indicate an abnormal state or disease.

Systemic circulation The path or circulation of the blood through the entire body except the lungs, which are served by the pulmonary circulation. Systemic blood begins in the left ventricle and passes through the arteries, capillaries and veins, which return the blood to the right atrium.

Systole The phase of each cardiac beat during which the ventricles are actively contracting and ejecting blood and receive no blood from the atria.

Tachycardia Abnormally rapid heart rate. A heart rate over 100 at rest.

Tetralogy of Fallot A congenital cardiac defect consisting of four anatomic abnormalities: ventricular septal defect, abnormal location of the aorta that receives blood from both the right and left ventricles, pulmonic stenosis, and right ventricular enlargement.

Thrombectomy Removal of a thrombus (clot) from a blood vessel.

Thrombolytic agent A substance that dissolves blood clots within the blood vessel.

Thrombophlebitis Simultaneous inflammation and blood clot formation in a vein.

Thrombosis The process of thrombus (clot) formation.

Thrombus The semi-solid material produced by clotting, or thrombosis, of blood.

Transducer A device used during cardiac catheterization to convert mechanical energy of pressures in the heart and blood vessels into electrical signals that can be recorded for analysis.

Tricuspid valve The valve, consisting of three cusps, between the right atrium and ventricle, which prevents backflow of blood from ventricle to atrium.

Unsaturated fat A fat the chemical structure of which can accept additional hydrogen atoms. Unsaturated fats tend to be liquids (oils) of vegetable origin. They usually contain less cholesterol than saturated fats of animal origin.

Vagus nerves Two nerves that are major components of the parasympathetic nervous system. Vagus nerve stimulation decreases the heart rate.

Valvular insufficiency Impaired function of a cardiac valve resulting in a leak, allowing backward flow of blood.

Vasodilator An agent or influence that relaxes blood vessels, reducing their resistance to blood flow and lowering blood pressure, and increasing blood flow. Vasodilator drugs are used to treat hypertension and to treat heart failure.

Vectorcardiography Determination and recording of the spatial direction and magnitude of the electrical forces of the heart. Performed by a specialized apparatus designed for this purpose.

Vein One of the blood vessels that returns deoxygenated blood to the heart from the body. The pulmonary veins are exceptions, returning oxygenated blood from the lungs to the left atrium.

Vena cava The superior and inferior venae cavae are the largest veins in the body and empty directly into the right atrium. The superior vena cava is the common channel through which blood is returned to the heart from the head, neck and chest; the inferior vena cava conveys blood from the abdomen and legs to the heart.

Venous blood Blood that is found within the veins. It is deoxygenated in all veins in the body except in the pulmonary veins. (See Vein.)

Ventricle One of the two large muscular pumping chambers of the heart. The right ventricle pumps blood to the lungs and the left ventricle pumps blood to the remainder of the body.

Venules The smallest veins.

SELECTED BIBLIOGRAPHY

Ad hoc Committee of the Steering Committee for Medical and Community Programs of the American Heart Association. "The Value and Safety of Diet Modification to Control Hyperlipidemia in Childhood and Adolescence. A Statement for Physicians." *Circulation*, 58:381A, 1978.

Amsterdam, E.A., et al. "Physiologic Approach to the Medical and Surgical Treatment of Angina Pectoris," in Naughton J., Hellerstein, H.K. (eds): *Exercise Testing and Exercise Training in Coronary Heart Disease*. New York: Academic Press, Inc., 1973.

Amsterdam, E.A., Wilmore, J.H., and DeMaria, A.N., eds. *Exercise in Cardiovascular Health and Disease*. New York: Yorke Medical Books, 1977.

Arteriosclerosis. A Report by the National Heart and Lung Institute Task Force on Arteriosclerosis. National Institute of Health, DHEW Publication No. (NIH) 72-137, Vol. 1, June, 1971.

Benson, H. with Klipper, M.Z. *The Relaxation Response*. New York: Avon Books, William Morrow & Co., 1975.

Berrytsson, C. et al. "Social Factors, Stress Experience, and Personality Traits in Women with Ischaemic Heart Disease, Compared to a Population Sample of Women." *Acta Medica Scand*, [Suppl.] 549:82-92, 1973.

Biron, P. et al. "Familial Aggregation of Blood Pressure in Adopted and Natural Children." *Circulation*, 49, 50 (Suppl. III): 111-106, 1974 (Abstract).

Blacker, R.S., and Levine, H.J. "The Language of the Heart." Commentary. *JAMA*, 236(15): 1699, 1976.

Bradley, D.D., et al. "Serum High-Density-Lipoprotein Cholesterol in Women Using Oral Contraceptives, Estrogens and Progestins." *N Engl J Med*, 299: 17-24, 1978.

Children With Heart Disease. A Guide for Teachers. Dallas: American Heart Association, 1971.

Cobb, S. and Rose, R.M. "Hypertension, Peptic Ulcer, and Diabetes in Air Traffic Controllers." *JAMA*, 224:489, 1973.

Collaborative Group for the Study of Stroke in Young Women. "Oral Contraceptives and Stroke in Young Women. Associated Risk Factors." *JAMA*, 231:718-722, 1975.

Committee on Exercise. *Exercise Testing and Training of Individuals with Heart Disease or at High Risk for Its Development: A Handbook for Physicians*. Dallas: American Heart Association, 1975.

Conti, R.C. "Influence of Myocardial Revascularization: Controversies in Cardiology, Part II." *Am J Cardiol*, 42:330-332, 1978.

Engel, G.L. "Sudden and Rapid Death During Psychological Stress. Folklore or folk wisdom?" *Ann Intern Med*, 74(5): 771-782, 1971.

European Cooperative Study Group for Streptokinase Treatment in Acute Myocardial Infarction. "Streptokinase in Acute Myocardial Infarction." *N Engl J Med*, 301:797-802, 1979.

Enos, W.F., et al. "Coronary Disease Among United States Soldiers Killed in Action in Korea." *JAMA*, 153: 1090, 1953.

Friedman, M., and Rosenman, R.H. *Type A Behavior and Your Heart*. Greenwich, Conn: Fawcett Publ., 1974.

Gordon, T., et al. "Coronary Heart Disease, Atherothrombotic Brain Infarction, Intermittent Claudication—A Multivariate Analysis of Some Factors Related to Their Incidence: Framingham Study 16-Year Follow-Up," in *U.S. National Heart Institute: The Framingham Study, An Epidemiological Investigation of Cardiovascular Disease*. Section 27, Washington, DC, U.S. Dept. of Health, Education and Welfare, 1971.

Gordon, T., et al. "Menopause and Coronary Heart Disease, The Framingham Study." *Ann Int Med*, 89:157-161, 1978.

Graham, J.D.P. "High Blood Pressure After Battle." *Lancet*, 1:239, 1945.

Harlik, R.J., and Feinleib, M., eds. *Proceedings of the Conference on the Decline in Coronary Heart Disease Mortality*. U.S. Dept. of Health, Education and Welfare, PHS, NIH Publication No. 79-1610, National Institutes of Health, Bethesda, Md., May 1979.

Hartung, G.H., et al. "Relation of Diet to High-Density-Lipoprotein Cholesterol in Middle-Aged Marathon Runners, Joggers, and Inactive Men." *N Engl J Med*, 302(7):357-361, 1980.

"Heart Facts 1981." Dallas: American Heart Association, 1980.

Heller, R.F., and Jacobs, H.S. "Coronary Heart Disease in Relation to Age, Sex, and the Menopause." *Br Med J*, 1:472-474, 1978.

Heyden, S., et al. "Elevated Blood Pressure Levels in Adolescents, Evans County, Georgia." *JAMA*, 209 (11):1683-1887, 1969.

Hurst, J.W., et al. "Value of Coronary Bypass Surgery: Controversies in Cardiology: Part I." *Am J Cardiol*, 42:157-160, 1978.

"Hypertension and Oral Contraceptives." *Br Med J*, June 17, 1978.

Jenkins, C.D. "Recent Evidence Supporting Psychologic and Social Risk Factors for Coronary Disease (First of Two Parts)." *N Engl J Med*, 294(18): 987-994, 1976.

Jenkins, C.D. "Recent Evidence Supporting Psychologic and Social Risk Factors for Coronary Disease (Second of Two Parts)." *N Engl J Med*, 294(19): 1033-1038, 1976.

Jick, H., Dinan, B., and Rothman, K.J. "Oral Contraceptives and Nonfatal Myocardial Infarction." *JAMA*, 239(4): 1403-1406, 1978.

Jick, H., et al. "Myocardial Infarction and Other Vascular Diseases in Young Women." *JAMA*, 240:2548-2552, 1978.

Johnson, A.L., et al. "Influence of Race, Sex and Weight on Blood Pressure Behavior in Young Adults." *Am J Cardiol*, 35:523-530, 1975.

Kannel, W.B. "Role of Blood Pressure in Cardiovascular Morbidity and Mortality." *Progress in Cardiovascular Disease*, XVII:5-24, 1974.

Kannel, W.B. "Some Lessons in Cardiovascular Epidemiology from Framingham." *Am J Cardiol*, 37:269-282, 1976.

Kannel, W.B., and Sorlie, P. "Hypertension in Framingham," in *Epidemiology and Control of Hypertension*, P. Oglesby, ed. Miami: Symposia Specialists, 1975, pp. 553-92.

Kannel, W.B., et al. "Components of Blood Pressure and Risk of Atherothrombotic Brain Infarction: The Framingham Study." *Stroke*, 7:327-331, 1976.

Kannel, W.B., et al. "Role of Blood Pressure in the Development of Congestive Heart Failure. The Framingham Study." *N Engl J Med*, 287: 781-787, 1972.

Kannel, W.B., et al. "Systolic Versus Diastolic Blood Pressure and Risk of Coronary Heart Disease. The Framingham Study." *Am J Cardiol*, 27:335-346, 1971.

Keys, A. *Coronary Heart Disease in Seven Countries*. New York: The American Heart Association, 1970.

Keys, A., et al. *Epidemiological Studies Related To Coronary Heart Disease: Characteristics of Men Aged 40-59 in Seven Countries*. Tampere: Acta Medica Scandinavica, 1966.

Koskenvuo, K., et al. "Death From Ischemic Heart Disease in Young Finns Aged 15 to 24 Years." *Am J Cardiol*, 42:114-118, 1978.

Loop, F.D., et al. Editorial, "Coronary Bypass Surgery Weighed in the Balance." *Am J Cardiol*, 42:154-156, 1978.

Mann, G.V. "Diet-Heart: End of an Era." *New Engl J Med*, 297: 644-650, 1977.

Marmot, M.G., et al. "Epidemiologic Studies of Coronary Heart Disease and Stroke in Japanese Men Living in Japan, Hawaii and California: Prevalence of Coronary and Hypertensive Heart Disease and Associated Risk Factors." *Am J Epidemiol*, 102:514-525, 1975.

McNamara, J.J., et al. "Coronary Artery Disease in Combat Casualties in Vietnam." *JAMA*, 216:1185, 1971.

McQueen, E.G. "Hormonal Steroid Contraceptives: A Further Review of Adverse Reactions." *New Ethicals and Medical Progress*, October, 1978, pp. 133-158.

Murphy, M.L., et al. "Treatment of Chronic Stable Angina." A Preliminary Report of Survival Data of the Randomized Veterans Administration Cooperative Study. *N Engl J Med*, 297:621-627, 1977.

National Heart and Lung Task Force on Arteriosclerosis. "Arteriosclerosis." Department of Health, Education, and Welfare (NIH 72-137), Vol. 1, June 1971.

Nutrition Committee of the Steering Committee for Medical and Community Programs of the American Heart Association. "Diet and Coronary Heart Disease." Dallas: American Heart Association, 1978.

Ory, H.W. "Association Between Oral Contraceptives and Myocardial Infarction. A Review." *JAMA*, 237: 2619-2622, 1977.

Paffenbarger, R.S., Jr., and Wing, A.L. "Chronic Disease in Former College Students. X. The Effects of Single and Multiple Characteristics on Risk of Fatal Coronary Heart Disease." *Am J Epidemiol*, 90(6): 527-535, 1968.

"Prospective Randomised Study of Coronary Artery Bypass Surgery In Stable Angina Pectoris." 2nd Interim Report by the European Coronary Study Group. *Lancet*, Sept. 9, 1980 p. 491.

Ramcharan, S., et. al. "The Walnut Creek Contraceptive Drug Study. A Prospective Study of the Side Effects of Oral Contraceptives." *J Reprod Med*, 25:6 (suppl), 355-368, 1980.

Ratie, R.H., et al. "Subjects' Recent Life Changes and Coronary Heart Disease in Finland." *Am J Psychiatr*, 130:1222-1226, 1973.

"Recommendations from the Findings by the RCGP Oral Contraceptive Study on the Mortality Risks of Oral Contraceptive Users." *Br Med J*, 2:947, 1977.

"Report of the Committee on Stress, Strain and Heart Disease. American Heart Association." *Circulation*, Vol. 55 (May 1977).

Rhoads, G.G., et al. "Serum Lipoproteins and Coronary Heart Disease in a Population Study of Hawaii Japanese Men." *New Engl J Med*, 294:293-298, 1976.

Royal College of General Practitioners, Oral Contraception Study. "Mortality Among Oral-Contraceptive Users." *Lancet*, 2:727-730, 1977.

Ruskin, A., et al. "Blast Hypertension: Elevated Arterial Pressures in the Victims of the Texas City Disaster." *Am J Med*, 4:228, 1978.

Schmeck, H.M. "A Decade After the First Heart Transplant: The Fanfare Has Died But At Least 85 Live." *The New York Times*, Dec. 2, 1977.

Schoenberger, J.A., et al. "Current Status of Hypertension Control in an Industrial Population." *JAMA*, 222:559-562, 1972.

Select Committee on Nutrition and Human Needs. *Dietary Goals for the United States*. U.S. Senate: February 1977.

Shekelle, R.B., et al. "Diet, Serum Cholesterol, and Death from Coronary Heart Disease. The Western Electric Study." *N Engl J Med*, 304:65-70, 1981.

Sloane, D., et al. "Relation of Cigarette Smoking to Myocardial Infarction in Young Women." *N Engl J Med*, 298: 1273-1276, 1978.

Smoking and Health, a Report of the Surgeon General. U.S. Dept. of Health, Education, and Welfare, DHEW Publication No. (PHS) 79-50066, U.S. Govt. Printing Office, Wash., D.C., 1979.

"Special Correspondence—A Debate on Coronary Bypass." *N Engl J Med*, 297: 1464-1470, 1977.

Stamler, J.S. "Can We Stop the Coronary Epidemic?" *Coronary Artery Disease*,

New York, Medcom, Inc., 1972.

Stamler, J.S., et al. "Hypertension Screening of 1 Million Americans. Community Hypertension Evaluation Clinic (CHEC) Program, 1973 through 1975." *JAMA*, 235: 2299-2306, 1976.

"Standards and Guidelines for Cardiopulmonary Resuscitation (CPR) and Emergency Cardiac Care (ECC)." *JAMA*, 244(5): 453-509, 1980.

U.S. National Heart Institute. *The Framingham Study, An Epidemiological Investigation of Cardiovascular Disease*. Sections 1-26, Washington, D.C., U.S. Dept. of Health, Education and Welfare, 1968-70.

Veterans Administration Cooperative Study Group on Antihypertensive Agents. "Effects of Treatment on Morbidity in Hypertension. II. Results in Patients With Diastolic Blood Pressure Averaging 90 through 114 mm Hg." *JAMA*, 213: 1143-1152, 1970.

Veterans Administration Cooperative Study Group on Antihypertensive Agents. "Effects of Treatment on Morbidity in Hypertension. III. Influence of Age, Diastolic Pressure, and Prior Cardiovascular Disease; Further Analysis of Side Effects." *Circulation*, 45:991, 1972.

Walker, W.J. "Editorial. Changing United States Life-Style and Declining Vascular Mortality: Cause or Coincidence?" *N Engl J Med*, 297: 163-165, 1977.

Waters, D.D., et al. "Coronary Artery Disease in Young Women: Clinical and Angiographic Features and Correlation With Risk Factors." *Am J Cardiol*, 42:41-47, 1978.

Zohman, L.R. *Beyond Diet...Exercise Your Way to Fitness and Heart Health.* Mazola Corn Oil, CPC International Inc., 1974.

INDEX